Study Guide to Accompany

Porth's Essentials of Pathophysiology: Concepts of Altered Health States

SECOND EDITION

Kathleen Schmidt Prezbindowski, PhD, MSN
Professor, Department of Biology
College of Mount St. Joseph
Cincinnati, OH

 Lippincott Williams & Wilkins
a Wolters Kluwer business

Philadelphia · Baltimore · New York · London
Buenos Aires · Hong Kong · Sydney · Tokyo

Managing Editor: Timothy Reiley
Senior Production Editor: Debra Schiff
Director of Nursing Production: Helen Ewan
Manufacturing Coordinator: Karin Duffield

9 8 7 6 5 4

ISBN-13: 978-0-7817-7228-0
ISBN: 0-7817-7228-1

Care has been taken to confirm the accuracy of the information presented and to describe generally accepted practices. However, the authors, editors, and publisher are not responsible for errors or omissions or for any consequences from application of the information in this book and make no warranty, express or implied, with respect to the content of the publication.

The authors, editors, and publisher have exerted every effort to ensure that drug selection and dosage set forth in this text are in accordance with the current recommendations and practice at the time of publication. However, in view of ongoing research, changes in government regulations, and the constant flow of information relating to drug therapy and drug reactions, the reader is urged to check the package insert for each drug for any change in indications and dosage and for added warnings and precautions. This is particularly important when the recommended agent is a new or infrequently employed drug.

Some drugs and medical devices presented in this publication have Food and Drug Administration (FDA) clearance for limited use in restricted research settings. It is the responsibility of the health care provider to ascertain the FDA status of each drug or device planned for use in his or her clinical practice.

Introduction

This second edition of the *Study Guide to Accompany Porth's Essentials of Pathophysiology: Concepts of Altered Health States* is designed for use in conjunction with the Essentials version of Carol Mattson Porth's text. Like the text, this *Study Guide* broadens students' understanding of normal anatomy and physiology by exploring causes, alterations and adaptations, manifestations, and resolution of disease states. The emphasis in this guide is on active learning, not passive reading, as students bridge the gap from objectives to integration and application of knowledge. Examining concepts through a variety of approaches, students are helped not simply to study, but to learn, correlate, and apply to clinical settings.

The 45 chapters of the *Study Guide* parallel those of the text. Students will find that the following features in each chapter enhance the effectiveness of this excellent text.

- Review Questions in each *Study Guide* chapter are grouped into sections according to those in the text chapter. References to text figures, tables, and charts encourage students to fully utilize the text.

- Review Questions include a variety of approaches to learning, such as multiple-choice, matching, arrange-in-correct-sequence, fill-in, discussion, and figure completion exercises. These exercises help students to "handle" concepts, almost as if they are working with clay, to achieve a depth of learning that comes through active participation.

- Answers to Review Questions are located at the end of the *Study Guide*, where they can be bookmarked for easy access.

- Clinical correlations introduce application especially relevant for students in nursing and other areas of health science. These are based on my own experiences as an RN/MSN and on discussions with colleagues. Because Porth's text addresses a multitude of pathologies, clinical studies include many brief examples rather than just a few detailed case studies. These challenging exercises allow students to relate pathogenesis to actual clinical settings.

Acknowledgments

I appreciate my students and colleagues for their ongoing support of teaching, learning, and clinical practice. Special thanks to Laurie Prezbindowski and Rachel Simmons for many months of thorough and accurate editorial assistance. I am grateful to all of my family for their constant encouragement and caring: Maureen Schmidt Thielens and Alexis Thielens; Laurie and Amy Prezbindowski; and Joost, Stephanie, and Nicholas Claeys. Thanks to Lippincott Williams & Wilkins editor, Timothy Reiley, for his expertise and patience.

About the Author

Kathleen Schmidt Prezbindowski holds a PhD in biological sciences, Purdue University, and MSNs in Gerontological Nursing and Psychiatric/Mental Health Nursing, University of Cincinnati. Over the past 35 years, she has taught pathophysiology, anatomy and physiology, and biology of aging at Columbia Basin College, the College of Mount St. Joseph, and the University of Cincinnati. Dr. Prezbindowski is a professor of biology at the College of Mount St. Joseph, where she has been named Distinguished Professor of the Year. Through a grant from the U.S. Administration on Aging, Dr. Prezbindowski produced the first video series and training manual designed to help older persons understand the aging human body and maintain wellness. She is a delegate to the Health Promotion Institute of the National Council on the Aging. Dr. Prezbindowski has also authored four learning guides in anatomy and physiology and one other guide to pathophysiology.

Contents

CHAPTER 1

Cell Structure and Function

■ Review Questions

A. FUNCTIONAL COMPONENTS OF THE CELL

A1. Explain why the study of cells is critical to understanding pathophysiology.

_____

_____

A2. Arrange the chemical components of cells (carbohydrates, lipids, proteins, water) from highest to lowest concentration:

_____, _____,

_____, _____

A3. Match the following cell components with their characteristics:

Carbohydrates   Potassium   Lipids
Sodium   Proteins   Water

(a) Insoluble in water, this category of chemicals includes cholesterols and triglycerides: _____

(b) Form only a small amount of body tissues; are used primarily for cellular fuel: _____

(c) The major cation within cells (in intracellular fluid): _____

(d) Constitute(s) more than 70% of cells: _____

A4. List two or more functions of proteins synthesized by cells.

_____

_____

_____

A5. Circle the correct answer within each statement.

(a) The type of RNA that moves amino acids to proteins that are forming on ribosomes is (messenger? ribosomal? transfer?) RNA.

(b) Ribosomal RNA is transcribed in (ribosomes? the nucleolus?).

A6. Describe two methods by which cells actively involved in transcription (copying of DNA by mRNA) preceding cell division can be differentiated from inactive cells.

(a) _____

(b) _____

A7. Match the names of the following organelles with their descriptions:

Golgi   Lysosomes   Mitochondria
Peroxisomes   Rough ER   Smooth ER

(a) Proteins (the major components of enzymes) are synthesized here: _____

(b) Lipids are synthesized here: _____

(c) Carbohydrates that help form glycoproteins are made here: _____

(d) Located close to the nucleus, these organelles modify proteins to prepare them for export from the cell: _____

(e) The inactive form of insulin is activated within these organelles in pancreatic cells: _____

(f) Liver cells conduct their detoxification activities through these organelles: _____

(g) Enzymes that digest microbes are found in these sacs in phagocytic white blood cells: _____

(h) These organelles normally destroy harmful free radicals: _____

(i) These organelles contain their own DNA (inherited from the mother), so they can self-replicate: _____

(j) These organelles extract energy from chemicals in foods and store the energy in ATP; large numbers are found in muscle cells that require much energy: _____

(k) Sarcoplasmic reticulum (SR) that releases calcium to activate muscle cells is a form of this organelle: _____

A8. Circle all of the sentences that are true:

(a) Lipofuscin accumulates in lysosomes of aging cells.

(b) Pigments used in tattoos are retained in lysosomes of cells.

(c) Lysosomes are called "powerhouses of the cell."

(d) Lysosomes normally produce an enzyme that is missing in babies with Tay-Sachs disease.

A9. Choose an answer from the following list to fill in the blank.

The components of the cytoskeleton are involved primarily with _____ the cell.

(a) Shape and movements of

(b) Secretion by

(c) Protein synthesis within

A10. Match the following cytoskeletal structures with their related descriptions.

Actin and myosin   Basal bodies
Centrioles   Cilia   Flagella

(a) Provide motility for sperm: _____

(b) Move mucus and debris along respiratory membranes: _____

(c) Thin and thick filaments involved in muscle contraction: _____

(d) Form the mitotic spindle required for mitosis: _____

(e) Form the microtubules found in cilia and flagella: _____

A11. Write brief descriptions of the roles of microtubules in these clinical cases.

(a) Mrs. Jefferson has diabetes (which alters microtubules); she has frequent respiratory infections.

_____

_____

(b) The autopsy of Sister Agnes's brain reveals the presence of neurofibrillary tangles associated with Alzheimer disease.

_____

_____

A12. Circle the two true statements about the cell (plasma) membrane. (Pay particular attention to whether the **bold-faced** word or phrase makes the statement true or false.)

(a) The bilayer of this membrane is composed of **lipid,** through which lipid-soluble chemicals can be transported.

(b) The "tails" of the phospholipid molecules in this membrane are **hydrophilic.**

(c) Most of the specific functions of the cell membrane are carried out by **proteins,** including channels for transport of non–lipid-soluble chemicals.

(d) **Peripheral** proteins extend from the inside to the outside of the membrane.

A13. Circle the correct answer within each statement.

(a) The A antigens that cause Katisha to have type A blood are found in the *(cell coat? cell membrane?)* of her red blood cells.

(b) The cell coat *(is? is not?)* involved in cell recognition.

B. CELL METABOLISM AND ENERGY SOURCES

B1. Circle the correct answer or fill in the blanks within each statement about metabolism.

(a) Synthesis of proteins from amino acids is an example of *(anabolism? catabolism?).*

(b) ATP contains *(one? two? three?)* phosphates and *(one? two? three?)* high-energy bonds. *(ADP? ATP?)* contains more energy.

(c) Glycolysis is a process that *(does? does not?)* require oxygen. This process *(begins? completes?)* the catabolism of glucose, which is converted into *(pyruvate? CO_2 and H_2O?)*. In the process, *(large? small?)* amounts of energy are captured in ATP. In addition, hydrogen atoms (H) removed during glycolysis are transferred to _____.

(d) In the absence of oxygen, pyruvate is converted to _____ acid. Many cells that lack oxygen can convert this acid back to _____ acid, which can later be used to form glucose or for energy when oxygen is available.

(e) Aerobic metabolism is a process that *(does? does not?)* require oxygen. In this process, products of glycolysis move through the Krebs (or _____ acid) cycle within the *(cytoplasm? mitochondria?)*. This cycle begins when acetyl coenzyme A (derived from _____ acid by removal of a CO_2) combines with _____ acid to form citric acid.

(f) Within the many steps of the Krebs cycle, hydrogen atoms are removed from citric acid and other chemicals and ionized so that their electrons can be conveyed along carriers in the electron _____ system (ETS). Hydrogen atoms attached to NAD (as NADH), which were products of _____, are also ionized and utilized now. The ETS taps energy from all of these electrons to convert ADP to ATP by a process of oxidative _____. The chemical _____ causes death by poisoning the enzymes involved in oxidative phosphorylation.

(g) Products of protein and fat digestion *(can? cannot?)* contribute to energy supply. Explain how, or why not.

_____

(h) Aerobic metabolism provides sufficient ATP molecules to supply *(30? 60? 90?)%* of the body's energy needs. The hydrogen and carbon atoms from the original glucose combine with oxygen to form two by-products of aerobic metabolism: _____, which is exhaled, and _____.

C. CELL MEMBRANE TRANSPORT, SIGNAL TRANSDUCTION, AND GENERATION OF MEMBRANE POTENTIALS

C1. Explain why an understanding of cell membrane permeability is integral to the study of pathophysiology. _____

_____

_____

C2. *(Active? Passive?)* transport processes of movement across membranes require expenditure of energy. Passive transport moves chemicals *("downhill" with? "uphill" against?)* the chemical or electrical gradient.

List three examples of passive transport processes.

(a) _____

(b) _____

(c) _____

C3. Select the answer that fits each description of transport processes.

Diffusion　　Facilitated diffusion　　Osmosis

(a) Movement of molecules or ions (related to their kinetic energy) from regions of high to low concentration of those chemicals: _____

(b) A process by which molecules such as glucose are transported because they are not lipid soluble and are too large to pass through protein pores: _____

(c) A process that requires a transport protein (carrier) but not ATP: _____

C4. Circle the correct answer within each statement about cell membrane transport.

(a) Lipid-soluble molecules such as O_2 and CO_2 gases, alcohol, and fatty acids pass across the *(phospholipid bilayer? proteins with pores?)* portions of cell membranes.

(b) In osmosis, water moves from the region in which *(water molecules? other particles?)* are most concentrated to regions where they are less concentrated.

C5. Circle the correct answer or fill in the blank within each statement about active transport.

(a) Pinocytosis refers to cell *(eating? drinking?)*.

(b) After phagocytosis, the ingested particle is transported to a *(mitochondrion? lysosome?)*, where it is digested.

(c) One type of cell that engulfs bacteria by phagocytosis is a _____.

(d) Removal of cell debris is carried out by *(endo? exo?)*cytosis.

C6. Choose the two true statements about active transport mechanisms. (Pay particular attention to whether the **bold-faced** word or phrase makes the statement true or false.)

(a) Active transport mechanisms **do** require an energy source such as ATP.

(b) The Na^+/K^+ pump is responsible for keeping the concentration of Na^+ 14 times greater **inside** of the cell membrane than **outside**.

(c) Cotransport uses energy derived from **secondary** active transport.

(d) In countertransport systems, sodium and a second chemical are transported in **opposite** directions.

C7. Circle the correct answer within each statement about ion channels embedded in the cell membrane.

(a) Ion channels are composed of *(phospholipids? integral proteins?)*. Some of these channels open only upon stimulation; these are known as *(gated? nongated or leakage?)* channels.

(b) Voltage-gated channels respond to *(electrical changes? presence of ligands?)* in the membrane.

(c) A neurotransmitter such as acetylcholine normally attaches to a receptor on a nerve or muscle cell. The *(acetylcholine? receptor?)* is known as a ligand and it is a chemical that has a *(high? low?)* affinity for a receptor.

C8. List four mechanisms involving chemicals by which cells can communicate with each other.

(a) _____

   _____

   _____

(b) _____

   _____

   _____

(c) _____

   _____

   _____

(d) _____

   _____

   _____

C9. Which mechanism that you listed for Question C8 is the process by which protein or peptide hormones (as well as neurotransmitters) activate cells? *(a? b? c? d?)* This process is known as signal _____; it involves proteins that can change shape (conformation) with the help of proteins known as

_____.

C10. Circle the correct answer or fill in the blanks within each statement about receptors involved in cell-to-cell communication.

(a) When excessive chemical messengers (for example, a particular type of hormone) are present, the body will normally *(up? down?)*-regulate by *(increasing? decreasing?)* the number of cell membrane receptors for that chemical (hormone).

(b) Receptors on nerve or muscle cells that respond to neurotransmitters are _____ channels, such as for sodium ions (Na^+).

(c) The microbial toxin that initiates the severe diarrhea of cholera acts as a *first messenger* that activates a(n) _____ protein and results in production of the second messenger, named _____.

(d) Insulin is a *(protein? lipid?)* hormone. Its receptor activates mechanisms that lead to the uptake of _____ by a cell.

(e) Because they are lipids, steroid hormones *(can? cannot?)* pass across cell membranes. They activate *(cAMP? the nucleus?)*, causing synthesis of proteins that alter cell function.

C11. Circle the correct answers or fill in the blanks within each statement related to membrane potentials.

(a) The cell membranes of nerve or muscle cells in the resting state *(are? are not?)* polarized. Typically, the inside of the resting membrane is more *(positive? negative?)*. This membrane difference (or charge or potential) is measured in *(volts? millivolts?)*.

(b) Two main factors contribute to the membrane excitability. These are the concentration of _____ on the inside and outside of the membrane, as well as changes in membrane _____.

(c) A nerve impulse begins when the membrane becomes more permeable to (K^+? Na^+?), which causes the inside of the nerve cell to become more (*positive*? *negative*?).

D. BODY TISSUES

D1. Name the four basic types of tissues. Which of these develops mainly from ectoderm?

(a) _____

(b) _____

(c) _____

(d) _____

D2. Choose the two true statements about epithelium. (Pay particular attention to whether the **bold-faced** word or phrase makes the statement true or false.)

(a) Cells are held **tightly** together with **many** cell junctions.

(b) Epithelium is **highly vascular.**

(c) Simple squamous epithelium consists of a **single layer of cube-shaped cells** resting on a basement membrane.

(d) Glands (such as sweat glands and salivary glands) are composed of **epithelium.**

D3. Circle all answers that contain a type of epithelium and a correct location of that type of epithelium.

(a) Simple cuboidal: lines the intestine

(b) Keratinized stratified squamous: forms the epidermis of the skin

(c) Ciliated pseudostratified: lines the upper respiratory tract

(d) Transitional: forms the kidneys

D4. Circle the correct answer or fill in the blank within each statement.

(a) Glands that produce sweat or milk are classified as _____ crine glands.

(b) Glands that produce hormones are known as _____ crine glands.

(c) Which glands are ductless because they empty secretions directly into the bloodstream. (*Endocrine? Exocrine?*)

D5. Match the type of cell junction that fits each description:

Adhering junctions   Continuous tight junctions

Gap (nexus) junctions   Hemidesmosomes

(a) Communication channels that allow small chemicals to pass directly from cell to cell: _____

(b) Found only in epithelium, they seal adjacent cells together: _____

(c) Prevent separation of cardiac muscle cells: _____

(d) Found at the base of epithelial cells, they help to attach epithelium to underlying tissue: _____

D6. Circle the correct answer or fill in the blanks within each statement.

(a) Of the many types of cells in connective tissue, which type forms fibers? _____

(b) Which type of connective tissue (*dense? loose? reticular?*) forms a supportive framework for the liver and for blood-forming tissues?

(c) Tendons and ligaments are (*loose? dense regular? dense irregular?*) connective tissue.

(d) Periosteum is (*loose? dense regular? dense irregular?*) connective tissue that covers (*cartilage? bone?*).

(e) Adipose tissue is the technical name for _____ tissue.

(f) Glycosaminoglycans (GAGs) form much of the extracellular _____. GAGs are composed of _____ and _____.

(g) Which protein is the most abundant protein in the body and it forms strong fibers that allow tendons to resist stretching? _____ Which protein is abundant in structures that do stretch well, such as the aorta and ligaments? _____

D7. Choose the two true statements about muscle tissue. (Pay particular attention to whether the **bold-faced** word or phrase makes the statement true or false.)

(a) **Smooth** muscle is found in the walls of blood vessels, stomach, urinary bladder, and in the iris of the eye.

(b) Skeletal muscle tissue is **avascular.**

(c) Endomysium surrounds a **larger** amount of muscle than epimysium does.

(d) It is the arrangement of **actin** and **myosin** that accounts for the striated appearance of skeletal and cardiac muscle.

D8. Circle all answers that match a term with a correct description about skeletal muscle contraction.

(a) Sarcolemma: forms sarcoplasmic reticulum

(b) Myosin: thick, dark-staining myofilaments that form cross-bridges with actin

(c) Sarcomere: extends from one H zone to another

(d) Skeletal muscle cells: have many nuclei per cell

(e) T tubules: convey action potentials from sarcolemma into the interior of muscle cells

(f) Tropomyosin: binds Ca^{2+} so that myosin can form cross-bridges with actin

(g) Ca^{2+}: ions must be inside of sarcoplasmic reticulum for muscle cells to contract

(h) Actin and myosin filaments: shorten during muscle contraction

(i) Breakdown of ATP: provides the energy required to activate a myosin head so it can form a cross-bridge with actin

D9. Circle the correct answer within each statement about smooth muscles.

(a) Smooth muscle contraction is *(voluntary? involuntary?).*

(b) Smooth muscle cells have *(one nucleus? many nuclei?)* per cell.

(c) Arrangement of actin and myosin *(does? does not?)* produce cross-striations in smooth muscle cells.

(d) Smooth muscle contraction depends on a supply of Ca^{2+} from *(sarcoplasmic reticulum? extracellular fluid?).*

(e) The calcium-binding regulatory protein in smooth muscle is *(troponin? calmodulin?).*

D10. Answer the following questions about structures that make up the nervous system.

(a) Circle the structures that form the central nervous system (CNS):

Spinal cord   Brain
Cranial nerves   Spinal nerves

(b) *(Neurons? Glial cells? Satellite cells?)* conduct nerve impulses.

(c) Motor neurons are known as *(afferent? efferent?)* neurons.

D11. Circle the correct answer within each statement about neurons.

(a) The nucleus of a neuron is located in the *(axon? dendrite? cell body?).*

(b) Nissl bodies contain *(chromosomes? mitochondria? ribosomes?).*

(c) A(n) *(axon? dendrite?)* carries nerve impulses away from a cell body. Most neurons have *(one? many?)* axon(s) with *(no? some?)* branches.

D12. Select the supporting cells of the nervous system that fit descriptions of their functions.

Astrocytes   Ependymal cells
Microglia   Oligodendrocytes
Satellite cells   Schwann cells

(a) Line ventricles of the brain which are spaces that contain cerebrospinal fluid (CSF): _____

(b) Phagocytic "clean-up" cells: _____

(c) Form myelin around neuronal processes of the brain and spinal cord: _____

(d) Form myelin around axons and dendrites of the PNS: _____

(e) Surround and protect cell bodies in ganglia of the PNS: form myelin around axons of the brain and spinal cord:

_____

(f) Most abundant of the neuroglia; they bind blood vessels to neurons and help form the barrier (blood-brain barrier) that protects the brain: _____

CHAPTER 2

Cellular Responses to Stress, Injury, and Aging

■ Review Questions

A. CELLULAR ADAPTATION

A1. Explain why cells adapt.

_____

_____

_____

Circle the type of genes most involved in adaptations.

(a) "Differentiating" genes

(b) "Housekeeping" genes

A2. Choose the term or phrase that best fits each description of atrophy.

Decrease in hormones   Denervation   Disuse
Ischemia   Poor nutrition

(a) Decrease in breast size and thinning of vaginal lining in elderly women: _____

(b) Lack of adequate blood flow: _____

(c) Immobilization of a fractured leg: _____

A3. Choose the term that best fits each description of cellular adaptation.

Atrophy   Hypertrophy
Hyperplasia   Dysplasia
Metaplasia

(a) Enlargement of a tissue or an organ related to increase in cell number:_____

(b) Enlargement of a tissue or an organ related to increase in cell size: _____

(c) Reversible conversion of ciliated columnar epithelium lining the respiratory tract into stratified squamous epithelium in response to chronic irritation of smoking: _____

(d) Enlargement of biceps brachii as a result of exercise: _____

(e) Increase in thickness of the heart wall in response to increased workload caused by hypertension: _____

(f) Formation of calluses on hands as a result of work with hands; wart formation; wound healing: _____

(g) The cellular adaptation that is considered most "deranged" and most likely to lead to cancer: _____

(h) Decreased brain size that accompanies aging: _____

A4. Removal of a large amount (up to 85%) of liver tissue (partial hepatectomy) *(will never? may?)* be followed by regrowth of most of the liver tissue. *Circle the correct answer in the preceding sentence and explain why.*

_____

_____

_____

A5. Explain why benign prostatic hyperplasia/ hypertrophy (BPH) might lead to hypertrophy of the bladder wall.

_____

_____

_____

A6. Select the condition from the following list that fits the related description.

Alzheimer disease   Black lung disease
Fatty liver   Jaundice
Lead poisoning   von Gierke disease

(a) Associated with accumulation of abnormally folded proteins: _____

(b) May be related to alcoholism, starvation, or diabetes: _____

(c) Involves accumulation of excessive amounts of glycogen in the liver: _____

(d) Indicated in adults by formation of a blue line along gum margins: _____

A7. List three or more possible causes of jaundice (icterus).

_____

_____

_____

A8. What does lipofuscin mean?

_____

Is it known to be harmful to cells? *(Yes? No?)*

A9. Name an occupation that is at high risk for causing black lung disease: _____ What exactly accumulates in the lungs of these workers? _____

A10. Contrast *dystrophic* calcification with *metastatic* calcification by writing those terms next to descriptions that fit.

(a) Mrs. Simonson has hypercalcemia caused by bone breakdown associated with immobilization of her fractured femur: _____

(b) Mr. Orbach's hyperparathyroidism and high blood calcium level are related to his renal failure: _____

(c) X-rays of Col. Brunswick's lungs show calcifications at sites of healed tuberculosis lesions: _____

(d) Mrs. Porter's aortic stenosis involves calcification of this valve: _____

B. CELL INJURY AND DEATH

B1. Cellular swelling and accumulation of fat are likely to be examples of *(reversible? irreversible?)* cellular injury. Name two organs in which fatty accumulation tends to occur: _____ and _____. Cellular swelling may be associated with impairment of the _____ pump and with excessive movement of Na⁺ ions *(into? out of?)* cells.

B2. Circle the correct answer or fill in the blanks within each statement to describe two major effects of hypoxia on cells.

(a) One product of anaerobic metabolism is _____ acid. Its accumulation in

cells causes pH there to *(increase? decrease?)*, possibly damaging the nucleus and other cellular structures.

(b) *(Much? Little?)* ATP is produced by anaerobic metabolism, and ATP is especially needed for "fueling" the _____/_____ pump. When that pump fails due to hypoxia, excessive *(Na⁺? K⁺)* builds up in cells; this also affects osmosis of water, so that cells *(shrink? swell?)* dramatically. As a result, cell membrane permeability *(increases? decreases?)* including membranes of lysosomes (that may release _____ enzymes).

B3. Choose from the following list to identify the category or cause of cell injury in each case.

Biological agents   Chemical injury
Electrical injury   Hypoxia
Ionizing radiation   Mechanical forces
Nutritional imbalances Temperature extremes

(a) Frostbite in which ice crystals form in body tissues: _____

(b) Lead or alcohol toxicity; tobacco smoke and other air pollutants: _____

(c) Respiratory disease, anemia, or carbon monoxide poisoning (which prevents red blood cells from carrying oxygen): _____

(d) Lightning; or electrocution caused by turning on a hair dryer while standing in a pool of water: _____

(e) Fever of 107°F; or being trapped in a burning building: _____

(f) A fall from a high bridge: _____

(g) Viruses that incorporate into human DNA and lead to production of billons more viruses; bacteria that release toxins: _____

(h) Anticancer drugs and immunosuppressant drugs taken by transplant patients: _____

(i) Radiation treatment for cancer that also destroys some healthy tissue: _____

(j) Protein-calorie starvation: _____

B4. Circle the correct answer within each statement.

(a) Cold temperatures cause injury by *(vasoconstricting? vasodilating?)* blood vessels in skin.

(b) Heat tends to *(increase? decrease?)* metabolic rate.

(c) With injuries caused by lightning, the injury tends to be most severe in *(skin at entrance and exit sites? internal organs?)*.

(d) *(Alternating current [AC]? Direct current [DC])?)* is more likely to cause serious electrical injuries.

B5. Circle the correct answer or fill in the blank within each statement about lead (Pb) toxicity.

(a) Children are most likely to be exposed to lead by _____.

(b) Lead *(can? cannot?)* cross the placenta to affect a developing fetus.

(c) Lead toxicity can affect *(blood cell formation? gastrointestinal tract? kidneys?)*.

(d) Lead toxicity in children *(is? is not?)* likely to affect the nervous system and reduce intelligence.

B6. Stanley attempts suicide by ingesting an entire bottle (100 tablets) of acetaminophen. Which of his organs is likely to be irreversibly damaged?

_____

B7. Circle the two true statements about radiation injuries. (Pay particular attention to whether the **bold-faced** word or phrase makes the statement true or false.)

(a) Nonionizing radiation is considered **more** lethal than ionizing radiation.

(b) Most radiation injury is related to exposure to **whole body irradiation.**

(c) Rapidly dividing cells (such as those in bone marrow or the lining of the GI tract) are **more** vulnerable to radiation than cells that undergo little or no mitosis (such as those in bone or muscle).

(d) The initial response to radiation is **edema** and **reddening of skin.**

B8. In Questions B2 through B7, you have considered many different categories of agents that can cause cell injury. Now fill in the

blanks about three major mechanisms by which these agents can inflict their cell injury.

(a) Depletion of _____, often caused by hypoxia or toxins. As a result cells are likely to *(shrink? swell?)*, ___-creasing permeability of the cell membrane. (See Questions B1 and B9.)

(b) _____ formation. (See Questions B10 and B11.)

(c) Disruption of intracellular _____ homeostasis. (See Question B12.)

B9. Dr. Benton writes "elevated serum levels of CPK, LDH, and GOT" on a patient's chart. What does this phrase suggest diagnostically?

_____

_____

_____

B10. Fill in the blanks in this exercise about free radicals.

(a) A free radical has one or more single, unpaired _____.

(b) State the major source of free radicals in humans. _____

_____

(c) List one or more source(s) of free radicals that you can avoid: _____

_____

(d) List three examples of antioxidants that can provide some protection against free radicals. _____ _____ _____

B11. Identify the type of chemical (DNA, lipid, or protein) that is damaged when the following cell parts are exposed to free radicals.

(a) Enzymes: _____

(b) Genes: _____

(c) Bilayer of cellular membranes: _____

B12. Circle the correct answers within each statement about other effects of hypoxia on cells.

(a) Normally, intracellular calcium ion (Ca^{2+}) levels are kept *(high? low?)* by *(active? passive?)* transport mechanisms.

(b) Hypoxia tends to cause *(increase? decrease?)* of intracellular Ca^{2+}, which tends to *(activate? inhibit?)* enzymes that break down cell structure.

B13. Contrast two types of cell death, apoptosis and necrosis, by completing this exercise.

(a) A pathological, unregulated digestion of living cells with release of cell contents, and initiation of an inflammatory response: _____

(b) Controlled destruction of worn out cells that helps maintain a balance between cells produced and cells lost; the process does not initiate inflammation:

_____

B14. Describe three or more examples of apoptosis in normal human function.

_____

_____

_____

B15. Apoptosis *(does? does not?)* appear to be involved in some pathologic conditions. List several examples.

_____

_____

_____

B16. Circle all answers in which the term is correctly defined.

(a) Hypoxia: low blood level, possibly to the entire body

(b) Ischemia: low blood flow to certain tissues

(c) Infarction: tissue death when tissue is deprived of arterial blood

(d) Necrosis: reversible cell injury

(e) Edema: tissues with excessive fluid that increases diffusion distance between blood and cells

B17. *(Like? Unlike?)* apoptosis, necrosis involves destruction of the cell membrane with release of cell contents that initiates an inflammatory response. Necrosis *(fosters? interferes with?)* tissue regeneration.

Match the type of necrosis with the descriptions below.

Caseous   Coagulative   Liquefactive

(a) Tissue develops the consistency of cottage cheese; normally occurs in lungs after tuberculosis: _____

(b) Occurs when enzymes pour out of dead tissue and digest that tissue, leaving a "hole" or abscess; can occur in brain or skin: _____

(c) Occurs as a result of ischemia, as in the heart following a myocardial infarction (heart attack): _____

B18. Gangrene refers to a *(small? large?)* mass of necrotic tissue. Circle all of the following characteristics that are associated more with *moist gangrene* than with *dry gangrene*.

(a) Mr. Taylor, who has diabetes, has gangrene of four toes of the right foot; the tissue is black and swollen with blebs full of fluid on the surface of toes; amputation may be required.

(b) The gangrene on Ms. Jenkins's left leg has a slowly advancing pace with a clear line of demarcation of healthy versus gangrenous tissue.

(c) Nurse Hathaway notes that Ms. Jenkins's gangrene has no odor whatsoever.

(d) Dr. Carter finds during surgery that the patient's colon feels cold to the touch, is swollen, and has no pulse.

(e) Rev. Davis's gangrene is caused by disruption of blood flow through the anterior tibial artery to her right leg.

B19. Answer these questions about gas gangrene.

(a) Which odoriferous gas is released and causes much of the malodor of gas gangrene?

(1) Nitrous oxide

(2) Methane

(3) Carbon dioxide

(4) Carbon monoxide

(5) Hydrogen sulfide

(b) Which microorganism lives in soil that may infect necrotic tissue and produce this gas? _____

(c) Name four locations in the body where gas gangrene tends to occur.

_____, _____,

_____, _____

(d) Given that clostridia are *(aerobic? anaerobic?)* bacteria, treatment may involve exposure to *(high? low?)* levels of oxygen within a hyperbaric chamber.

C. AGING CHANGES

C1. Indicate whether each of the following factors tends to increase or decrease with normal aging.

 (a) Kidney function as indicated by glomerular filtration rate: _____

 (b) Synthesis of nucleic acids and structural proteins: _____

 (c) Muscular strength: _____

 (d) The amount of air that can be exhaled after a maximal inhalation (vital capacity): _____

C2. Contrast different theories of aging by circling the correct answers or fill in the blanks within each statement.

 (a) "Programmed change" theories of aging propose that aging changes are *(genetically? environmentally?)* determined.

 (b) Werner syndrome is a(n) *(autosomal? X-linked?)* genetic disorder in which aging takes place at a *(faster? slower?)* than normal rate.

 (c) Define the "stochastic theories" of aging: _____ _____. Now list three examples of stochastic theories of aging. _____ _____ _____

 (d) Telomeres are *(sections of DNA? enzymes?)*. The presence of telomerase causes telomeres to *(maintain their length? shorten?)*. As a result, the rate of aging is *(accelerated? slowed down?)*. Absence of telomerase *(accelerates? slows down?)* aging.

CHAPTER 3

Genetic Control of Cell Function and Inheritance

■ Review Questions

A. GENETIC CONTROL OF CELL FUNCTION

A1. Circle the correct answer or fill in the blank within each statement.

(a) A gene is a section of _____ that codes for synthesis of a single _____ .

(b) *(Transcription? Translation?)* is the first step in protein synthesis.

(c) The type of RNA formed by transcription of DNA is *(messenger? ribosomal? transfer?)* RNA.

(d) The DNA in liver cells is *(the same as? different from?)* the DNA in skin cells. The cells' difference in structure relates to their transcribing *(all? only part?)* of their DNA.

A2. The organelles within the cytoplasm that contain DNA are named _____. Name one disorder that involves matrilineal inheritance transmitted by DNA in these organelles: _____

A3. Circle the correct answer or fill in the blanks within each statement about DNA.

(a) A DNA nucleotide consists of one _____, one _____, and one _____.

(b) The "backbone" of DNA consists of alternating _____ and _____, with bases attached to *(deoxyriboses? phosphates?)*.

(c) In DNA, the base adenine is paired with *(guanine? thymine?)*, whereas cytosine is paired with _____.

(d) Enzymes known as _____ases separate the double-stranded DNA when DNA is to be duplicated or transcribed. In transcription, *(only one strand is? both strands are?)* copied.

(e) Histones are *(RNA? proteins?)* that help to control the structure of DNA strands.

A4. Circle the correct answers or fill in the blanks within each statement related to RNA and protein synthesis.

(a) A codon is a series of *(one? two? three? four?)* bases found in *(mRNA? tRNA?)*. The codon indicates where a specific *(amino acid? rRNA?)* should be positioned.

(b) The codons A A A and A A G code for placement of *(leucine? lysine?)*. *(Hint: see Table 3-1 in Essentials of Pathophysiology.)* These two codons are called _____ because they code for the same amino acid.

(c) RNA and DNA differ in that *(RNA? DNA?)* is single stranded, RNA contains the sugar named _____, and RNA contains the base *(thymine? uracil?)*. During transcription, the triplet A T C in DNA would be transcribed as _____ in mRNA.

(d) The enzyme _____ is required for the transcription process. The sections of transcribed RNA that are spliced out before translation are known as *(exons? introns?)*. The mRNA molecules that result when one section of DNA is spliced *(will be identical? may differ?)*. As a result, *(only one? many different?)* proteins can be produced based on information in a single DNA gene.

(e) Transfer RNA (tRNA) is the *(largest? smallest?)* type of RNA. At least *(80? 64? 20?)* tRNAs exist, one for each type of amino acid. Each transfer RNA has a site that recognizes one amino acid and another that recognizes _____.

(f) Ribosomal RNA makes up *(most? a small part?)* of ribosomes. This type of RNA is synthesized in the _____ and combined with protein. The entire ribosome is formed in the *(cytoplasm? nucleus?)*. Once sent out to the cytoplasm, each ribosome then attaches to _____, where mRNA is "read" in the process of *(transcription? translation?)*.

(g) Polypeptides formed by translation each contain about *(10–30? 100–300? 1,000–3,000?)* amino acids.

A5. Circle all of the sentences that are true. (Pay particular attention to whether the **bold-faced** word or phrase makes the statement true or false.)

(a) **All** genes are active in every cell.

(b) Gene expression is increased by gene **repression.**

(c) Throughout most of life, induction is promoted by some **external** influence.

A6. Circle the correct answer or fill in the blank within each statement about mutations.

(a) Mutations are errors in _____, specifically in the *(base? phosphate? sugar?)* portion of a nucleotide.

(b) Most changes in base pairs *(do? do not?)* result in serious mutations.

(c) Mr. Jensen has one brown eye and one blue eye, an example of a poly_____ that *(can? cannot?)* be transmitted to his children because it results from a *(somatic? germ?)* cell mutation.

B. CHROMOSOMES

B1. Circle the two true statements about human chromosomes. (Pay particular attention to whether the **bold-faced** word or phrase makes the statement true or false.)

(a) Of the 23 pairs of chromosomes, 22 are known as **autosomes.**

(b) Autosomes of females appear **significantly different** from autosomes of males.

(c) Normally, **females** receive an X chromosome from the mother and a Y chromosome from the father.

(d) A **Barr body** is an **inactive X** chromosome, meaning that it **does not** control genetic traits and is present in **females** but not in males.

B2. Answer these questions related to Barr bodies.

(a) Describe the Lyon principle described by geneticist Mary Lyon.

_____

(b) Typically, how many Barr bodies are present in somatic cells of males? _____

(c) Indicate the number(s) of each type of sex chromosome in a child born with Klinefelter syndrome:

(1) Active X chromosome(s): ___

(2) Inactive X chromosome(s) (Barr body): ___

(3) Y chromosome(s): ___

B3. Write *meiosis* or *mitosis* after each description that fits that type of cell division.

(a) The process is preceded by replication of DNA (so that the 46 chromosomes are doubled): _____

(b) Involves two divisions: _____

(c) Includes pairing of homologous chromosomes (in tetrads or bivalents): _____

(d) Results in two identical cells: _____

(e) Occurs only in ovaries or testes: _____

B4. Describe one process in meiosis that leads to the possibility of an almost infinite variety of sperm or ova.

_____

_____

_____

B5. Answer these questions about chromosome structure.

(a) What is the division of genetics that studies the structure and characteristics of chromosomes? _____

(b) What is the source of human cells typically examined for chromosome structure?

_____

(c) What is a karyotype?

_____

(d) What is an acrocentric chromosome?

_____

(e) How is the short arm of a chromosome designated? _____ Regions on chromosomes are identified by being numbered from *(long end of a chromosome inward? centromere outward?).*

(f) What is the function of telomeres? (*Hint:* See study guide Chapter 2, Question C2 [d].)

_____

C. PATTERNS OF INHERITANCE

C1. Use each of the following answers once to fill in the blanks below.

Allele	Genotype	Locus
Multiple-gene	Multifactorial	Penetrance
Phenotype	Single-gene	

(a) "Type A" blood is a _____ , whereas "Ao" is the related _____.

(b) That 50% of people with a particular genotype will have the related phenotype is known as _____ of that gene.

(c) The specific location on a chromosome is known as the _____ of that gene, whereas the possible forms of genes at that site (such as A, B, or O for blood type) are known as _____s.

(d) Most human traits are determined by _____ inheritance; Mendelian laws govern _____ inheritance. _____ inheritance incorporates environmental effects.

C2. Briefly describe Gregor Mendel's work in genetics by circling correct answers and filling in blanks in this paragraph.

Mendel's work was published in the *(19th? 20th?)* century. He studied inheritance in *(beans? eggplant? peas?)*. In Mendel's work, "A" referred to *(round? wrinkled?)* peas. The possible combinations that can result from "crossing" single-gene traits can be described in a _____ square.

C3. Circle the correct answers within each statement. (Statements a–d involve two parents, Katie and John, with the following genotypes: Katie is AA and John is Aa.)

(a) *(A? a?)* is the recessive gene.

(b) *(Katie's? John's?)* genotype is homozygous dominant. Which genotype is heterozygous?

_____

(c) A carrier is *(homozygous? heterozygous?)* and *(does? does not?)* express the trait.

_____

(d) A graphic portrayal of Katie and John's family inheritance is known as a *(karyotype? pedigree?)*.

D. GENE TECHNOLOGY

D1. Describe the Human Genome Project and explain why it was an enormous undertaking.

_____

_____

_____

D2. Describe research efforts to map genes that determine the following traits:

(a) Color blindness _____

(b) Duffy blood group _____

D3. In the "transcript mapping" method used in most genome mapping, *(DNA? mRNA? tRNA?)* is isolated immediately after transcription. From this information, both the complementary DNA and the resultant gene product (_____) can be identified.

D4. Circle the correct answers within each statement about linkage studies.

(a) Linkage studies look at genes that are located on *(the same? different?)* chromosomes. They are located *(close together? far apart?)*, so they *(are? are not?)* likely to be linked during crossing-over of DNA in meiosis I.

(b) Two genes that are likely to be linked are genes for hemophilia and color-blindness, both located on the *(X? Y?)* chromosome. Because males have *(only one? two?)* X chromosome(s), males are *(more? less?)* likely to inherit these conditions. Males are known as *(hemizygous? homozygous? heterozygous?)* for sex-linked traits.

D5. Using dosage studies in which the amount of an enzyme is measured, it is possible to determine whether _____ gave the gene to the child.

D6. Fill in the blanks in the following statements about hybridization studies.

(a) Somatic cell hybridization studies involve fusion of human somatic cells with cells of _____. These studies can identify the location of a specific _____ on a particular chromosome that codes for a specific enzyme.

(b) In situ hybridization uses "probes" consisting of _____ that can identify the location of a specific _____.

D7. Fill in the blanks in the following statements about recombinant DNA.

   (a) Name two hormones that are available for pharmaceutical use as a result of recombinant DNA technology: _____ and _____

   (b) This technology involves the use of restriction enzymes (derived from _____) that cut _____ into many sections, a first step in isolating the _____ of interest.

   (c) Ultimately, this DNA is introduced into a culture of _____ that express the gene by producing large amounts of the gene product (such as insulin).

D8. Describe how gene therapy can be used for persons with cystic fibrosis.

_____

_____

_____

D9. Explain how DNA fingerprinting can be used in forensics.

_____

_____

_____

CHAPTER 4

Genetic and Congenital Disorders

■ Review Questions

A. GENETIC AND CHROMOSOMAL DISORDERS

A1. Be sure that you understand the meaning of the following terms discussed in the last chapter: *single-gene, multifactorial inheritance; locus, allele; homozygous, heterozygous; genotype, phenotype; dominant, recessive.*

A2. Circle the two true statements. (Pay particular attention to whether the **bold-faced** word or phrase makes the statement true or false.)

   (a) Signs and symptoms of **all** genetic defects **are** apparent at birth.

   (b) Birth defects are the **leading** cause of infant deaths.

   (c) Congenital defects may be due to **either** genetic or nongenetic factors.

   (d) A single-gene disorder (such as Marfan syndrome) **will always affect only one part** of the body.

A3. Which of the following is the most common category of single-gene disorder?

   (a) Autosomal dominant

   (b) Autosomal recessive

   (c) Sex-linked

A4. Refer to the pedigree chart in Figure 4-1 in *Essentials of Pathophysiology,* which depicts three generations of a family with an autosomal dominant disorder such as Huntington disease (HD). Circle the correct answer within each statement about this family.

   (a) The grandparents (first generation) have *(2? 4? 6?)* children, of whom *(1? 2? 3?)* are male (squares) and *(1? 2? 3?)* are female (circles).

   (b) In the second generation, *(2? 4? 6?)* individuals appear to be single; the other

two are partnered, and each of these couples has *(2? 4?)* of their own children.

   (c) Each individual receives chromosomes from each of his/her parents. Genes on maternal chromosomes are represented by small *(circles? squares?)*; genes on paternal chromosomes are shown by small *(circles? squares?).*

   (d) Given that the small colored circle represents the mutant autosomal dominant gene, the history of the HD gene in this family can be traced back to the *(grandmother? grandfather?),* who inherited the mutated gene from her/his own *(mother? father?).*

   (e) Do any of the four children in the second generation have the HD gene? *(Yes? No?)* If so, who? _____

   (f) Can HD be transmitted from a mother to a son, or from a father to a daughter? *(Yes? No?)* Explain.

   _____

   _____

   _____

A5. Name two disorders *other than* HD that involve autosomal dominant inheritance. (Note that the pedigree chart in Figure 4-1 could apply to these disorders as well.)

   (a) _____

   (b) _____

A6. Circle the correct answer or fill in the blank within each statement about autosomal dominant disorders.

   (a) For children to inherit autosomal dominant disorders, *(only one parent? both parents?)* must have the defective gene.

   (b) It is probable that *(100%? 50%? 25%? 0%?)* of the children of a parent with an autosomal dominant disorder will inherit the condition.

(c) Asymptomatic individuals *(can? cannot?)* transmit autosomal dominant disorders to their children, thereby "skipping a generation."

(d) If different family members of a family with the HD gene exhibit different signs or symptoms of HD, this is an example of variable _____.

A7. Circle the correct answers or fill in the blanks within each statement about the autosomal dominant disorders Marfan syndrome and neurofibromatosis.

(a) Marfan syndrome is a _____ tissue disorder that primarily affects three systems, namely the *(skin? skeletal? muscular? cardiovascular? endocrine? special senses [eyes]?)*. Most life-threatening are effects on the _____ system. One readily observable effect is the *(short, obese? tall, thin?)* stature. Marfan syndrome has been mapped to a gene that codes for the connective tissue protein named _____ on chromosome _____.

(b) Neurofibromatosis (NF) exists in *(two? three?)* forms located on *(the same? different?)* chromosome(s). *(NF-1? NF-2?)* involves skin lesions arising from peripheral nerves and also flat skin lesions known as *(café-au-lait spots? Lisch nodules?)*. Also affected are *(eyes? ears?)* and skeleton. NF-2 affects *(vision? hearing?)*. The occurrence of NF-2 is much *(more? less?)* common than that of NF-1.

A8. Circle the three true statements about disorders of autosomal recessive inheritance. (Pay particular attention to whether the **bold-faced** word or phrase makes the statement true or false.)

(a) For children to inherit an autosomal recessive disorder, **both parents** must have the defective gene.

(b) Carriers of autosomal recessive disorders **always** manifest signs or symptoms.

(c) Autosomal recessive disorders typically involve **deficiencies of enzymes** rather than **structural abnormalities.**

(d) Phenylketonuria is an autosomal recessive disorder that, if untreated, leads to **mental retardation.**

(e) **Both PKU and Tay-Sachs disease** can be treated effectively by a special diet.

(f) Tay-Sachs disease results from faulty **mitochondrial** function.

A9. Circle the correct answer within each statement.

(a) Cystic fibrosis, sickle cell anemia, and Tay-Sachs disease are all autosomal *(dominant? recessive?)* disorders.

(b) All sex-linked disorders are carried on the *(X? Y? X or Y?)* chromosome, and in most cases the gene for the disorder is *(dominant? recessive?)*. Sex-linked disorders affect more *(females? males?)*.

(c) Men with hemophilia *(can? cannot?)* transmit the defective gene for hemophilia to their sons.

A10. Determine the probability of phenotypes (and, where indicated, genotypes) of children of the following couples. Refer to Figures 4-1, 4-2, and 4-3 below.

(a) Mr. Perez has the genotype for the autosomal dominant disorder achondroplasia, and Mrs. Perez does not. (Note: A = dominant, a = recessive for achondroplasia.) (Figure 4-1)

(b) Both Janet and Phillip are carriers for cystic fibrosis (CF). (Note: C = dominant, c = recessive for CF.) Complete the Punnett square. (Figure 4-2)

(c) Mimi is a carrier for hemophilia A; Patrick does not have the mutant gene for hemophilia A. (Note: H = dominant, or normal gene, h is recessive gene for hemophilia A.) (Figure 4-3)

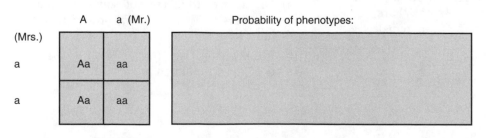

FIGURE 4-1

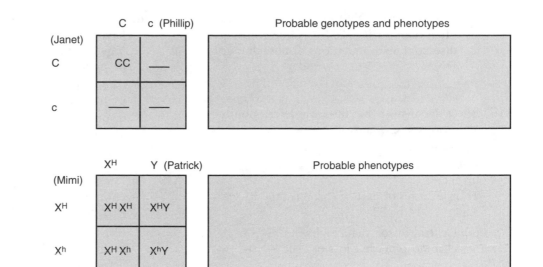

FIGURE 4-2

FIGURE 4-3

A11. Circle the correct answer or fill in the blanks within each statement about a male who has fragile X syndrome.

(a) He *(can? cannot?)* transmit this disorder to his sons.

(b) What percentage of his daughters are likely to be carriers? (Assume that their mother is normal for fragile X.) *(0%? 25%? 50%? 100%?)*

(c) Individuals with fragile X syndrome are likely to be *(highly intelligent? mentally retarded?)*.

(d) List three typical manifestations of this genetic disorder.

(a) _____

(b) _____

(c) _____

A12. Circle the disorders that are attributed to multifactorial inheritance.

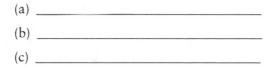

Pyloric stenosis	Fragile X syndrome
Clubfoot	Diabetes mellitus
Tay-Sachs disease	Congenital heart disease
Congenital hip dislocation	Coronary artery disease

A13. Defend or dispute this statement about Marya, who is 3 months pregnant: "Because Marya's first cousin just gave birth to a baby with cleft palate, Marya is at increased risk for giving birth to a baby with cleft palate."

_____

_____

_____

A14. Circle the true statements about cleft lip and cleft palate. (Pay particular attention to whether the **bold-faced** word or phrase makes the statement true or false.)

(a) Cleft lip is one of the most **common** birth defects.

(b) Cleft lip is more common among **girls,** and cleft palate is more common among **boys.**

(c) Cleft lip or cleft palate is a developmental defect that has its origin during the **second** month of gestation.

(d) Cleft lip and cleft palate are caused by hereditary **but not** environmental effects.

(e) Typically, correction of bilateral cleft lip, gums, and nasal deformity take place in a **series of staged surgeries.**

A15. Circle the correct answers or fill in the blanks in the following statements about mitochondrial gene disorders.

(a) DNA is located within the nucleus *(and also? but not?)* the mitochondria of a cell.

(b) Mitochondria contain *(3.7 million? 3,700? 37?)* genes. This DNA is inherited from *(mother? father? both mother and father?)*. These genes code for products (polypeptides) that take part in processes that lead to production of _____ and also help to regulate cell death by *(apoptosis? necrosis?)*.

(c) Mitochondrial DNA mutates *(more? less?)* often than nuclear DNA. Name two diseases due to mutations of mitochondrial DNA. _____ and _____

A16. Select the answer that fits each description of alterations in chromosome structure.

Deletion
Robertsonian translocation
Inversion
Translocation of part of chromosome 21 with part of 14 or 22

(a) Central fusion that results in only 45 chromosomes but loss of little DNA: _____

(b) A chromosomal rearrangement in which the number of chromosomes is still 46, but there is a trisomy of part of chromosome 21: _____

(c) A piece of a chromosome is broken off: _____

A17. Circle the two true statements. (Pay particular attention to whether the **bold-faced** word or phrase makes the statement true or false.)

(a) Shorthand for a **female** with Down syndrome is 47,XY, +21.

(b) **Aneuploidy** refers to an abnormal chromosome number in cells.

(c) **Nondisjunction** is one cause of Down syndrome.

(d) The term *mosaicism* means that one individual has **fewer than normal chromosomes in every cell.**

A18. Circle the correct answers or fill in the blanks in the following statements about Down syndrome.

(a) Cells of people with Down syndrome typically contain a total of _____ chromosomes. In most cases this number results from an extra chromosome number _____.

(b) Down syndrome is a *(rare? common?)* chromosomal disorder. Incidence of Down syndrome *(increases? decreases?)* with the age of the mother.

(c) Children with Down syndrome tend to have a *(larger? smaller?)* than normal head with a *(larger? smaller?)* than normal tongue.

(d) People with Down syndrome are likely to have *(stronger? weaker?)* than normal muscles, a condition known as *(hypertonia? hypotonia?)*.

(e) Children with Down syndrome have a 10 to 20 times greater risk of the blood disorder _____. They are also at greater risk for _____ disease later in life.

A19. Answer the following questions about the detection of Down syndrome.

(a) Circle the three words or phrases that are components of the triple-screen performed on maternal blood that can accurately detect 60% of fetuses with Down syndrome:

Amniocentesis	Human chorionic
Chorionic villi	gonadotropin
sampling (CVS)	(HCG)
Percutaneous	Alpha-fetoprotein (AFP)
umbilical blood	Unconjugated estriol
sampling	

(b) Which answers above are tests that can detect 100% of fetuses with Down syndrome?

_____

A20. Select the answer that fits each description of a chromosomal disorder.

Fragile X syndrome   Klinefelter syndrome
Turner syndrome

(a) Monosomy X (or 45,X/0), a chromosomal disorder in which the female has only one X chromosome; she lacks ovaries and has other anatomical disorders: _____

(b) Polysomy X: males with extra X chromosome(s), such as genotype XXY or XXXY: _____

(c) A disorder that causes mental retardation, large testicles (macroorchidism), and highly flexible joints: _____

B. DISORDERS DUE TO ENVIRONMENTAL INFLUENCES

B1. Choose the two true statements. (Pay particular attention to whether the **bold-faced** word or phrase makes the statement true or false.)

(a) Formation of organs (organogenesis) normally occurs during the **middle** trimester (months **4 to 6**) of pregnancy.

(b) Development of the brain and the heart begin during the **third** week of human development. (*Hint:* Refer to Figure 4-11 in *Essentials of Pathophysiology.*)

(c) Teratogens are **cancer**-causing agents.

(d) Thalidomide is an infamous teratogen that is known to cause **phocomelia** (failure of the **extremities** to develop normally).

B2. Circle the correct answers within each statement.

(a) There *(is? is not?)* evidence that diagnostic levels of radiation cause congenital abnormalities.

(b) *(Most? Few?)* developmental defects are known to be caused by specific drugs or environmental agents.

(c) *(Water? Lipid?)*-soluble drugs such as alcohol and those with *(small? large?)* molecular weight are more likely to cross the placenta and expose the fetus.

(d) In the Food and Drug Administration's classification of drugs that may harm the fetus, those in class *(A? C? X?)* are contraindicated because they are known teratogens.

(e) Doses of vitamin A greater than *(1,000? 10,000?)* IUs should be avoided by women who may be pregnant.

(f) Maternal consumption of alcohol should be avoided *(only after the first three months of? at any time during?)* pregnancy.

B3. List the three clinical findings associated with a diagnosis of fetal alcohol syndrome (FAS).

(a) _____

(b) _____

(c) _____

B4. Choose an answer from the following list to fill in the blank. The U.S. Surgeon General's office recommends that pregnant women drink _____ servings of wine or beer per day.

(a) No more than four

(b) No more than two

(c) No

B5. Fill in the blanks within each statement.

(a) Increase in folic acid intake (such as 0.4 mg/day prenatally and more during pregnancy) has been found to decrease incidence of _____ defects such as _____.

(b) Folic acid is found in foods such as:

_____

(c) The antibiotic tetracycline is associated with defects in _____ development.

B6. Circle the correct answers within each statement about TORCH-caused fetal anomalies.

(a) *TORCH* refers to *(chemicals? microorganisms?)* that are teratogenic.

(b) The *T* in *TORCH* stands for the *(bacterial? fungal? protozoan?)* disorder *toxoplasmosis,* which may be found in the excrement of *(dogs? cats?)*.

(c) *R* represents the *(bacterial? viral?)* infection *(mumps? German measles?)*, known as *rubella*.

(d) *H* stands for *(hepatitis? herpes?)* infections.

CHAPTER 5

Neoplasia: A Disorder of Cell Proliferation and Differentiation

■ Review Questions

A. CONCEPTS OF CELL GROWTH

A1. Circle the two true statements. (Pay particular attention to whether the **bold-faced** word or phrase makes the statement true or false.)

(a) **Cancer** is currently the leading cause of death in the United States.

(b) The term **proliferation** means specialization of cells.

(c) The G_0 phase is the **least active** phase of the growth cycle.

(d) **Apoptosis** is an attempt by the body to regulate cell number and type.

A2. Cell proliferation refers to increase in *(numbers? specialization?)* of cells, whereas differentiation refers to increase in *(numbers? specialization?)* of cells.

(a) Circle terms that best fit descriptions related to cell proliferation.

(1) Blood-forming tissue and cells lining the gastrointestinal tract are classified as *(labile? permanent? stable?)* cells.

(2) Neurons and heart muscle are classified as *(labile? permanent? stable?)* cells.

(b) Circle the term that best fits the description of cell differentiation. As cells become more differentiated, they *(lose? increase?)* their ability to divide.

A3. Arrange these cell categories from most to least differentiated. ___ ___ ___

(a) Pluripotent stem cells, as in bone marrow

(b) Adult stem cells

(c) Highly specialized cells such as neurons

A4. Arrange in correct sequence these phases of the growth cycle that follow the "M" phase:

G_1 G_2 S

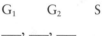

A5. Methotrexate, a type of drug used in chemotherapy, interferes with the replication of DNA required to double chromosome numbers before cell division occurs. This drug attacks cancer cells while they are in the

_____.

(a) G_1 or G_2 phase

(b) M phase

(c) S phase

A6. Describe factors that regulate the cell cycle by filling in blanks. Choose from these answers: cyclins, cyclin-dependent kinases (CDKs), and inhibitors.

(a) _____ are enzymes that phosphorylate specific proteins

(b) _____ and _____ form complexes that regulate specific phases of the cell cycle.

(c) _____ function as tumor suppressors and at least one is controlled by the p53 gene.

A7. Explain how "checkpoints" between cell cycle phases G1 and S and between phases G2 and M relate to cancer. _____

B. CHARACTERISTICS OF BENIGN AND MALIGNANT NEOPLASMS

B1. Circle the correct answer within each statement.

(a) *(Parenchymal? Stroma?)* cells determine the character and naming of a tumor.

(b) *(Parenchymal? Stroma?)* cells carry blood supply that supports survival of the tumor.

B2. Circle the two true statements. (Pay particular attention to whether the **bold-faced** word or phrase makes the statement true or false.)

(a) **All** tumors are cancerous.

(b) Sarcomas are cancers that derive from **epithelial** tissues.

(c) Leukemias are **malignant** tumors of **blood.**

(d) A leiomyosarcoma is a **malignant** tumor of **smooth muscle.**

B3. Write *M* for malignant or *B* for benign next to each description.

(a) An osteoma: ____

(b) More likely to be encapsulated: ____

(c) Tumor grows by crab-like infiltration and is likely to metastasize: ____

(d) Cells are poorly differentiated: ____

(e) Hemangiosarcoma: ____

(f) Not likely to cause death unless its size or location interferes with vital functions: ____

(g) Likely to differentiate normally but proliferate excessively: ____

B4. Circle the correct answers or fill in the blanks within each statement.

(a) When cancer cells mutate early in differentiation, they are likely to be *(more? less?)* malignant than cancer cells that mutate late in differentiation.

(b) Highly anaplastic cells are likely to resemble *(each other? cells from the site of origin?)*. A neoplasm classified as grade *(I? IV?)* is more indicative of anaplasia.

(c) Malignant cells exhibit a *(greater? lesser?)* degree of contact inhibition than normal cells. This is one reason why cancer cells have *(increased? decreased?)* cohesiveness and tend to *(stay in one place? infiltrate other regions?)* in the body. Another factor that contributes to the spread of cancer is the cancer cells' release of _____, which break down the matrix between cells.

(d) The shedding of fetal antigens by cancer cells serves as _____ for cancer and indicates that these cells are *(more? less?)* differentiated than normal cells.

(e) Cancer cells may produce chemicals that are not normally made by cells in this part of the body. List two examples:

_____   _____

B5. Mrs. Wren has a chest x-ray that reveals a lesion. A biopsy of the lesion identifies these cells as cancer cells that originated in Mrs. Wren's kidney. Explain.

_____

_____

_____

B6. Mrs. Chan's endometrial cancer has metastasized to several sites in her large intestine.

(a) Explain how this is likely to have occurred.

_____

_____

_____

(b) Cancer cells that spread into her lymph vessels and nodes are more likely to gain access to blood in *(arteries? veins?)*. Why?

_____

_____

B7. Ms. Lennon has a "sentinel lymph node" biopsied after she is diagnosed with breast cancer. Explain the significance of this node.

_____

B8. Which cancer is more likely to metastasize to the **liver** and which to the **lungs?** Explain why.

(a) Mr. Thomas's testicular cancer:

_____

_____

(b) Mr. Chase's colon cancer:

_____

_____

B9. Write an essay detailing the challenging journey that a cancer cell must undertake in order to metastasize via the bloodstream from a primary to a secondary site. Include these terms in your essay: *enzymes, extracellular matrix, tumor emboli, laminin receptors, angiogenesis,* and *transferrin.*

B10. Answer the following questions about tumor growth.

(a) Circle the answer that is true of cancer cells.

(1) They have a shorter cell cycle, so divide at a faster rate.

(2) They live longer than normal cells because they do not die on schedule.

(b) A tumor is normally undetectable until it contains more than _____ cells.

C. ETIOLOGY OF CANCER

C1. *Onco-* refers to _____. Define *oncogenesis.* _____

C2. List four types of genes that are related to development of cancer.

_____

_____

C3. Explain how the following therapies are related to etiological factors in the development of cancer.

(a) The drug trastuzumab (Herceptin)

_____

(b) Kinase inhibitors (See Question A6[a].)

_____

(c) Antiangiogenic therapy (See Question B9.)

_____

C4. Circle the two true statements about carcinogenesis. (Pay particular attention to whether the **bold-faced** word or phrase makes the statement true or false.)

(a) Most cancers are probably caused by **one** factor.

(b) Proto-oncogenes are sections of DNA that have the potential of being transformed into **cancer-causing** sections of DNA called **oncogenes.**

(c) **Most** cancers are known to be caused by viruses.

(d) Because p53 protein normally **suppresses** tumor growth, mutations of the p53 gene **increase** the risk of certain cancers such as breast and lung cancer.

C5. Circle the three true statements about carcinogenesis. (Pay particular attention to whether the **bold-faced** word or phrase makes the statement true or false.)

(a) The initiation step in carcinogenesis is a **reversible** mutation of DNA.

(b) The **initiation** step in carcinogenesis must precede the promotion step in carcinogenesis.

(c) Promotors do **not** alter DNA but change its expression.

(d) Promotion **is not** reversible, even if the promotor is removed.

(e) The progression step of carcinogenesis is **the same as** the promotion step.

(f) **Complete** carcinogens both initiate and promote.

C6. BRCA1 and BRCA2 refer to genes that increase a person's risk for _____ cancer. About (*10% to 20%? 70% to 80%?*) of all breast cancers are familial.

C7. Circle the type(s) of immune cells that can fight against cancer cells.

CD4$^+$ helper T cells   CD8$^+$ cytotoxic T cells
Natural killer (NK)   B lymphocytes
 cells

C8. In each of the following pairs, circle the name of the person who is likely to be at greater risk for cancer:

(a) Emily, age 77, compared with her 47-year-old daughter, Michelene

(b) Julia, who has taken immunosuppressants for 12 years following a kidney transplant, compared with Evelyn, who has taken no immunosuppressants

(c) Robert, who was diagnosed with AIDS two years ago and has received no treatment, compared with Daniel, whose AIDS has been treated

C9. *Carcinogenic* means:

(a) RNA

(b) Blood-vessel-forming

(c) Cancer-causing

(d) DNA

(e) Cachectic (cachexia-causing)

C10. Circle the correct answer within each statement.

(a) Inheritance of retinoblastoma (RB), a rare childhood tumor of the retina, tends to follow autosomal (*dominant? recessive?*) patterns.

(b) Children with inherited RB *(are? are not?)* likely to develop other cancer.

(c) Unique tumor-specific antigens are found *(only on tumor cells? on tumor cells and on normal cells?)*.

(d) The first association between environmental agents and causation of cancer linked *(coal soot and scrotal cancer? radiation and leukemia? tobacco and lung cancer?)*.

(e) Direct-acting carcinogens *(do? do not?)* require activation by the body to become carcinogenic.

(f) Smoking has been associated with *(only lung? many?)* cancers.

(g) Most known dietary carcinogens are found naturally occurring in *(plant? animal?)* food sources or are produced during food preparation.

C11. Jimmy, age 42, is having a history and physical taken. He states to the nurse that he "live(s) on hot dogs and barbecued pork, fries, beer, cigarettes, and playing cards and having some smokes with my buddies." Describe the aspects of Jimmy's lifestyle that increase his risk for cancer.

_____

_____

_____

C12. Match the type of cancer with the patient likely to be at greatest risk for it.

Leukemia   Lung   Skin   Thyroid   Vaginal

(a) Julia's mother took diethylstilbestrol (DES) while she was pregnant with Julia: _____

(b) Jesse, age 38, has done fieldwork in southern Arizona since he was a child; he experienced three severe sunburns between ages 7 and 10: _____

(c) Henry, age 68, is a survivor of the bombing of Hiroshima: _____

C13. Match the virus with the correct description below.

Epstein-Barr virus   Hepatitis B virus
Human T-cell   Human papillomavirus
  leukemia virus-1

(a) Associated with liver carcinoma as well as cirrhosis and hepatitis B: _____

(b) An RNA virus carried in CD4 cells and associated with a form of leukemia: _____

(c) More than 60 different types include those that cause warts (papillomas) and squamous cell carcinomas of the cervix: _____

(d) Associated with four human cancers, including some lymphomas: _____

D. CLINICAL FEATURES

D1. Explain how Mrs. Garcia's signs and symptoms of her end-stage colon cancer may be caused by the pathogenesis of cancer:

(a) Severe constipation with impaction and blood in the stool

_____

(b) Difficulty urinating

_____

(c) Severe abdominopelvic pain

_____

(d) Weight loss of 50 pounds even though she retains large amounts of fluid in her abdomen

_____

D2. Mr. Feinstein, age 55, was admitted to the Emergency Department with a fractured right hip resulting from a fall last evening. He also reports severe pain in his right calf. The ED nurse notes that Mr. Feinstein was diagnosed 15 months ago with multiple myeloma. Lab work indicates that Mr. Feinstein's serum calcium level is 13.0 mg/dL (high). Write rationales for Mr. Feinstein's clinical manifestations.

(a) Fractured hip:

_____

(b) Calf pain:

_____

D3. Mr. Eversen, age 40, was diagnosed nine months ago with small cell carcinoma of the lung. He tells the nurse, "I can hardly move my right arm and leg and I never had problems like this until recently." Explain.

_____

E. DIAGNOSIS AND TREATMENT

E1. Answer these questions about early detection of cancer.

   (a) Explain why cervical dysplasia cells are more likely to shed and be detected during a Papanicolaou (Pap) smear than normal cells are.

   _____

   _____

   _____

   (b) List several methods besides the Pap smear that are methods of secondary prevention (screening) for cancer.

   _____

   _____

   _____

E2. Mr. Rhodenberger's nurse practitioner discusses with her patient that his PSA level is higher than it was 3 months ago. What information is the nurse practitioner conveying?

   _____

   _____

   _____

E3. Match the antigens (tumor markers) with the types of cancer with which they are linked.

   Alpha-fetoprotein   Carcinoembryonic antigen
   Human chorionic   Prostate-specific antigen
     gonadotropin

   (a) Associated with most colorectal and pancreatic tumors, and many gastric and breast tumors: _____

   (b) Normally formed in the fetal liver and yolk sac, this antigen may also be elevated with primary liver cancers:
   _____

   (c) Normally produced by the placenta, elevated levels can indicate tumors related to pregnancy: _____

E4. Identify whether the following results of diagnostic tests on Mr. Rhodenberger's chart (from Question E2) are indicative of grading (G) or staging (S) of his cancer. Also answer the related questions by filling in the blanks. It may help to refer to Chart 5-2 in *Essentials of Pathophysiology*.

   (a) T2, N3, M1: ____ *N* of *N3* refers to involvement of _____. Has Mr. Rhodenberger's tumor spread to tissues or organs distant from the primary (original) site? ____

   (b) Moderately undifferentiated cells: ____ Which carries a worse prognosis: grade I or grade IV? _____

   (c) To what does pTNM refer? _____

E5. Sherrie had radiation, then surgery, and then chemotherapy for her synovial sarcoma. Explain why this sequence of treatments was used.

   _____

E6. Answer these questions about the ionizing radiation used to treat Ms. Bonner's breast cancer.

   (a) Her radiation especially targets *(slowly? rapidly?)* dividing cells. Fast-growing, poorly differentiating cancer cells are typically more *(radiosensitive? radioresistant?)* than slower-growing normal cells.

   (b) Ms. Bonner is likely to receive *(one large dose? multiple fractionated doses?)*. Explain why.

   _____

   (c) Explain why Ms. Bonner has bouts of nausea and vomiting and hair loss, and why her blood counts are checked frequently.

   _____

E7. Circle the correct answers or fill in the blank within each statement about the use of chemotherapy for cancer patients.

   (a) Explain why multiple courses of treatment are required for effective chemotherapy.

   _____

   (b) *(Combination? Single drug?)* chemotherapy is generally most effective.

   (c) Methotrexate is a cell-cycle *(specific? nonspecific?)* anticancer drug. It is most effective during the *(G_1? M? S?)* phase of the cycle. It is a component of the *(CHOP? CMF?)* drug regimen for breast cancer.

E8. Define biotherapy.

_____

_____

_____

Contrast the two major categories of cancer biotherapy by writing *A* for active or *P* for passive forms of immunotherapy.

(a) Introduction of antigens such as BCG that stimulate the patient's immune system: ___

(b) Vaccines composed of antigens derived from the patient's own tumor cells that activate immune responses: ___

(c) Introduction of natural killer (NK) cells activated by lymphokines such as interleukin-2 (IL-2); these directly attack cancer cells (as well as normal cells): ___

(d) Use of T cells taken from the person's tumor (tumor-infiltrating lymphocytes or TIL cells) and grown to form large numbers before reinfusion; TILs attack tumor cells but not normal cells: ___

E9. Match the biologic response modifiers (BRMs) with the descriptions below.

Hematopoietic growth factors	Interferons
	Interleukins
	Monoclonal antibodies

(a) Mrs. Jordan is receiving CSFs and erythropoietin to reverse the side effects of her radiation and chemotherapy drugs:

_____

(b) These antibodies were used to detect the presence of Mrs. Jordan's ovarian cancer classified as "targeted therapy":

_____

(c) Matthew's Kaposi sarcoma (KS) is treated by these BRMs that stimulate his own NK cells and T lymphocytes to combat this AIDS-related cancer: _____

(d) Mrs. Kern received this class of chemicals to activate many aspects of her immune system to attack metastasizing cells from her kidney tumor: _____

F. CHILDHOOD CANCERS

F1. Circle the two true statements about childhood cancers. (Pay particular attention to whether the **bold-faced** word or phrase makes the statement true or false.)

(a) Cancer is the **leading** cause of death among children.

(b) Most childhood cancers involve cells of **epithelial** origin.

(c) Families with one child with cancer are at **increased** risk of having another child who develops cancer.

(d) Children with hereditary disorders such as Down syndrome have an **increased** risk for developing cancer.

F2. List several warning signs of childhood cancers.

_____

_____

_____

F3. Circle the correct answers within each statement about childhood cancers.

(a) Cancer is *(more? less?)* frequently found among children than adults, contributing to the *(ease of? difficulty in?)* diagnosing childhood cancer.

(b) Sequelae of radiation treatment on growth and cognitive development are greater if the child is *(of preschool age? of school age or older?)* when the treatment is given.

(c) Radiation and chemotherapy *(virtually never? are known to?)* cause damage to heart and lungs.

CHAPTER 6

Disorders of Fluid, Electrolyte, and Acid-Base Balance

■ Review Questions

A. COMPOSITION AND COMPARTMENTAL DISTRIBUTION OF BODY FLUIDS

A1. Match the body fluids with the descriptions that follow.

Intracellular fluid   Interstitial fluid
Plasma or serum

(a) Fluid within cells; comprises about two thirds of body fluids: _____

(b) Contains a high level of potassium and small amounts of sodium and chloride: _____

(c) Fluid that is measured clinically (because of its accessibility): _____

(d) Extracellular fluids (ECF): _____ and _____

A2. Answer the following questions about body fluids and electrolytes.

(a) Circle the anion(s) in this list:

Bicarbonate   Chloride   Glucose
Potassium   Protein

(b) Which of the answers in A2(a) is a/are nonelectrolyte(s)? _____

(c) *(Diffusion? Dissociation? Osmosis?)* is the movement of water across a semipermeable membrane.

(d) Almost all of the osmotic pressure in extracellular fluids (ECF) is the result of:

   (1) Na^+, Cl^-, and HCO_3^-

   (2) BUN and glucose

(e) A 0.9% NaCl solution is *(hyper? iso? hypo?)* tonic to human cells.

(f) Human cells placed in hypotonic solutions are likely to *(shrink? swell?)*.

(g) Name two or more "transcellular spaces": _____, _____.
Accumulation of fluids here is known as _____-spacing.

A3. Timothy, a healthy 12-year-old, weighs 100 pounds. His body weight contains about ___ pounds of fluid. This fluid includes ___ pounds of fluid within cells (ICF) and ___ pounds of ECF. Most of his ECF is likely to be *(blood plasma? interstitial fluid?)*.

A4. Edema is most likely to result from any of the following factors. Give examples of causes in each case.

(a) An increase in *(capillary? tissue?)* filtration pressure that is a force that *(pushes out of? pulls into?)* blood vessels.

(b) Decrease in *(capillary? tissue?)* colloidal osmotic pressure (COP), a force that normally *(pushes out of? pulls into)* vessels.

(c) *(Increase? Decrease?)* in capillary permeability. _____

(d) Blockage of _____ flow.

A5. Circle the correct answer in the following questions about edema.

(a) Mrs. Sella has dependent edema. This is most likely to be caused by:

   (1)   Hypoalbuminemia

   (2)   Congestive heart failure

(b) Renal failure is more likely to lead to large amounts of _____ in urine.

   (1)   Albumin

   (2)   Fibrinogen

(c) Which edema is typically life threatening? Edema of:

   (1)   Larynx or lungs

   (2)   Ankles and feet

(d) Edema increases the risk of tissue breakdown (as in pressure ulcers) because edema _____ the distance between blood vessels and cells.

  (1)   Increases

  (2)   Decreases

(e) Mrs. Kuczkowski has +3 pitting edema that indicates that blood proteins such as fibrinogen _____ accumulated in tissues.

  (1)   Have

  (2)   Have not

(f) A weight gain of 9 pounds associated with edema indicates a water gain of about ___ liters.

  (1)   2

  (2)   4

  (3)   9

(g) Ascites refers to "third-spacing" of fluid in the _____ cavity.

  (1)   Pleural

  (2)   Pericardial

  (3)   Peritoneal

B. SODIUM AND WATER BALANCE

B1. List three important functions of sodium in the body.

_____

_____

_____

B2. List the major route by which sodium (Na$^+$) typically enters the body. _____

List two sources of sodium besides dietary intake: _____ and _____. Most sodium loss is typically through the *(kidneys? skin? gastrointestinal tract?)*.

B3. Circle the correct answer to indicate whether each of the following factors will cause the body to save or lose sodium (Na$^+$).

(a) Vasoconstriction of renal arteries with decreased glomerular filtration rate (GFR): *Save Na$^+$ Lose Na$^+$*

(b) The renin-angiotensin mechanism: *Save Na$^+$ Lose Na$^+$*

(c) Vomiting or diarrhea: *Save Na$^+$ Lose Na$^+$*

(d) Aldosterone: *Save Na$^+$ Lose Na$^+$*

B4. In healthy adults, total body water (TBW) normally ranges from about ___% to ___ % of body weight. Circle the persons more likely to have a higher proportion of total body water (TBW).

60-year-old woman	20-year-old woman
Lean person	Obese person
Person with body temperature of 104°F	Person with body temperature of 99.0°F
2-month-old infant	2-year-old child

List several reasons why.

_____

_____

B5. Refer to Table 6-2 in *Essentials of Pathophysiology* and answer these questions about fluid exchange.

(a) The body typically gains about 90% of its daily fluids through _____. The remainder comes from the _____ of foods.

(b) Normally, kidneys eliminate about _____ mL of urine per day (or ____ mL/minute).

(c) In association with GI infections, more fluid is likely to be lost through *(exhalations? GI tract? kidneys? skin?)*. During vigorous exercise, more fluid is likely to be lost through _____.

B6. Thirst is a(n) *(early? late?)* sign of hemorrhage or other fluid volume deficits. Circle the correct answers or fill in the blanks within each statement about how thirst helps maintain fluid volume. (*Hint:* refer to Figure 6-7 in *Essentials of Pathophysiology.*)

(a) The "thirst center" is located in the _____, which is located just *(inferior? superior?)* to the pituitary gland. Cells here shrink when the body is *(de? over?)*hydrated and send the message to drink water. List several other locations of thirst receptors.

_____

_____

(b) Hypothalamic cells also contribute to the maintenance of fluid level by secreting *(ADH? aldosterone? renin?)*, which is stored and released from the _____terior pituitary.

B7. Circle the correct answer or fill in the blank within each statement about alterations in thirst.

   (a) Mrs. Litwin, age 89, states "I don't drink much water; I just don't feel thirsty anymore." She is likely to have *(hypo? poly?)*dipsia.

   (b) Mr. Le Sourd, age 38, is an inpatient in a psychiatric unit. He has been drinking 2 to 3 gallons of water a day to "cleanse the evil demons." He is a 2-pack-a-day cigarette smoker. Name his thirst disorder: _____.

   (c) Mrs. San Domenico, age 70, is a person with diabetes whose blood glucose is 420 mg/dL. She has an increased urine output and is thirsty. Her thirst disorder is classified as _____ thirst. (Choose the correct answer from the following:)

      (1) False

      (2) Inappropriate

      (3) True or symptomatic

B8. Visualize the hypothalamus when blood passing through it is slightly "thicker" or more concentrated than normal. These cells secrete ADH, which has the following effects. (Circle the correct answers or fill in the blank.)

   (a) ADH stimulates kidney tubule cells to become *(more? less?)* permeable to water. In other words, ADH tells kidneys to "save the water!" ADH *(increases? decreases?)* blood volume (blood becomes "less thick") as urine output is *(increased? decreased?)*. The name antidiuretic hormone (ADH) indicates that its effects are *(similar to? opposite of?)* the effects of diuretics.

   (b) ADH is also known as a vaso_____ because it can vaso*(constrict? dilate?)* blood vessels to raise blood volume and blood pressure.

B9. Urinary output is likely to increase considerably after Ray drinks large quantities of beer. One reason is that beer contains a high percentage of water; the other is that alcohol *(increases? decreases?)* ADH production.

B10. Circle the correct answers or fill in the blanks within each statement about two disorders of ADH.

   (a) Dr. Tony has diabetes insipidus (DI).

      (a1) Her body produces too *(much? little?)* ADH. Without treatment she is more likely to produce *(15? 0.5?)* L of urine each day, causing her thirst to *(increase? decrease?)* as her blood is *(concentrated? diluted?)*. Treatment typically involves administration of ADH.

      (a2) In DI, the large urine output is *(sugary? nonsugary?)*, which accounts for the term "insipidus." In diabetes mellitus, a person produces a *(large? small?)* amount of urine that is *(sugary? nonsugary?)* because of a decrease in effective _____.

      (a3) Dr. Tony's DI is *(central or neurogenic? nephrogenic?)*. In nephrogenic DI, a person produces *(adequate? inadequate?)* ADH, and kidneys *(do? do not?)* respond to it.

   (b) Marc has SIADH.

      (b1) His condition involves *(over? under?)*production of ADH. Fluid *(retention? deficit?)* occurs, leading to *(dehydration? edema?)*, dilution of solutes such as sodium (which causes _____natremia), and dilution of red blood cells (_____).

      (b2) List several factors that can lead to SIADH.

      _____

      _____

See Table 6-1, on page 31; also refer to Tables 6-3 and 6-4 in Essentials of Pathophysiology *as you complete Questions B11 through B14. Circle the correct answers or fill in the blank within each statement.*

B11. Alterations in fluids and electrolytes are closely linked because body fluids contain electrolytes. The major electrolyte in plasma (or serum) is *(K+? Na+?)*. Two major categories of fluid and sodium disorders include the following:

   (a) Gains or losses of water. Some of these disorders were discussed in Question B10 because they involve imbalances in *(ADH? aldosterone?)*. For example, as much water is lost in diabetes insipidus (DI), serum sodium concentration *(increases? decreases?)* above the normal range of _____ mEq/L. (See also Questions B12 to B14.)

   (b) Excess or deficit in *both* sodium and water (isotonic fluids). The hormone most likely to be involved in these imbalances is *(ADH? aldosterone?)*. (See Questions B12 to B14.)

Table 6-1. Alterations in Fluid Volume and Sodium Concentration: Causes and Manifestations

Disorder	Causes	Manifestations
a. Fluid volume deficit (FVD) or isotonic fluid volume loss	**↑ Na⁺ and H₂O loss caused by:** GI loss (vomiting, diarrhea) Skin loss (fever, burns), ↑ exercise Third-spacing (burns, ascites) *Addison disease (↓ aldosterone) *Excess use of diuretics **↓ Na⁺ and H₂O intake (↓ thirst)**	Serum Na⁺ normal, thirst, ↑ pulse, ↓ BP, ↓ weight, ↓ skin turgor, depressed fontanels ↓ UO in all cases except * (in which ↑ UO)
b. Fluid volume excess (FVE) or isotonic fluid volume gain	**↓ Na⁺ and H₂O loss caused by:** Renal failure, heart failure ↑ aldosterone as in Cushing syndrome or primary aldosteronism or use of steroids *↑ **Na⁺ and H₂O intake (IV overload)**	Serum Na⁺ normal, edema and pulmonary edema with dyspnea, weight gain, bounding pulse, ↓ hematocrit. ↓ UO in all cases except * (in which ↑ UO)
c. Hyponatremia (dilutional)	**↑ Na⁺ loss with pure water replacement** (exercise) **↑ Pure water intake or retention caused by:** Psychogenic polydipsia *SIADH (↑ ADH) due to pain, stress	Serum Na⁺ <135 mEq/L, water intoxication, fingerprint edema, ↓ hematocrit, ↓ BUN (dilutional), muscle cramps ↑ UO except * (in which ↓ UO)
d. Hypernatremia	**↑ H₂O loss caused by:** Watery diarrhea *Diabetes insipidus (↓ ADH) **↓ H₂O intake caused by:** Impaired thirst Lack of acess to H₂O	Serum Na⁺ >145 mEq/L, thirst, ↑ pulse, ↓ BP, dry mouth, headache, ↑ hematocrit ↓ UO except in * (in which ↑ UO)

BP, blood pressure; UO, urine output.

B12. Circle the correct answers.

(a) Which one cause of fluid volume deficit (FVD) listed below will result in an increased urine output?

(1) Addison disease

(2) Burns

(3) Inability to access fluids

(4) Diarrhea

(5) Fever

(b) Which one cause of hypernatremia will manifest an increase in urine output (polyuria)?

(1) Impaired thirst

(2) Diabetes insipidus

(3) Fever

(4) Watery diarrhea

(5) Excessive sweating

(c) Circle the condition with manifestations most similar to FVD:

(1) Fluid volume excess (FVE)

(2) Hyponatremia

(3) Hypernatremia

(d) Circle the condition with manifestations most similar to FVE:

(1) FVD

(2) Hyponatremia

(3) Hypernatremia

(*Hint:* To remind yourself of these similarities, draw arrows on Table 6-1 between FVD and hypernatremia and also between FVE and hyponatremia.)

B13. Match the disorder with the appropriate description.

Fluid volume deficit   Fluid volume excess
 (FVD)   (FVE)
Hyponatremia   Hypernatremia

(a) Serum sodium level is 152 mEq/L; hematocrit is 52; thirst: _____

(b) Caused by increase in aldosterone:

_____

(c) Caused by increase in ADH (SIADH): _____

(d) Caused by chronic renal failure (CRF): _____

(e) Manifestations most resemble those of FVD: _____

(f) Most likely to be accompanied by hypotension and tachycardia: _____, _____

(g) Most likely to affect brain cells and cause altered personality and behavior: _____, _____

B14. Identify the disorder described in each case. Use the answers listed in Question B13.

(a) Mr. Evanston has congestive heart failure, both pulmonary and generalized edema, and venous distension; a sodium-restricted diet is prescribed for him: _____

(b) Ms. Annenburg has been diagnosed with adrenal insufficiency (Addison disease): _____

(c) Mr. Leon, age 55, has severely limited mobility related to his Huntington disease, but he still lives in his own house. In July, he fell and was unable to get up from the floor for 40 hours while temperatures in his house reached 105°F. His eyes were sunken; his skin turgor and capillary refill were both diminished: _____

(d) Dr. Tony, who has diabetes insipidus (and was discussed in Question B10[a]), is injured in a fall; she becomes unconscious and does not get her medication. Her pulse is 120 beats/minute, her skin and mucous membranes are dry, and her reflexes are decreased. She produces copious amounts of urine: _____

(e) Kathryn has been exercising and sweating on a hot, humid day. She has drunk more than 1.5 liters of water. She begins to feel weak, becomes nauseated, vomits, and faints: _____

(f) Todd, age 5 months, is in the children's burn unit with extensive second- and third-degree burns acquired in an automobile accident. His anterior fontanel is depressed: _____

(g) Sammy, age 2 months, has had diarrhea for 3 days. His weight has decreased from 14 pounds to 13 pounds. He is at greatest risk for (two answers): _____, _____

(h) Mr. Le Sourd, mentioned in Question B7(b), has added tap-water enemas to his psychogenic polydipsia in attempts to "cleanse his body of demons." The resulting "water intoxication" adds to signs of his psychosis. Fingerprint edema is manifested over his sternum: _____

C. POTASSIUM BALANCE

C1. Refer to Figure 6-1 when answering the following questions about potassium in the body. Circle the correct answers or fill in the blanks within each statement.

(a) Almost all potassium ions (K^+) are located within *(ICF? ECF?)*. Show this by writing (K^+) within the cell on Figure 6-1A. Circle the normal range for serum K^+: *(134 to 145 mEq/L? 22 to 27 mEq/L? 3.5 to 5.0 mEq/L?)*. Write this value on the leader line drawn to the blood vessel on Figure 6-1A.

(b) The main source of potassium is typically through diet. List several good sources of this electrolyte. _____

(c) Figure 6-1B shows that the hormones insulin and epinephrine facilitate movement of K^+ *(into? out of?)* cells. Severe exercise and cell trauma (including burns or excessive GI activity) move K^+ *(into? out of?)* blood.

(d) The major route by which healthy persons lose potassium each day is through the *(GI tract? kidneys? skin?)*. Aldosterone *(increases? decreases?)* tubular secretion of K^+ into urine. On Figure 6-1C, identify other actions of this hormone.

(e) Hyperkalemia tends to cause acidosis and vice versa, as a result of K^+-H^+ exchange mechanisms demonstrated in Figures 6-1 D and E. High blood levels of K^+ cause kidney tubules to secrete K^+ into urine and reabsorb another cation (___) back into blood (Figure 6-1D). During acidosis (Figure 6-1E), cells buffer H^+ and then give up K^+ to blood in exchange. An acidosis that lowers serum pH from 7.4 to 7.3 will typically raise serum K^+ by ____ mEq/L.

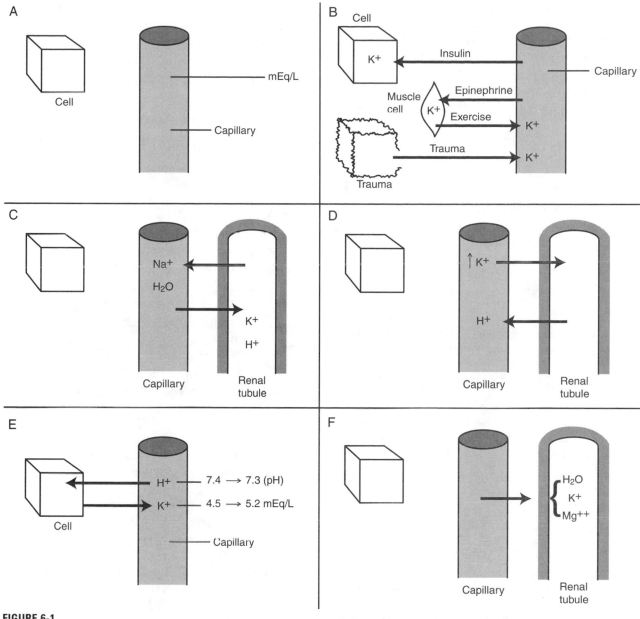

FIGURE 6-1

(f) The most common cause of excessive K+ loss occurs by use of _____, shown in Figure 6-1F. Such medications also cause loss of ____.

C2. Apply the alterations in K+ regulation just discussed in Question C1 to these cases of hypokalemia or hyperkalemia. Circle the correct answers or fill in the blanks within each statement.

(a) Ms. Annenburg (Question B14[b]) with Addison's disease has *(deficient? excessive?)* production of aldosterone. She is more likely to develop *(hypo? hyper?)*kalemia.

(b) Sammy (Question B14[g]) has lost a lot of fluid during his prolonged diarrhea. He is at risk for _____kalemia.

(c) Todd (Question B14[f]) has extensive burns and other tissue trauma resulting from his accident. His damaged cells are likely to release K+, initially causing _____kalemia. Over time the K+ in his ECF may leak out of his burned skin or exit in urine, leading to _____kalemia.

C3. Mr. Evanston (Question B14[a]) takes a thiazide diuretic and also digoxin for his congestive heart failure (CHF). Answer these questions about his case.

(a) He is at increased risk for _____kalemia because of the diuretic. The most serious effects of hypokalemia are those affecting the _____ system, particularly if serum K^+ drops below ____ mEq/L.

(b) The drug digitalis is likely to *(ameliorate = make better? exacerbate = make worse?)* the situation. Both hypokalemia and digoxin tend to cause *(brady? tachy?)*cardia.

(c) Hypokalemia *(increases? decreases?)* resting cell membrane potential, leading to *(increase? decrease?)* in muscle and nerve activity. Write examples of such manifestations.

_____

(d) List several approaches to increasing Mr. Evanston's serum K^+ level.

_____

_____

_____

(e) If he does require IV, what assessment should be made first? Explain.

_____

_____

_____

C4. Hye-Sun, age 35, (Chapter 25, Question B11) has end-stage renal disease (ESRD) with her glomerular filtration rate (GFR) currently less than 5 mL/min. Circle the correct answers or fill in the blank within each statement about her case.

(a) Her serum K^+ is 6.3 mEq/L, indicating *(hyper? hypo?)*kalemia. Decreased renal function is a *(rare? common?)* cause of hyperkalemia. Hyperkalemia is *(common? rare?)* among healthy persons.

(b) Hye-Sun *(is? is not?)* likely to manifest neuromuscular changes related to her hyperkalemia. Explain.

_____

(c) Many manifestations of hyperkalemia are similar to those of hypokalemia (see Table 6-5 in *Essentials of Pathophysiology*). Write two distinguishing manifestations of hyperkalemia.

_____

(d) The fact that her blood pH level is currently 7.1 is likely to *(ameliorate? exacerbate?)* her electrolyte disorder. Explain.

_____

(e) Interventions for Hye-Sun *(should? should not?)* include use of salt substitutes.

D. CALCIUM AND MAGNESIUM BALANCE

D1. Virtually all of the body's calcium ions (Ca^{2+}) are located within *(bones? blood?)* (see Figure 6-12 in *Essentials of Pathophysiology*). However, other tissues require these ions also. Fill in the blanks or circle the correct answer within each statement about how the body controls locations of these electrolytes.

(a) Two major factors that regulate these ions are vitamin ___ and the hormone ____.

(b) Vitamin D is activated by several organs, namely _____, _____, and _____, under the influence of the hormone _____.

(c) PTH is produced by the four parathyroid glands. What is their normal location? _____ *(Hyper? Hypo?)*calcemia serves as the major stimulus for secretion of PTH. Name an electrolyte also needed for normal PTH function. _____

D2. Circle the correct answers or fill in the blanks within each statement about PTH.

(a) An increase in PTH leads to a(n) *(increase? decrease?)* in serum Ca^{2+}. PTH either directly or indirectly "pulls" Ca^{2+} from three sources. Name them: _____, _____, _____

(b) PTH also influences PO_4^{-3} levels of blood. The hormone *(increases? decreases?)* blood PO_4^- levels by pulling the ion from bones, but *(increases? decreases?)* blood PO_4^{-3} by triggering _____ excretion of this ion. The latter effect is greater, so PTH tends to *(increase? decrease?)* serum PO_4^{-3}.

(c) PTH also increases blood _____ levels by pulling the ion from bones.

D3. List several causes of hypoparathyroidism.

_____

_____

_____

D4. Explain how renal failure can lead to the following conditions.

(a) Hyperparathyroidism

_____

_____

_____

(b) Bone demineralization

_____

D5. List several functions of calcium in the body.

_____

_____

D6. Circle the correct answers or fill in the blank within each statement about calcium.

(a) A serum level of 10.9 mg/dL is *(high? normal? low?)*.

(b) List several calcium-rich foods:

_____

(c) Dietary deficiency of calcium exerts more effects on Ca^{2+} levels in *(blood? bone?)*. Hypocalcemia due to inadequate dietary Ca^{2+} or vitamin D is *(common? rare?)* in the United States.

(d) The main route by which the body normally loses Ca^{2+} is *(feces? skin? urine?)*.

(e) The form of Ca^{2+} that is free to leave blood and take part in cell functions is the form that is *(complexed or chelated? ionized? protein-bound?)*.

(f) *(Hyper/Hypo?)*calcemia occurs in as many as 70% to 90% of patients in intensive care units.

D7. Write *hyper* or *hypo* next to factors that are likely to cause hypercalcemia or hypocalcemia.

(a) Failure to activate vitamin D due to liver or kidney disease: _____

(b) Leg immobilization for 2 months following a tibial fracture: _____

(c) Production of high levels of osteoclastic chemicals from tumor cells: _____

(d) Magnesium deficiency: _____

(e) Use of lithium to treat bipolar disorders and use of thiazide diuretics: _____

D8. *(Rapid? Slow?)* blood transfusions are more likely to lead to hypocalcemia. Explain.

_____

_____

_____

D9. Circle the correct answers or fill in the blanks within each statement about Hye-Sun, age 35, (Question C4) who has end-stage renal disease (ESRD). (*Hint:* See Question D4.)

(a) Her failing kidneys eliminate *(more? less?)* than normal PO_4^{-3} and *(more? less?)* than normal Ca^{+2}. Hye-Sun's serum calcium is more likely to be *(7.0? 11.5?)* mg/dL, indicating _____calcemia.

(b) Hye Sun's bones are soft and painful and prone to fracture. Explain.

_____

_____

(c) The nurse practitioner performs a Chvostek's sign on Hye-Sun. This involves *(inflating a blood pressure cuff on the arm? tapping on the face?)*. Describe a positive Chvostek's sign.

_____

_____

(d) Hye-Sun's behavior exhibits signs of psychoses and dementia. Explain.

_____

_____

(e) She experiences tingling known as _____ around her mouth and in extremities, as well as spasms of wrists and ankles (_____ spasms). Spasms of the _____ would exert potentially fatal effects.

(f) What treatments may improve Hye-Sun's condition?

_____

_____

D10. Write *hyper* or *hypo* next to signs or symptoms of hypercalcemia or hypocalcemia.

(a) Decreased neuromuscular activity as indicated by muscle weakness and atrophy, constipation, lethargy, stupor, and coma: _____

(b) Damage to kidneys which leads to inability of kidneys to concentrate urine and to polyuria and thirst:_____

(c) Cardiovascular alterations: _____

D11. Write *hyper* or *hypo* next to causes of hypermagnesemia or hypomagnesemia.

(a) Diarrhea or laxative abuse: _____

(b) Alcoholism (with associated malnutrition): _____

(c) Chronic use of magnesium-containing antacids or supplements: _____

D12. A normal range for serum level of magnesium is _____ mg/dL. Explain why adequate magnesium levels are critical to normal body function.

_____

_____

D13. Manifestations of hypomagnesemia mimic *(hyper? hypo?)*calcemia, for example with tetanic contractions and *(positive? negative?)* Chvostek's or Trousseau's signs. Hypermagnesemia is more likely to manifest with muscle *(weakness? spasticity?)* and *(hyper? hypo?)*tension.

E. ACID-BASE BALANCE

E1. Circle the two true statements. (Pay particular attention to whether the **bold-faced** word or phrase makes the statement true or false.)

(a) An acid is a molecule that can **accept** a hydrogen (H^+) ion.

(b) Most of the body's acids, such as carbonic acid, are **weak** acids.

(c) A pH of 7.5 is **more** acidic than a pH of 7.4.

(d) **Carbonic** acid is classified as a volatile acid because exhalation can eliminate it.

(e) Almost all of the CO_2 in blood is transported **attached to hemoglobin.**

E2. Write the chemical reactions that show formation and dissociation of carbonic acid. Write *CA* (carbonic anhydrase) above the reaction that is accelerated 5,000 times by this enzyme.

_____

Note that if bicarbonate (HCO_3^-) combines with H^+, carbonic acid (H_2CO_3) results. But bicarbonate can also combine with another cation (Na^+ in ECF or K^+ in ICF) to form sodium bicarbonate ($NaHCO_3$) or potassium bicarbonate ($KHCO_3$), respectively.

E3. Name two or more acids in each category that are produced by metabolism.

(a) **Organic** _____

(b) **Inorganic** _____

E4. Circle the correct answers or fill in the blanks within each statement about maintaining blood pH.

(a) Arterial blood pH is normally maintained at about *(7.2? 7.3? 7.4?)*, or within a range of pH _____ to _____.

(b) Refer to the reactions in Question E2. To maintain a pH of 7.4 in the plasma (ECF) of arterial blood, a ratio of Na.HCO_3 to H.HCO_3 ($NaHCO_3$ to H_2CO_3) of ___: ___ must be maintained. This is determined by the _____-_____ equation. *Note: If one of these values increases, then the other value must also increase to maintain the ratio.*

(c) The concentration of bicarbonate in plasma is within the range of _____ to _____ mEq/L, or a mean of about _____ mEq/L. (*Hint:* see Table 6-1 in *Essentials of Pathophysiology.*)

(d) Because H_2CO_3 cannot be measured directly, it is determined by the amount of CO_2 dissolved in plasma. This is calculated by multiplying PCO_2 by 0.03 (the solubility coefficient of CO_2). Venous blood contains $45 \times 0.03 =$ _____ mEq/L of dissolved CO_2 and arterial blood contains _____ $\times 0.03 =$ _____ mEq/L. It is logical that arterial blood contains a little *(more? less?)* dissolved CO_2 than venous blood.

(e) Calculate the normal ratios that must be maintained for acid-base balance:

(e1) Ratio in venous blood

$$\frac{NaHCO_3}{H_2CO_3 = \text{dissolved } CO_2} = \underline{\quad} \text{ mEq/L} = \frac{20}{1}$$

(e2) Ratio in arterial blood

$$\frac{NaHCO_3}{H_2CO_3 = \text{dissolved } CO_2} = \underline{\quad} \text{ mEq/L} = \frac{20}{1}$$

(f) Calculate an acid-base *imbalance* in which hypoventilation causes retention of CO_2 so that the level of dissolved CO_2 doubles from 1.2 to ____ mEq/L. $NaHCO_3$ will need to *(increase? decrease?)* to ____ mEq/L to maintain a 20:1 ratio. So, as one value increases, the body compensates by causing the other value to *(increase also? decrease?)*. (See Question E4[b].) Complete the new ratio.

$$\frac{NaHCO_3}{H_2CO_3 = \text{dissolved } CO_2} = \frac{24 \text{ mEq/L}}{1.2} = \frac{\underline{\quad}}{2.4}$$

(g) Bicarbonate ($NaHCO_3$) levels fluctuate widely in the body because this chemical is expended in buffering acids produced by metabolism. For example, lactic acid released during vigorous muscle metabolism decreases plasma levels of bicarbonate because the bicarbonate is being used as a buffer. Therefore metabolic acid-base imbalances are reflected by altered *($NaHCO_3$? H_2CO_3 = dissolved CO_2?)*. Respiratory acid-base imbalances result from a respiratory condition that alters *($NaHCO_3$? H_2CO_3 = dissolved CO_2?)*. The disorder in Question E4(f) is an example of a compensated *(metabolic? respiratory?)* acid-base imbalance.

E5. List the three major mechanisms that work to maintain acid-base balance.

(a) _____

(b) _____

(c) _____

Arrange them in correct sequence from fastest- to slowest-acting in responding to acid-base imbalances: _____,

_____, _____

E6. Visualize buffers as tiny sponges floating around in plasma. Fill in the blanks within each statement about the carbonic acid–bicarbonate buffer system.

(a) The buffer consists of an anion (in this case, _____)— the "sponge" that can either absorb or eject different cations such as Na^+ or H^+. Typically, there are ____ bicarbonates attached to Na^+ for every ___ bicarbonate attached to H^+ (the 20:1 ratio).

(b) When the body develops acidosis and needs to buffer a strong acid such as HCl, the Na^+ ions are "squeezed out" of the

"sponge" (HCO_3^-) so that the H^+ ions can enter the sponge and form the weaker acid, _____. The remaining Na^+ ions combine with ____. Complete the reaction: $HCl + NaHCO_3 \rightarrow$ _____ + _____

E7. Choose the buffer system that fits each description below.

Ammonia   Bicarbonate–carbonic acid
Protein   Transcellular H^+/K^+ exchange

(a) The most common buffer system in cells (ICF); albumin is a major buffer of this type: _____

(b) Involves the acid formed from $CO_2 + H_2O$: _____

(c) This system allows kidneys to increase elimination of H^+: _____

(d) Allows kidneys to eliminate ammonia, H^+ and Cl^-, in the form of ammonium chloride (NH_4Cl): _____

(e) The result of this system is that when plasma H^+ increases (acidosis), K^+ will increase, as will Ca^{2+}, and vice versa (see Question C1[e] and related Figures 6-1D and 6-1E about shifts of H^+ and K^+): _____

E8. Fill in the blanks or circle the correct answer within each statement about renal and respiratory mechanisms that regulate acid-base balance.

(a) Kidneys regulate acid-base balance by altering their tubular secretion of _____ or elimination of a _____ ion over several days. Several mechanisms are employed.

(a1) H^+ ions are removed in urine by the carbonic anhydrase–mediated system that causes kidneys to retain _____ and _____.

(a2) H^+ ions are removed in urine by the _____ buffer system that again involves kidney retention of _____ and _____.

(a3) H^+ ions are removed in urine by the _____ buffer system. In this system, ammonia (_____) combines with H^+ to form ammonium (_____) that is excreted as NH_4Cl while again kidneys retain _____ and _____.

(a4) All these systems allow acid to be eliminated and alkaline $Na^+HCO_3^-$ to be retained. How else are the different buffers helpful?

_____

(b) Slight acidosis stimulates hyperventilation that will tend to *(raise? lower?)* blood pH because, as the person exhales, less CO_2 is available for formation of _____ acid and free hydrogen ions.

E9. Fill in the blanks within each statement about other mechanisms that help regulate pH.

(a) Hyperkalemia (high levels of _____) tends to cause acidosis (high levels of _____) and vice versa (see Figures 6-1D and 6-1E). Conversely, hypokalemia leads to _____osis.

(b) High aldosterone levels cause kidneys to retain _____ and _____ and to secrete _____ and _____ (see Figure 6-1C). Thus, primary aldosteronism tends to lead to _____osis (and hypokalemia), whereas Addison disease leads to _____osis (and hyperkalemia).

(c) During a meal, the stomach secretes gastric juices including the acid _____. In response, the body will retain another anion (_____) to maintain electrochemical balance. Then, after a meal (postprandially), _____osis occurs briefly.

E10. Teri, age 42 and a lifelong smoker, is in early stages of emphysema. Blood is removed from her left radial artery for testing of arterial blood gases (ABGs). Circle "yes" or "no" to indicate whether each result is normal.

(a) Her arterial PO_2 is 88 mm Hg.   Yes No

(b) Her arterial PCO_2 is 48 mm Hg.   Yes No

(c) Her arterial pH is 7.30.   Yes No

(d) Her arterial HCO_3^- is 36 mEq/L.   Yes No

(e) Her arterial base excess is   Yes No
3.3 mm Hg.

E11. Larry completed a 15-mile run 2 hours ago. Look at his arterial blood gases (ABGs) and serum electrolyte values and determine his anion gap. Is this high, low, or normal?

Na^+: 136 mEq/L   Arterial PCO_2: 44 mm Hg

Cl^-: 86 mEq/L   Arterial PO_2: 86 mm Hg

HCO_3^-: 34 mEq/L Arterial pH: 7.35

Explain your answer.

_____

_____

_____

F. ALTERATIONS IN ACID-BASE BALANCE

F1. Identify whether a correction or a compensation is taking place in each case.

(a) Mr. Hershey has increased blood levels of BUN, creatinine, K^+, and H^+ as a result of acute renal failure caused by nephrotoxic drugs. ECG changes, abdominal cramping, and diarrhea result from his hyperkalemia. His doctor changes his prescription to one that is not toxic to kidneys:

_____

(b) Mrs. Litzinger is hyperventilating during labor and delivery. She begins involuntary wrist and ankle movements (carpopedal spasms). Her kidneys start producing more highly alkaline urine: _____

F2. Circle the correct answers or fill in the blanks within each statement about the effects of altered pH on the central nervous system (CNS).

(a) In acidosis, H^+ *(increases? decreases?)*, pH *(increases? decreases?)*, and CNS activity *(increases? decreases?)*. (*Hint:* as pH goes down, so does CNS activity.) Write typical signs and symptoms:

_____

_____

(b) In alkalosis, H^+ *(increases? decreases?)*, pH *(increases? decreases?)*, and CNS activity *(increases? decreases?)*. Write typical signs and symptoms:

_____

_____

F3. Identify the source of the signs or symptoms in Question F1.

(a) Signs of the primary disorder:

_____

(b) Signs of altered pH:

_____

(c) Signs of a compensatory mechanism:

_____

F4. Indicate which of the four categories of acid-base imbalances is most likely to occur as a result of each condition.

Metabolic acidosis   Metabolic alkalosis
Respiratory acidosis   Respiratory alkalosis

(a) Mr. Hershey (Question F1[a]) during his acute renal failure: _____

(b) Teri (Question E10) with emphysema: _____

(c) Myocardial infarction: _____

(d) Suzanne, who is on a ketogenic 400 cal/day diet for weight reduction: _____

(e) Severe diarrhea with loss of pancreatic secretions (high in HCO_3^-): _____

(f) Diuretics that cause potassium loss: _____

(g) Primary aldosteronism: _____ (See Question E9[b].)

(h) Loss of gastric juices (with hypochloremia) by nasogastric suction: _____ (See Question E9[c].)

F5. Circle the correct answers or fill in the blank within each statement about acid-base imbalances.

(a) Mary Emma, age 11, has diabetes and is currently in ketoacidosis. She is breathing as if she just finished running hard. This is known as _____ breathing and is a classic compensatory sign of *(metabolic? respiratory?)* acidosis. The pH of her urine is likely to be *(5.0? 7.0?)*. Acidosis *(can? does not?)* affect Mary Emma's skeletal growth.

(b) Emily has purging bulimia. Her plasma pH is 7.54, PCO_2 is 52 mm Hg, and HCO_3^- is 36 mEq/L. Her breathing is slow and shallow. Explain why KCl is administered.

_____

(c) Mr. Feinberg cannot breathe deeply after fracturing a rib 3 days ago. His blood pH is 7.33, PCO_2 is 52 mm Hg, and HCO_3^- is 36 mEq/L. His bicarbonate has *(increased? decreased?)* as a compensatory mechanism because PCO_2 is increased; this is an attempt to maintain the 20:1 ratio between these two chemicals. (See Questions E4[b and f].) The change in bicarbonate level happens *(quickly? slowly?)*. State the clinical significance.

_____

_____

_____

(d) Julia has a panic attack and is in the psychiatric emergency department. Her hyperventilation is likely to lead to an arterial pH of *(7.3? 7.5?)* with *(hyper? hypo?)*excitability of her nervous system. Describe one simple method that can help to reverse her acid-base imbalance.

_____

F6. How can you determine the type of acid-base imbalance when values for PCO_2 and HCO_3^- are similar, as for Emily and Mr. Feinberg in Question F5(b and c)?

_____

_____

_____

CHAPTER 7

Stress and Adaptation

■ Review Questions

A. HOMEOSTASIS

A1. Match these theorist researchers with the descriptions of their work.

Claude Bernard   Hans Selye   Walter Cannon

(a) Identified the *milieu intérieur* as the fluid environment around cells: _____

(b) Described homeostasis as a stable internal environment achieved by mechanisms that resist various disturbances that he described as "fight or flight" responses: _____

(c) In the early 1930s, he described mechanisms of adaptation to stress: _____

A2. Circle the correct answers within each statement about control mechanisms of the human body.

(a) When David runs a mile, his muscles release heat, which causes his body temperature to increase. In efforts to return his temperature back to normal, his sweat glands are likely to *(increase? decrease?)* secretions, and blood vessels of his skin are likely to *(dilate? constrict?)*. These mechanisms are examples of *(positive? negative?)* feedback control mechanisms because they alter a parameter such as temperature in the *(same? opposite?)* direction as it had originally been changed.

(b) Most control systems of the body are *(positive? negative?)*. They introduce *(stability? instability?)* into a system. An example is release of the pancreatic hormone insulin in response to *(elevated? decreased?)* blood glucose level. The effect of insulin is to *(raise? lower?)* blood glucose level.

A3. Contrast allostasis and homeostasis in Mary Ann, who experiences stress associated with fibromyalgia.

(a) Homeostasis is an attempt to achieve stability through *(processes that oppose change? change?)*. Allostasis is an attempt to achieve stability through _____.

(b) Allostasis *(does? does not?)* involve Mary Ann's previous experiences with pain and her perception of her condition now. Mary Ann's comparison of her life with fibromyalgia versus the pain-free life she had envisioned for herself is known as the _____ *activation theory of stress.*

B. STRESS

B1. Briefly describe possible roles of stress in disease causation.

_____

_____

_____

B2. List the three specific anatomic changes that Hans Selye described in rats exposed to various stressors.

_____

_____

_____

B3. Spell out the acronym GAS described by Hans Selye:

G _____ A_____ S_____.

Use these words to answer the following questions about the GAS.

Alarm   Exhaustion   Resistance

(a) Arrange in correct sequence the three phases of the GAS: _____, _____, _____

(b) Which phase involves action of pituitary and both adrenal medulla and adrenal cortex hormones, as well as sympathetic nerves? _____

(c) In which phase does the body try to fight back or "resist"? _____ But if these mechanisms fail, then the stage of _____ (with possible death) occurs.

B4. List several conditions likely to result from emotional disturbances (stress) and the body's adaptive mechanisms.

_____

_____

_____

B5. Discuss stressors and their impact by circling the correct answers or filling in the blank in these statements about Mrs. Robinson, whose daughter's wedding is this week.

(a) The stressors associated with planning the wedding are _____genous stressors.

(b) Mrs. Robinson is recovering from hip replacement and her husband has prostate cancer. These are likely to be *(internal? external?)* conditioning factors that *(increase? decrease?)* her adaptive capacity.

B6. Identify the three major systems that interact in response to stressors.

_____

_____

_____

B7. Match the parts of the brain with the stress-related functions that follow.

Cerebral cortex   Hypothalamus
Locus ceruleus   Limbic system
  norepinephrine pathway   Thalamus
Reticular activating system

(a) Conveys sensory information about stressors to different parts of the brain: _____

(b) Facilitate mental alertness and vigilance during stress responses (two answers): _____, _____

(c) Involved primarily with emotional aspects of stress responses: _____

(d) Coordinate autonomic and endocrine responses to stressors: (two answers): _____, _____

(e) A site of neurons in the brain stem that release norepinephrine (NE): _____

(f) CRF made here stimulates release of ACTH that triggers adrenal cortical production of cortisol: _____

B8. Fill in the blanks within each statement about relationships between neuroendocrine and immune function.

(a) Two classes of hormones that inhibit immune function are _____ and _____. The fact that at least eight hormones influence lymphocytes is evidenced by the presence of _____ for these hormones on lymphocytes.

(b) It is known that cytokines such as interleukins released by _____ activate the hormones of the HPA system. This system includes cells of the hypothalamus as well as the _____ and _____ glands.

B9. Consider how each of the following factors would be likely to have an impact on your own adaptation to the stress of your being diagnosed with an illness such as diabetes, multiple sclerosis, or a brain tumor. Select one diagnosis and discuss with a friend or a colleague.

(a) Your life experiences
(b) Your nutritional patterns and status
(c) Your overall health status
(d) Your hardiness

B10. Circle the person who is likely to adapt better in each case. Then identify from the following list the type of factor involved in each case of adaptation. Write the factor on the line provided.

Age   Health status
Psychosocial factors   Timing of onset

(a) Loss of 25% of total blood volume in:
(1) Jeanette, by arterial hemorrhage within a period of 3 minutes
(2) Irma, by bleeding from a peptic ulcer over the course of 3 months

_____

(b) Prolonged diarrhea in:
(1) Jamie, who is 2 months old
(2) Cassandra, who is 20 years old

_____

(c) A respiratory infection in:
(1) Terrence, who has cystic fibrosis
(2) Paula, whose lungs are healthy

_____

(d) Diagnosis of HIV-positive status in:

   (1) Lee, who has a supportive significant other and caring siblings

   (2) Sandy, who is homeless and suffers from alcoholism

_____

B11. Contrast these two sleep disorders: *insomnia* and *increased somnolence*.

_____

_____

_____

C. DISORDERS OF THE STRESS RESPONSE

C1. Identify the pattern of stressors in each case.

   Acute time-limited   Chronic intermittent
   Chronic sustained

   (a) Jamal, age 5, has had middle ear infections four times in the past 2 years: _____

   (b) Chris, age 40, was diagnosed with amyotrophic lateral sclerosis (ALS, or Lou Gehrig disease) when he was 37. He can still speak and swallow, but most of the rest of his body is paralyzed: _____

   (c) Steffy develops a respiratory infection that leads to pneumonia within the first few days after she begins attending day care during a viral epidemic: _____

C2. Mr. Clement, who has diabetes and significant renal impairment, is involved in an auto accident and brought to an emergency room. His blood pressure is 192/112 mm Hg. Speculate about the impact of this acute stress on him.

_____

_____

_____

C3. Mrs. Delany, age 78, is caring for her older sister who has Alzheimer disease. List several physical indicators of stress for which Mrs. Delany is at higher risk.

_____

_____

_____

C4. Janelle, age 48, was working at the World Trade Center on September 11, 2001. She survived with no physical injuries but with major psychological trauma. Janelle has since been diagnosed with PTSD. Write the meaning of this acronym:

   P_____ T_____ S_____
   D_____

C5. Jennifer, age 19, is the only survivor of a boating accident 3 months ago in which both her fiancé and her brother drowned. Write the related sign or symptom next to each of Jennifer's statements that characterize her PTSD. Select from these terms:

   Avoidance   Alcohol or drug abuse
   Depression   Intrusions
   Memory problems   Sleep disturbances
   Survival guilt

   (a) "I just want to be alone and drink; I shouldn't even be alive."

   _____

   (b) "Three nights this week I woke up and lived it all over again."

   _____

C6. Answer the following questions about PTSD.

   (a) List several other events besides boating accidents that might lead to PTSD.

   _____

   _____

   _____

   (b) Physiologic mechanisms of PTSD include activation of _____-related systems in several brain parts, for example the _____ and the _____. The function of the _____ in memory is thought to contribute to the intrusive nature of PTSD recollections.

   (c) Additional physiologic mechanisms of PTSD include exaggerated *(sympathetic? parasympathetic?)* nerve responses and *(increased? decreased?)* levels of catecholamines such as _____.

   (d) Persons with PTSD manifest *(increased? decreased?)* levels of cortisol and a(n) *(increased? decreased?)* dexamethasone suppression test. These factors *(mimic? differ from?)* typical stress responses.

   (e) Studies suggest that strong family relationships may *(increase? decrease?)* risk for PTSD among children exposed to violent events.

(f) List several methods other than antidepressant or antianxiety medications that may be used in the treatment of PTSD.

_____

_____

_____

C7. One example of biofeedback therapy is based on the finding that during stress, temperature *(increases? decreases?)* in fingers or toes, as a result of sympathetic vaso*(constriction? dilation?)* of blood vessels in the extremities. Such changes can be monitored by the patient as a result of *(electromyodermal? electrodermal? electrothermal?)* detection.

CHAPTER 8

Alterations in Body Nutrition

■ Review Questions

A. REGULATION OF FOOD INTAKE AND ENERGY METABOLISM

A1. Describe how the adage "You are what you eat" applies to pathophysiology.

_____

_____

_____

A2. Arrange these food types from greatest to least caloric value:

Alcohol   Carbohydrates or proteins   Fats

_____, _____, _____

A slice of bread is likely to contain about 100 *(calories? kilocalories?)*.

A3. Answer the following questions about adipose tissue.

(a) More than ___% of body energy (or fuel) is stored within adipose tissue. _____ is the process in which fats (or other chemicals) are broken down, transformed, or otherwise converted into energy for cells.

(b) List three or more functions of adipose tissue.

_____

_____

_____

(c) People born with large numbers of adipocytes *(do? do not?)* have increased risk of becoming obese.

(d) The antidiabetic drugs in the TZD class (thiazolidinediones) can *(stimulate? inhibit?)* formation of new fat cells, allowing uptake of glucose by these cells. The ultimate effect is a(n) *(increase? decrease?)* in blood glucose levels.

(e) HAART (highly active antiretroviral therapy) drugs taken by persons infected with the HIV virus cause a(n) *(increase? decrease?)* in numbers of fat cells, leading to the HIV-associated condition known as

_____.

(f) Most fat in adults is *(brown? white?)* fat. Write one advantage of the presence of brown fat in infants and also in hibernating animals.

_____

A4. Circle the correct answer to complete each statement about nutritional needs.

(a) The RDA (recommended daily allowance) refers to an amount of a nutrient required for _____ healthy persons of a specific group.

   (1) Almost all

   (2) Half of

(b) The _____ is the maximum intake that is judged unlikely to pose a health risk in almost all healthy persons in a specific group.

   (1) Adequate Intake

   (2) Tolerable Upper Intake Level

(c) The _____ indicates what percent of the FDA's daily value (for example, of saturated fat) is supplied by one serving of a specific food.

   (1) Estimated Average Requirement

   (2) Percent Daily Value (% DV)

(d) _____ are likely to require more kilocalories per kilogram of body weight.

   (1) Preschoolers

   (2) Fifth-graders

(e) _____ is likely to require more kilocalories per kilogram of body weight.

   (1) Maureen, not pregnant,

   (2) Norine, 7 months pregnant,

(f) _____ amino acids are classified as "essential."

   (1) 9

   (2) 20

(g) _____ fats tend to raise blood cholesterol.

(1) Polyunsaturated

(2) Saturated

(h) _____ carbohydrates are more recommended for the diet.

(1) Simple

(2) Complex

(i) Vitamins _____ directly provide energy.

(1) Do

(2) Do not

(j) Because _____ vitamins are stored in the body, it is more likely that excessive dietary amounts of these will lead to toxicity.

(1) A, D, E, K (fat soluble)

(2) B complex and C (water soluble)

(k) Calcium, phosphorus, and magnesium are all _____

(1) Macrominerals

(2) Trace minerals

(l) The daily dietary recommendation for cholesterol is less than _____ mg.

(1) 30

(2) 300

A5. Select the chemical category that best fits each of the following descriptions.

Carbohydrates   Fats   Proteins

(a) Glucose and glycogen are both examples: _____

(b) Insulates and protects organs: _____

(c) Contain about 16% nitrogen, so their adequacy is measured by positive or negative nitrogen balance: _____

(d) Composed of combinations of the 20 different amino acids sequenced correctly: _____

(e) Typically accounts for about one third of the calories in the U.S. diet; serves as carriers for vitamins A, D, E, and K: _____

(f) Typically accounts for one half to two thirds of the calories in the U.S. diet: _____

(g) Linoleic acid is the one chemical in this category that is required in the diet: _____

(h) The nervous system, including the brain, depends almost exclusively on this type of chemical as a fuel source: _____

(i) Form much of muscles and bones, as well as hemoglobin, antibodies, and enzymes: _____

A6. Defend or dispute this statement: "Because there is no specific daily requirement for carbohydrates, RDAs indicate that carbohydrates should be eliminated from the diet."

_____

_____

_____

A7. Complete this exercise about regulation of food intake.

(a) *(Hunger? Appetite?)* is the desire for a particular type of food. _____ refers to a feeling of fullness.

(b) In what part of the brain are centers for hunger and satiety? _____ List three categories of triggers that signal these centers.

_____

_____

_____

(c) In the space after each of the following descriptions of mechanisms that regulate food intake, write *S* for a mechanism that provides for short-term regulation and *IL* for a mechanism that provides intermediate- or long-term regulation.

(c1) Low blood levels of glucose that cause hunger: _____

(c2) Release of the hormone leptin (from fat cells with high fat content), which decreases appetite and increases metabolic rate: _____

(c3) Tasting, chewing, and swallowing, which have the effect of depressing appetite: _____

(c4) Stretch receptors in the walls of the stomach, which trigger vagus nerve impulses to depress appetite: _____

(c5) Cholecystokinin (CCK) released in response to the presence of fats in the duodenum and also glucagons like peptide-1: _____

A8. Kathy is on a weight-loss plan that involves checking for the presence of ketones in her blood or urine. Explain the reason for this test.

_____

_____

A9. Select the nutritional assessment methods that fit each of the descriptions that follow.

Biological impedance	BMI
Laboratory studies	MRI
Relative weight	Waist-to-hip circumference

(a) Determination of fat content in body tissues based on electrical resistance: _____

(b) Actual weight divided by desirable weight and multiplied by 100: _____

(c) Assessment of serum levels of albumin to assess protein status: _____

(d) Which of these methods are anthropometric measurements? _____

A10. Calculate your own body mass index (BMI).

(a) Your weight = _____ pounds divided by 2.2 pounds/kg = _____ kg.

(b) Your height = _____ inches × 2.54 cm/inch = _____ cm divided by 100 = _____ meters. Now square that number = _____ m².

(c) Calculate BMI. BMI equals your weight in kg (_____) divided by your height squared (_____ m²).

(d) A BMI of 32 kg/m² indicates that the person is *(underweight? normal weight? overweight? obese?)*. What does your BMI indicate about your weight?

_____

A11. Circle the correct answers related to body measurements.

(a) Circle the desirable percentage(s) of body fat for men:
7%   14%   21%   28%

(b) Circle the desirable percentage(s) of body fat for women:
7%   14%   21%   28%

(c) Physical exercise is likely to *(increase? decrease?)* lean body mass.

B. OVERNUTRITION AND OBESITY

B1. Circle the correct answer or fill in the blank within each statement about overnutrition and obesity.

(a) The World Health Organization describes "being overweight" as a BMI that exceeds *(25? 30? 35? 40?)*.

(b) About *(5? 15? 30?)*% of the U.S. population is estimated to be classified as obese, that is, with a BMI over _____.

(c) Obesity is more prevalent among people who *(are wealthy? live below the poverty level?)*.

(d) Obesity is attributed to *(genetic? environmental? both genetic and environmental?)* factors.

(e) List several medications that are likely to increase body weight.

_____

_____

_____

B2. Write a short essay about the factors that contribute to overnutrition and obesity. Include these terms: *automobile, computer, energy density, portions, anxiety,* and *comfort.*

_____

_____

_____

_____

_____

B3. Research indicates that *(presence of fat? fat distribution?)* may be the more important factor for morbidity and mortality. Mrs. Santangelo, age 58, weighs 225 lb. Her waist is 42 inches and her hips are 45 inches. Answer the following questions about her fat distribution.

(a) Her waist to hip ratio is *(0.8? 0.933? 1.07?)*, which indicates *(upper? lower?)* body obesity. After menopause, women are likely to develop *(upper? lower?)* body obesity. People with *(upper body or abdominal? lower body or gluteal-femoral?)* obesity are at higher risk for myocardial infarction, cerebrovascular accident, and death.

(b) Her excessive abdominal fat has a higher risk of impairing liver function if the fat is *(visceral? subcutaneous?)*. List several other

health conditions for which she is at
increased risk.

_____

_____

_____

B4. Theresa, age 24, who is Mrs. Santangelo's
daughter, weighs 155 lb. She consults the
nutritionist for ideas that may help keep her
from becoming obese. Make several suggestions.

_____

_____

_____

B5. Complete this exercise about Mr. Hastings, age
48, who is 6' tall and weighs 220 lb.

(a) Circle each of Mr. Hastings's characteristics
that is a health risk factor:

(1) His age

(2) His waist measurement: 41 inches

(3) HDL of 32 mg/dL and LDL of
184 mg/dL

(4) Blood pressure of 136/82 mm Hg

(5) He has never smoked

(6) He is able to exercise but limits his
activity to a golf game about once a
month.

(7) His BMI

(b) Mr. Hastings talks with a nutritionist about
his goal to lose 20 lb over the next 6
months. To do this, it is recommended that
he reduce caloric intake by (300–500?
500–1,000?) kcal/day. His diet should
contain less than (10%? 30%? 50%?) fat
calories.

(c) His exercise goal should include _____
hour(s) or more of moderate activity (once
a day? most days each week?).

(d) Suggest techniques for behavioral
modifications to help with Mr. Hastings's
weight loss.

_____

_____

_____

(e) Based on his BMI, Mr. Hastings (is? is not?)
a candidate for a surgical intervention for
his weight.

B6. Obesity is a (rare? common?) disorder among
children and adolescents. Currently, about
_____% of children in the United States
are overweight. One common method of
assessing childhood obesity is a measurement
weight for height of greater than _____%.

List two major concerns about childhood
obesity.

_____

_____

B7. Circle all of the following factors that put
children at risk for obesity. Having:

Active lifestyle   Highly educated parents
Parents in poverty   Obese parents
Many siblings

C. UNDERNUTRITION

C1. Match these causes of undernutrition with the
disorders that follow:

Lack of food   Physical health
  availability   problem
Willful eating behaviors

(a) Crohn disease: _____

(b) Anorexia nervosa: _____

(c) Kwashiorkor and marasmus:

_____

C2. Globally, it is estimated that the number of
children under 5 years of age who are
undernourished is about _____.
Kwashiorkor and marasmus are two forms of
undernourishment in children. Identify the
characteristics below that pertain to
kwashiorkor and those that pertain to
marasmus.

(a) Deficiency of both calories and protein:

_____

(b) The child looks wasted with stunted growth
but has relatively normal skin and hair:

_____

(c) This condition occurs when a child is
displaced from the mother's breast after the
birth of another child: _____

(d) The child manifests an enlarged abdomen
with hepatomegaly and distended abdomen,
edema, skin lesions, and profound apathy:

_____

C3. Antonio is in the final stages of AIDS. Describe the systemic effects of tissue wasting that are likely to affect Antonio.

_____

_____

C4. Julia is dying of ovarian cancer. Fill in the blanks within each statement about her case with one of these terms: carbohydrate, fat, or protein.

(a) Most of Julia's body's available sources of calories are likely to be those stored as

_____.

(b) Breakdown of large amounts of _____ is likely to cause Julia to develop ketosis.

(c) Loss of lean mass causing her "wasting" appearance results mostly from breakdown of _____, which also affects respiratory and cardiac muscle.

(d) Julia's net loss of this type of chemical in the postabsorptive state is matched by a net postprandial gain: _____

(e) Poor wound healing comes primarily from _____ deficiency.

C5. Treatment of severe protein-calorie malnutrition should be undertaken (_rapidly? slowly?_). Edema (_is? is not?_) likely to occur, and diuretics (_should? should not?_) be used.

C6. Circle the correct answer or fill in the blanks within each statement about eating disorders.

(a) The incidence of eating disorders is greater among (_females? males?_). About ____ of 1,000 cases of anorexia nervosa are fatal.

(b) Besides including an eating disorder, "female athlete triad" affects the _____ and _____ systems.

C7. Circle each of the characteristics below that would contribute to a DSM-IV-TR diagnosis of anorexia nervosa for Amelia, age 16.

(a) Amelia maintains her weight at 87% of the expected BMI for her height.

(b) She has an intense fear of gaining weight.

(c) Although she reached menarche at age 13, Amelia has not menstruated for the past 18 months.

(d) Amelia does not think that she has a problem with low body weight.

(e) She has fine body hair (lanugo).

(f) Her ECG result is abnormal, her BP is 76/46 mm Hg, and she has electrolyte imbalances.

C8. Explain how amenorrhea associated with anorexia can be linked to osteoporosis.

_____

_____

_____

C9. Fill in the blanks or circle the correct answers in the following questions about Marianne, age 21, who measures 5'2" and weighs 105 lb. She intentionally vomits several times a week after binge eating. Her teeth are severely eroded and her dentist has recommended extraction of all of her teeth with fitting for dentures. She has esophageal reflux with heartburn and has developed pneumonia twice this year.

(a) Which DSM-IV-TR criteria of bulimia nervosa does Marianne meet?

_____

_____

(b) Her bulimia is classified as (_purging? nonpurging?_).

(c) What is the likely cause of Marianne's dental problems and her heartburn?

_____

(d) How are her episodes of pneumonia likely to be related to her eating disorder?

_____

(e) Her body weight is more typical of (_bulimia? anorexia?_).

C10. List several therapy goals for binge eaters.

_____

_____

_____

CHAPTER 9

Disorders of White Blood Cells and Lymphoid Tissues

■ Review Questions

A. HEMATOPOIETIC AND LYMPHOID TISSUE

A1. Hematopoiesis means _____.
Fill in the blanks or circle the correct answers within each statement about hematopoiesis.

   (a) All blood cells—red cells, white cells, and platelets—form from _____ stem cells, and these can develop into two main types of cells known as common _____ stem cells and common _____ stem cells.

   (b) Common myeloid cells mature in *(bone marrow? lymphatic?)* tissue. Red blood cells, most white blood cells, and platelets develop from *(lymphoid? myeloid?)* stem cell pathways. *(Red blood cells? Most white blood cells? Platelets?)* are formed from large cells known as megakaryocytes.

   (c) Committed stem cells can form *(any? specific?)* blood cells. These cells are also known as CFUs, or _____ _____ _____.

   (d) Cytokines influence blood-forming cells to develop into specific cell types. For example, GM-CSF are chemicals that promote formation of white blood cells categorized as _____ and _____. Interleukins are cytokines that enhance production of _____. EPO is a cytokine that stimulates formation of _____.

A2. Circle the correct answers or fill in the blank to answer these questions about functions of lymphoid tissue.

   (a) Bone marrow is considered *(central? peripheral?)* lymphoid tissue. *(All? Most?)* lymphocytes originate here.

   (b) T cells mature and become competent in *(bone marrow? lymph nodes? the thymus?)*.

This is also where T cells that would attack "self" are normally eliminated.

   (c) Name several locations in the body where mature lymphocytes respond to foreign antigens.

_____

A3. Circle the correct answers within each statement about blood cells.

   (a) White blood cells are also known as *(thrombocytes? leukocytes?)*. Their function is *(carrying CO_2? infection control? clotting?)*.

   (b) The most common type of white blood cell is a *(neutrophil? lymphocyte?)*. State the basis for classifying neutrophils as "PMNs." _____

   (c) Neutrophils that line the inside of walls of small blood vessels are known as *(circulating? marginating?)* PMNs.

   (d) State the function of the granules in neutrophils and eosinophils when they encounter microbes such as bacteria or parasites. _____

   (e) Mature neutrophils spend about 4 to 8 *(hours? days? weeks?)* circulating in the bloodstream before they move into tissues. There they spend an average of 4 to 5 *(hours? days? weeks?)* before they die as a result either of their functions (phagocytosis) or of senescence (old age).

A4. Select the type of white blood cell (WBC) that fits the related description.

Basophils   Eosinophils   Lymphocytes
Monocytes   Neutrophils

   (a) Comprise 20% to 30% of WBCs; nucleus is spherical and takes up most of the cell; includes three main types (B, T, and NK); function in immunity: _____

(b) The largest WBCs, they become macrophages and function in chronic inflammations; known as microglial cells in the brain and Kupffer cells in the liver: _____

(c) Typically, the least abundant type of WBC; release the anticoagulant heparin and also the vasodilator histamine: _____

(d) Normally make up 1% to 3% of circulating WBCs; combat parasitic infections: _____

(e) Granulocytes (three answers): _____, _____ and _____

(f) Function during allergic responses (two answers): _____ and _____

A5. Describe lymphocytes by circling correct answers or filling in the blanks in this exercise.

(a) *(B? T? Natural killer?)* lymphocytes are most directly involved with antibody production that occurs in humoral immunity.

(b) These three main subsets of lymphocytes can be distinguished by markers known as CDs. Write the meaning of this acronym: C_____ D_____. "Helper T cells" express *(CD4+? CD8+)* molecules on their surfaces.

B. NON-NEOPLASTIC DISORDERS OF WHITE BLOOD CELLS

B1. Circle the correct answers or fill in the blanks within each statement about white blood cell (WBC) deficiency.

(a) A normal WBC count is *(600? 6,000? 60,000? 6 million?)*/mL. A low WBC count is known as *(leukocytosis? leukopenia?)*.

(b) Typically, more than 50% of WBCs are *(neutrophils? lymphocytes?)*. Deficiency of this category of WBC is a *(common? rare?)* form of leukopenia, a condition known as ____.

(c) Jenna's circulating neutrophil count of 180 cells/μL denotes *(agranulocytosis? neutropenia?)*. Which of Jenna's body systems is most likely to be the site of her most serious and fatal infection? _____ Jenna is treated with rhG-CSF, which refers to _____.

B2. Select the factor leading to neutropenia that matches the related description. One answer will be used twice.

Aplastic anemia
Bacterial or viral infection
Congenital neutropenia
Drugs that interfere with normal marrow function
Felty syndrome
Hemopoietic cancer
Metastatic solid tumor cancer

(a) A form of rheumatoid arthritis in which large amounts of neutrophils are destroyed in the spleen: _____

(b) Hereditary disorders such as Kostmann syndrome and cyclic neutropenia: _____

(c) Chemotherapy or irradiation: _____

(d) Cause of most cases of neutropenia: _____

(e) Condition that decreases production of RBCs, platelets, and most WBCs: _____

(f) WBCs used up faster than they can be replaced: _____

(g) Spread of breast carcinoma to bone marrow, which prevents normal marrow function: _____

(h) Leukemia in which normal bone marrow function is displaced by unregulated formation of immature (and useless) cancerous WBCs: _____

B3. Tiffany experienced an *idiosyncratic* drug reaction to a medication. Define this term.

_____

B4. Julie reports that her mother has been taking a series of chemotherapy treatments for cancer over the past 8 months. Her mother also has developed sores in her mouth that are so painful that she cannot eat and she has recurrent bouts of nausea and vomiting. As a result, Julie's mother is extremely tired and emaciated; her self-esteem is low related to loss of most of her body hair (alopecia). She has recurrent respiratory infections. Explain why she is likely to have these signs and symptoms.

_____

_____

_____

B5. Circle the correct answer or fill in the blanks within each statement about the pathophysiology of infectious mononucleosis (IM).

(a) The microbe that causes infectious mononucleosis (IM) is the EBV virus; this abbreviation stands for: _____ _____ _____.

(b) The EBV virus invades *(B? T?)* lymphocytes in tissues lining the mouth and pharynx. The virus may kill these cells or may incorporate into the cell's _____. These cells then circulate in the blood and release _____ antibodies into the blood. What is the basis of the naming of these antibodies?

_____

Presence of these antibodies in blood is a diagnostic sign of _____.

(c) Atypical ___-cell proliferation results from stimulation by infected B cells; these T cells are also useful diagnostically and they eventually _____ infected B cells.

B6. Arrange in correct sequence these phases in the pathogenesis of infectious mononucleosis (IM):

Incubation period (4 to 8 weeks)
Acute phase (2 to 3 weeks)
Prodromal phase (several days)
Recovery phase (2 to 3 months)

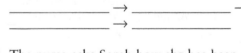

B7. The nurse asks Sarah how she has been feeling and Sarah makes the statements listed below. Circle the three statements that indicate the presence of the typical triad of manifestations of infectious mononucleosis (IM).

(a) "I have a pounding headache."

(b) "My glands are so swollen on both sides of my neck; I feel like I can hardly move my neck, and it hurts here in my groin."

(c) "My throat is killing me; it hurts to even *think* of talking."

(d) "My temperature was 102.5°F this morning."

(e) "I have terrific pain in my hip joints."

B8. In infectious mononucleosis, lymphocytes may proliferate so much that they account for 60% of the total WBCs. In normal blood, _____ % of all WBCs are lymphocytes.

B9. Explain why lymph nodes, spleen, and liver tend to enlarge in response to blood disorders such as IM (and also leukemia).

_____

_____

_____

B10. Circle the three true statements about infectious mononucleosis (IM). (Pay particular attention to whether the **bold-faced** word or phrase makes the statement true or false.)

(a) Infectious mononucleosis (IM) is most common **among welfare and Medicaid** patients.

(b) The virus that causes IM **can be transmitted** through saliva.

(c) IM more commonly affects **children** and **adolescents** than **old people**.

(d) Most persons who survive infectious mononucleosis **do** experience significant impairment after the disease.

(e) IM is spread **only** by patients with **current symptoms** of IM.

(f) Once infected with EBV, the person **is** likely to have asymptomatic IM **for life**.

C. NEOPLASTIC DISORDERS OF HEMATOPOIETIC AND LYMPHOID ORIGIN

C1. Select the type of cancer that originates from cells in each of the sites described below.

Leukemias   Lymphomas   Multiple myeloma

(a) Lymph nodes or lymphoid tissues: sites of B-cell and T-cell maturation

_____

(b) Bone marrow where B cells differentiate into plasma cells: _____

(c) Hematopoietic stem cells in bone marrow:

_____

C2. Contrast the two major types of lymphomas by writing *HL* (Hodgkin lymphoma) or *NHL* for non-Hodgkin lymphoma.

(a) Begins with a **single** enlarged lymph node, usually above the diaphragm and typically in the neck: ___

(b) Begins with **several** enlarged lymph nodes in various locations: ___

(c) Enlarged lymph nodes are typically **painless:** _____

(d) Much more **common** and typically more **lethal** form of lymphoma: ___

(e) Diminishes **humoral** immunity more than cellular immunity: ____

(f) About 80% to 85% of such lymphomas are of **B-cell** (not T-cell) origin: ____

C3. Lymphomas are *(common? rare?)* forms of cancer. Discuss factors related to causes of lymphomas.

_____

_____

(a) Although the cause of lymphomas is unknown, some forms of lymphoma (such as Burkitt) have been associated with the _____ virus.

(b) List categories of persons who are at higher risk for developing lymphomas.

_____

C4. Diagnosis of Hodgkin lymphoma requires the presence of _____ cells in biopsy of lymph nodes. List other diagnostic techniques.

_____

_____

C5. (a) Explain why the staging of Hodgkin lymphoma is critical.

_____

_____

_____

(b) List several "B" symptoms associated with stage B lymphomas.

_____

C6. Describe the treatment for Hodgkin and non-Hodgkin lymphoma.

_____

C7. At age 27, Margaret was diagnosed with non-Hodgkin lymphoma. Massive radiation cured her lymphoma. At age 37, myocardial ischemia required a quadruple bypass. At age 47, she experienced a myocardial infarction (MI) and shortly thereafter went into clinical trials for an angiogenic medication to increase coronary perfusion (blood flow). Explain the

likely connection between the lymphoma and the cardiac disease.

_____

_____

_____

C8. Circle the correct answers within this statement: Whereas lymphomas are cancers initiated in *(bone marrow? lymph tissue?)*, leukemias primarily involve *(bone marrow? lymph tissue?)*.

C9. Summarize the basic problem in leukemia.

_____

_____

_____

Circle the correct answers within these statements: Leukemia occurs *(only in children? only in adults? in persons of all ages?)*. It is a *(common? rare?)* cause of cancer deaths in children.

C10. Circle the correct answers or fill in the blanks within each statement about leukemia.

(a) The A in ALL and AML stands for *(acquired? acute?)*. Chronic leukemias have a more *(sudden? gradual?)* onset than acute leukemia. *(Acute? Chronic?)* leukemias involve proliferation of well-differentiated myeloid or lymphoid cells.

(b) Lymphocytic leukemia involves accelerated production of immature _____ cells that infiltrate organs such as _____. *(Myelogenous? Lymphocytic?)* leukemia affects pluripotent stem cells in *(bone marrow? lymph tissue?)*, preventing normal hematopoiesis.

(c) Causes of leukemia *(are? are not?)* known. List several factors that are associated with an increasing incidence of leukemia.

_____

_____

(d) Manifestations of ALL *(are? are not?)* similar to those of AML. Both may lead to pancytopenia. Explain.

_____

(e) Write *R, W,* or *P* next to the following warning signs of acute leukemia to indicate whether the sign indicates deficiency in red blood cells, white blood cells, or platelets.

(1) Fatigue, lethargy, dyspnea, pallor: ___

(2) Repeated infections, such as genitourinary: _____

(3) Easy bruising and nosebleeds (epistaxis): _____

C11. Select the type of leukemia that fits the descriptions that follow.

ALL   AML   CLL   CML

(a) The most common type of leukemia in children and young adults, this form of leukemia now has a higher cure rate (70%) than other types of leukemia: _____

(b) Chiefly a cancer in adults, especially the elderly; also the type of leukemia most associated with Down syndrome; virtually all blast cells of this type of leukemia have CD33 antigens on them that MOA treatments can target. (See Question C6.)

(c) Almost all affected persons over 50 years of age; may be diagnosed by a complete blood count (CBC) because typically has no signs or symptoms at time of diagnosis; the slow course permits a normal life for many years; over time lymph nodes become considerably enlarged: _____

(d) Patients often present with a feeling of abdominal fullness related to splenomegaly; patients with high counts of leukocyte blast cells have a poor prognosis; the only available cure is bone marrow or stem cell transplantation: _____

C12. Write the pathophysiologic rationale for each of these factors related to acute leukemia or its treatment.

(a) "Blasts" forming 60% to 100% of circulating blood cells

_____

(b) Leukostasis requiring leukapheresis to prevent formation of leukoblastic emboli

_____
_____
_____

(c) Nausea and vomiting (especially with all), headache, papilledema, and possibly seizures or coma

_____
_____
_____

(d) High levels of uric acid in blood that can lead to renal damage

_____
_____
_____

(e) Tumor lysis syndrome

_____
_____

(f) Hepatomegaly, splenomegaly, and lymphadenopathy

_____
_____
_____

C13. Arrange in correct sequence, from first to last, these stages in chemotherapy treatment of leukemia:

Intensification   Induction   Maintenance

_____→_____→
_____

C14. Explain why the following regimens may accompany chemotherapeutic treatment of leukemia.

(a) Central nervous system (CNS) prophylaxis

_____
_____

(b) Antibiotic therapy

_____
_____

(c) Allopurinol

_____
_____

C15. Circle the correct answers or fill in the blanks within each statement about multiple myeloma.

(a) Multiple myeloma is the most common example of a dyscrasia (disorder) of _____ cells. The median age of persons with malignant melanoma is *(21? 71?)* years. List several risk factors for multiple myeloma.

_____

(b) The role of plasma cells is to excrete antibodies known as _____ (____). Eighty percent of cases of multiple myeloma involve excessive production of monoclonal antibodies—either Ig__ or Ig___; both of these Igs are categorized as ___ protein. However, production of normal Igs decreases, causing *(increased? decreased?)* risk of bacterial infection.

(c) In the remaining cases of this cancer, the plasma cells produce only abnormal proteins known as _____ _____ proteins that can be detected in serum or urine. Many of these proteins are toxic to _____, possibly leading to renal failure.

(d) Abnormal proliferation of plasma cells in multiple myeloma is *(enhanced? inhibited?)* by growth factors. Name several of these cytokines.

_____

(e) Myeloma cells secrete chemicals that stimulate *(osteoblasts? osteoclasts?)* that cause bone *(synthesis? destruction?)* and fractures. Bone pain is a(n) *(early? late?)* and *(common? rare?)* sign of multiple myeloma. Osteolysis leads to *(hyper? hypo?)*calcemia with possible kidney damage.

(f) Abnormal plasma cells can also secrete amyloid, which can cause damage to _____ and _____. Other abnormal proteins cause injury to _____ and can lead to chronic renal failure (CRF).

C16. Helen was diagnosed at age 42 with multiple myeloma. She had to go on disability from her job to undergo treatments with profound side effects. After 44 months of chemotherapy and/or radiation, she had to stop treatments because of the effects of *pancytopenia*. She experienced extreme *pain* in her back, hips, and extremities. She died at age 47 of complications of *chronic renal failure (CRF)*. Explain reasons for the *italicized* conditions.

_____

_____

_____

C17. MGUS is an acronym for a condition in which persons *(do? do not?)* have M proteins in serum *(and also? but do not?)* have other manifestations of multiple myeloma. About *(2? 20%? 80?)* of people with MGUS will develop a plasma cell dyscrasia.

CHAPTER 10

Alterations in Hemostasis

■ Review Questions

A. MECHANISMS OF HEMOSTASIS

A1. "Hemostasis" means _____ of blood flow. List the two main categories of disorders of hemostasis.

(a) _____

(b) _____

A2. Identify the four major factors that are required in order for hemostasis to take place adequately but not excessively by matching them with descriptions below.

    Anticoagulants produced by body cells

    Clotting factors in plasma

    Platelets

    Properties (such as smoothness) of blood vessel lining

(a) Normally 150,000–400,000/μL of blood, with one third stored in the spleen:

_____

(b) Formed in an inactive state; identified by Roman numerals (such as IV, VII, IX, or X); function in a cascade of steps:

_____

(c) Normally regulate clotting so that it is not excessive; examples are antithrombin III and proteins C and S:

_____

(d) Probably the most important factor in preventing excessive clotting; prevents adherence of platelets and clotting factors:

_____

A3. Circle correct answers or fill in the blanks within each statement about the first of these four factors, platelets.

(a) Platelets are derived from large bone marrow cells known as _____, and typically they have a life span of 8 to 9 days. Their production is regulated by the chemical *(erytho? thrombo?)*poietin. List three sources of this chemical:

_____

(b) List and state functions of chemicals found in the following structures of platelets:

(b1) Glycocalyx on platelet surface:

_____

(b2) a-granules:

_____

(b3) δ-granules (dense granules):

_____

(b4) Microtubules:

_____

(c) Each platelet *(does? does not?)* contain a nucleus and *(does? does not?)* contain mitochondria.

A4. Explain how the following aspects of coagulation afford protection to the body:

(a) Cascade effect

_____

(b) Inactive procoagulation factors normally present in blood at all times

_____

A5. Arrange the five steps/stages of hemostasis in correct sequence from first to last:

    Coagulation   Clot retraction

    Fibrinolysis   Platelet plug formation

    Vasospasm

_____, _____, _____,

_____, _____

A6. Circle the correct answers within each statement about the initial stages of hemostasis.

(a) In vasospasm, blood vessels *(constrict? dilate?)*, usually for *(less than a minute? several days?)* after the injury. *(Thromboxane A_2 [TXA_2]? Prostacyclin?)* is a vasoconstrictor released from *(platelets? the lining of blood vessels?)*.

(b) Platelet plug formation involves two steps: platelet *adhesion* and platelet _____. The outside of the platelet membrane is coated with glycoproteins that *(are? are not?)* likely to adhere to the normal vessel lining. When platelets bind to injured vessels, their receptors become *(smooth? spiny?)* so they adhere to exposed *(elastin? collagen?)* in the vessel by way of *(TXA₂? vWF?)*. This chemical is made by *(platelets? endothelial cells lining vessels?)*, and it circulates in blood as a carrier for coagulation factor *(III? VIII?)*.

(c) The platelet membrane also has glycoprotein receptors that bind _____ and link _____ together. Name two chemicals made by platelets that enhance platelet aggregation:

_____

(d) Platelet release of chemicals such as TXA₂ cause a "snowball effect" as platelet aggregation *(increases? decreases?)*. The platelet plug is later stabilized by *(fibrin? prothrombin?)* formed in the process of coagulation.

(e) Deficiency in platelet receptor sites or von Willebrand factor leads to excessive *(bleeding? platelet plug formation?)*.

A7. Blood clotting (coagulation) involves formation of *(fibrin? fibrinogen?)*. Fill in the blanks or circle the correct answers within each statement about the normal sequence of events in the clotting process.

(a) The intrinsic coagulation pathway begins *(within? outside of?)* blood, specifically when blood comes into contact with _____. This leads to activation of circulating *(factor XII? tissue factor?)*.

(b) How is the extrinsic coagulation pathway triggered? _____
This process occurs more *(rapidly? slowly?)* than the intrinsic pathway and leads to bleeding that is *(more? less?)* severe than that initiated by the intrinsic pathway.

(c) A vitamin necessary for normal blood clotting is vitamin ___.

(d) A mineral needed for normal blood clotting (coagulation) is _____.

A8. Match the coagulation factor with the correct description.
IV   VIII   X

(a) Citrate chelates this factor so that blood stored for transfusions will not clot: factor _____

(b) This is the end-product of both the intrinsic and extrinsic coagulation pathways: activated factor _____

(c) This factor is most often deficient in hemophilia; normally carried by the von Willebrand factor (vWF): factor _____

A9. Contrast the terms in each pair:
(a) Fibrinogen/fibrin

_____
_____
_____

(b) Thrombin/plasmin

_____
_____
_____

(c) An anticoagulant/a fibrinolytic agent

_____
_____
_____

(d) Antithrombin III/protein C

_____
_____
_____

A10. Match each chemical with the related description.
Heparin   Plasminogen
Plasminogen activator   Warfarin

(a) A vitamin K antagonist, it decreases prothrombin production; can be taken orally:

_____

(b) Produced naturally by some leukocytes (basophils) and by mast cells in connective tissues; helps to inactivate thrombin and factor Xa; oral form (low molecular weight) is injectable and inhibits only factor Xa: _____

(c) Typically found in blood; once activated, it causes breakdown of fibrin (fibrinolysis):

_____

(d) Made by liver, kidneys, plasma, and vascular endothelium: _____

A11. Classify these chemicals according to their functions; write answers on the lines provided. (Note: some chemicals fit into more than one category.)

Antithrombin III	Fibrinogen
Calcium ions (factor IV)	Protein C
Coagulation factors VII to XII	Heparin
Tissue-plasminogen activator	Thrombin
	Warfarin

(a) Procoagulation factors:

_____

(b) Anticoagulation factors:

_____

(c) Fibrinolytic agent:

_____

B. HYPERCOAGULABILITY STATES

B1. Respond to this statement: "Blood clotting is good news and bad news."

_____

_____

_____

B2. Circle the correct answer: Thrombi in (*arteries? veins?*) are composed of platelets.

List several factors that can lead to excessive clot formation caused by:

(a) Increased platelet function

_____

(b) Increase in clotting activity

_____

B3. Select the category of factors that leads to hypercoagulability associated with each

condition below. In some cases, more than one answer is appropriate.

Damaged blood vessel lining
Increased clotting factors
Platelet adhesiveness and aggregation
Stasis of blood flow
Deficiency of anticoagulant production

(a) Atherosclerosis:

_____

(b) Cancer:

_____

(c) Diabetes:

_____

(d) Thrombocytosis:

_____

(e) Sickle cell anemia:

_____

(f) Heart failure:

_____

(g) Pregnancy or use of oral contraceptives:

_____

(h) Decreased synthesis of antithrombin III:

_____

B4. Mr. Longstreth, age 72, 232 lb, is in an ER in Sarasota, Florida. He and his partner drove from Cincinnati to Florida within 24 hours, trying not to "dawdle" (Mr. Longstreth's term) along the way. Mr. Longstreth's chest pain, severe dyspnea (difficulty breathing), and rapid breathing suggest the presence of a pulmonary embolism (PE). Explain why Mr. Longstreth might be a candidate for a PE.

_____

_____

_____

B5. Write *A* (acquired) or *G* (genetic or inherited) to indicate the category of each of these hypercoagulability states.

(a) Ms. O'Loughlin, age 83, has been wearing an immobilizer since she fractured her tibia a month ago: _____

(b) Mrs. North has the Leiden mutation in which her factor Va cannot be inactivated:

_____

(c) Nancy is a smoker and is "on the pill":

_____

B6. List five or more categories of persons at increased risk for thromboses associated with antiphospholipid syndrome.

_____

_____

_____

C. BLEEDING DISORDERS

C1. Claudia has a platelet count of 18,000/mL. Circle the correct answer to complete these statements about Claudia's condition.

(a) This count:
  (1) Is normal
  (2) Indicates thrombocytosis
  (3) Indicates thrombocytopenia

(b) Claudia has petechiae on her arms; these are:
  (1) Large bruises
  (2) Pinpoint red areas

(c) She also has frequent occurrences of epistaxis, which is:
  (1) Abnormal menstrual bleeding
  (2) Bleeding from gums
  (3) Nosebleeds

C2. Explain probable mechanisms for low platelet counts in each patient.

(a) Mr. Lewis has cirrhosis of the liver.

_____

_____

(b) Ms. Schmidt has been taking sulfa drugs for an infection.

_____

_____

(c) Mr. Stanford is halfway through his chemotherapy protocol for cancer.

_____

_____

_____

(d) Mr. Ardmore has been on heparin for 10 days.

_____

_____

(e) Mrs. Fernandez has widespread thrombi in small vessels of her brain and kidneys; she has severe headaches and seizures. Mrs. Fernandez is undergoing plasmapheresis in which her plasma is replaced with fresh-frozen plasma.

_____

_____

_____

C3. Jennifer, the neonatal nurse, administers vitamin K to newborn baby Kareenya. Explain why Kareenya may require vitamin K.

_____

_____

_____

C4. Discuss the likely cause of bleeding in each case.

(a) Mr. Lewis (see Question C2[a]) has had alcoholism for more than 20 years.

_____

(b) In providing information for her history and physical, Mrs. Snyderman tells the nurse that she has taken "pain medicine" for her arthritis for many years. She notes that whenever she has a cut or she scratches a sore, she "bleeds forever."

_____

_____

(c) Terry has been taking antibiotics for recurrent infections.

_____

_____

(d) Timmy and Tommy, 10 years old, are identical twins who each have 1% of normal blood levels of factor VIII. Both boys have such sufficient damage to joints of their legs that their mobility is limited. Tommy has developed hepatitis C.

_____

_____

(e) Samantha's vWF deficiency was diagnosed after she had her wisdom teeth removed.

_____

_____

(f) Ms. Franer has received massive transfusions following extensive bleeding during childbirth.

_____

C5. Circle the factors in the following list that are likely to lead to hypocoagulability.

Aneurysm	Dehydration
Lack of factor VIII (as in the most common form of hemophilia)	Smoking
	Smoking and taking oral contraceptives
	Taking a baby aspirin each day
Splenomegaly	Lack of vitamin K
Diabetes mellitus	Heparin or coumadin

C6. DIC is an acronym for _____. Answer the following questions about the disorder.

(a) List several causes or triggers of DIC.

_____

_____

(b) Explain why DIC is called a "paradoxical" disorder.

_____

_____

(c) Which sign is more observable in DIC? _(Bleeding? Ischemia?)_ List several examples.

_____

(d) Which organs are likely to become necrotic as a result of ischemia?

_____

C7. Define these two forms of vascular disorders that may lead to bleeding.

(a) Telangiectasia

_____

(b) Senile purpura

_____

CHAPTER 11

The Red Blood Cell and Alterations in Oxygen Transport

■ Review Questions

A. THE RED BLOOD CELL

A1. What is the primary role of red blood cells (RBCs)?

_____

What is the secondary role of RBCs?

_____

Explain how the structural design of RBCs and the presence of spectrin aid the cells' functioning.

_____

_____

_____

A2. Circle the correct answers or fill in the blank within each statement about hemoglobin.

(a) Each hemoglobin molecule consists of a total of *(two? four? eight?)* polypeptide chains. Which portion of these chains contains an iron (Fe) atom to which oxygen can bind? *(Heme? Globin?)* Therefore, each hemoglobin molecule can transport a maximum of *(two? four? eight?)* oxygen molecules.

(b) Which type of hemoglobin is predominant in the fetus? *(HbA? HbF?)* This type of Hb consists of two beta and two *(alpha? gamma?)* chains. This structural difference causes fetal Hb to have *(higher? lower?)* affinity for oxygen. State the significance of this fact. _____

A3. Fill in the blanks or circle the correct answer within each statement about how iron (Fe) functions in the blood.

(a) Typically, most iron is ingested in foods such as _____. Iron is transported within plasma to bone marrow in the form of *(transferrin? ferritin?)* and stored in the liver as _____. Low levels of *(transferrin? ferritin?)* indicate a need for an iron supplement.

(b) At any given time, most of the Fe of the body is:

(1) Stored in the liver

(2) Suspended in plasma

(3) Present in hemoglobin

A4. Fill in the blanks or circle the correct answers to complete this exercise about erythropoiesis.

(a) Arrange these stages in the development of RBCs in correct sequence from first to last.

Erythroblasts   Erythrocytes
Pluripotent stem cells   Reticulocytes

_____ → _____ →
_____ → _____

(b) In which stage do most potential RBCs move out of bone marrow and into circulating blood?_____
This type of cell *(has? lacks?)* a nucleus. A normal reticulocyte for circulating blood is_____ %. (See Question A9.)

(c) Because RBCs live about ____ days, about ___% of RBCs are replaced each day. One reason that a mature RBC lives a relatively short life span is that it lacks a _____.

(d) Where is almost all erythropoietin produced within the human body? Circle the correct answer.

Bone marrow   Kidneys   Liver
Spleen   Thymus

(e) _____ serves as the trigger for production of erythropoietin.

A5. LaVerne Jackson, age 47, has had diabetes for 32 years. She manifests a common effect of long-term diabetes, renal failure, and takes dialysis treatments (to clean her blood). She feels debilitating fatigue much of the time. Her hemoglobin (Hb) level is currently 6.5 g/dL. Explain what is likely to cause her fatigue and what treatment may help.

_____

_____

_____

_____

A6. Mrs. Jackson's husband, Rev. George Jackson, has serious liver disease that causes jaundice, which is due to excessive _____ in the blood. The Reverend has black skin. How can the nurse best assess the presence of jaundice in Rev. Jackson?

_____

_____

_____

What other conditions besides liver disease can lead to jaundice?

_____

_____

_____

A7. Although erythrocytes transport oxygen, RBCs cannot use oxygen for ATP production (as virtually all other body cells do). Why not?

_____

_____

_____

RBCs therefore depend on *(aerobic? anaerobic?)* metabolism of glucose. Explain what happens to RBCs as a result of the hereditary deficiency of glucose-6-phosphate dehydrogenase (G6PD).

_____

_____

_____

A8. Select numbers from this list to fill in the blanks below.

1	2	4	6	9	14
20	42	75	98	120	

(a) Number of hemes (and also of Fe atoms) in each hemoglobin molecule: _____

(b) Typical hemoglobin value: _____ g/dL

(c) Normal RBC count for women: _____ million/μL

(d) A likely value for MCV in megaloblastic (macrocytic) anemia: _____ fL

(e) The percent of oxygen that is carried bound to hemoglobin: _____ %

A9. Susan F. gave birth to a healthy baby boy. However, Susan hemorrhaged so much that her hematocrit dropped to 12%. Answer the following questions related to her case.

(a) Write a value for a normal hematocrit: _____%.

(b) Susan receives treatment to stimulate RBC production. Which test is the best indicator of successful antianemic therapy? Circle the correct answer.

(1) Total RBC count

(2) Hematocrit

(3) Reticulocyte count

(c) Which value for this test most indicates success of the therapy? Circle the correct answer.

1   15   150   1200

A10. Choose the two true statements. (Pay particular attention to whether the **bold-faced** word or phrase makes the statement true or false.)

(a) Hypochromic anemia indicates a **lower** than normal concentration of Hb in blood.

(b) Jaundice is a classic sign of **anemia.**

(c) Overall, normal RBC values tend to be **higher** for women than for men.

(d) In general, the value for hemoglobin can be expected to be **one third** the value of hematocrit.

B. ANEMIA

B1. Fill in the blanks within each statement about the two major causes of anemia.

(a) Anemia can result from blood loss caused by, for example, _____ or _____.

(b) Anemia can be caused by inadequate replacement of normal RBCs, a result of, for example, _____ deficiency or _____ failure.

B2. The following statements describe major categories of signs and symptoms of anemia. Fill in the blanks or circle the correct answers.

(a) Hypoxia that may manifest by

_____.

Compensatory mechanisms lead to *(increased? decreased?)* heart rate; vasoconstriction of blood vessels in skin, nail beds, and gums, causing *(pallor? cyanosis?)*; and *(increased? decreased?)* RBC production, which may cause bone pain.

(b) Changes in RBC _____ as seen in microcytic or megaloblastic anemias, or in RBC color as in hypochromic anemias.

(c) Manifestations of the underlying cause of anemia, such as _____ accompanying hemorrhagic anemia resulting from an automobile accident.

B3. Circle the correct answers within each statement about different types of anemia.

(a) Hypovolemic shock is more likely to accompany *(acute? chronic?)* blood loss. Fluid shifts from intercellular spaces into blood plasma, causing blood to be more *(concentrated? diluted?)*. These RBCs have *(normal? reduced?)* hemoglobin level.

(b) Loss of blood due to gastric irritation associated with chronic aspirin use is more likely to lead to *(acute? chronic?)* anemia. This *(is? is not?)* iron-deficiency anemia. These cells have *(normal? reduced?)* hemoglobin level, so are said to be *(normochromic? hypochromic?)*.

(c) Identify whether the following descriptions pertain more to extravascular (E) or intravascular (I) hemolysis.

(c1) Premature breakdown of RBCs occurs in sinusoids of the spleen, especially when RBCs have decreased ability to deform: *(E? I?)*

(c2) RBC destruction accompanied by hemoglobinemia, hemoglobinuria, hemosiderinuria, and jaundice: *(E? I?)*

(c3) The more common type of hemolysis: *(E? I?)*

B4. Choose the two true statements about sickle cell anemia. (Pay particular attention to whether the **bold-faced** word or phrase makes the statement true or false.)

(a) Sickle cell anemia is classified as an **autosomal recessive** hereditary disorder.

(b) About 1 in 1,200 African Americans carries the sickle cell trait.

(c) A person with *sickle cell trait* is **more** likely than one with *sickle cell anemia* to experience sickle cell crises.

(d) Sickle cell anemia is likely to be a **progressive** ("gets worse over time") disease.

(e) Adults with sickle cell trait are likely to have about **90%** of their hemoglobin in the form of HbS.

B5. Answer these questions about sickle cell anemia (SCA).

(a) Describe sickle cell "crises."

_____

_____

_____

(b) List several situations that trigger hypoxia that patients with SCA should avoid.

_____

_____

(c) Circle what is typically the most serious complication of SCA.

(1) Fatigue

(2) Bleeding into joints with limitation of mobility and confinement to wheelchair

(3) Stroke (in as many of two thirds of affected children 1 to 15 years of age)

(4) Malaria

(d) Children with SCA typically start showing signs and symptoms at about age 4 to 6 _____. (Fill in the blank with an answer from the following list.)

(1) Hours

(2) Days

(3) Weeks

(4) Months

(5) Years

(e) Which organ is especially at risk for destruction in infants with SCA who are as young as 3 to 6 months of age? _____ How can such organ injury contribute to serious infections and septicemia? _____

_____

(f) Circle the correct answers. Currently there *(is? is not?)* a cure for SCA. Screening tests for SCA *(are? are not?)* available.

(g) _____ is a promising new treatment for sickle cell anemia. How does it work?

_____

(h) List several other approaches to managing sickle cell anemia.

_____

_____

_____

B6. Match the type of anemia with its related description.

Aplastic B_{12} deficiency
Chronic disease   Folic acid deficiency
Hemolytic   Hemorrhagic
Iron-deficiency   Sickle cell
Spherocytosis   Thalassemia

(a) Typically, a slowly developing megaloblastic anemia caused by gastritis with decreased production of intrinsic factor; accompanied by neurologic changes: _____

(b) A megaloblastic anemia associated with malnutrition, for example, in elderly people or people with alcoholism; not accompanied by neurologic changes:

_____

(c) A cause of acute anemia with risk of hypovolemic shock; cells are of normal size and color: _____

(d) End-stage renal failure, lupus, AIDS, or cancer are most likely causes of:

_____

(e) Accompanies menstrual blood loss as well as gastric irritation caused by chronic aspirin use for control of arthritis pain; red blood cells are microcytic and hypochromic:

_____

(f) RBCs are injured and destroyed, for example by transfusion reactions, toxins, medications, venoms, malaria, or by mechanical injury with burns or heart valve defects; RBCs are normal size and color:

_____

(g) Signs and symptoms include increased risk of bleeding, infections, and fatigue, because of failure to produce adequate red cells, white cells, or platelets; likely to occur in cancer patients taking chemotherapy or radiation treatments: _____

(h) Hereditary anemia affecting blacks; hemoglobin HbS causes abnormally shaped RBCs, which leads to hypoxia:

_____

(i) Hereditary anemia in various racial and ethnic groups; genetic errors result in absent or defective synthesis of hemoglobin chains;

children with the disorder may have severe growth retardation; homozygotes can have Hb Bart's hemoglobin that will not release oxygen and can lead to death _in utero:_

_____

(j) An autosomal dominant deficiency of membrane proteins such as spectrin that leads to formation of RBCs that are tight spheres and are easily destroyed in vessels of the spleen; may be treated by splenectomy: _____

B7. Worldwide, _(women? men?)_ are at greater risk for iron-deficiency anemia.

(a) Explain why.

_____

(b) List several categories of persons also at increased risk for this type of anemia.

_____

_____

_____

_____

B8. Circle the correct answer or fill in the blanks within each statement about two forms of nutritional anemias.

(a) Vitamin B_{12} deficiency decreases production of _____ cells as well as _____ surrounding neurons. Absorption of this vitamin requires production of intrinsic factor (IF) from the _____ lining. This is needed to "ferry" vitamin B_{12} through the GI tract to the ileum of the _(large? small?)_ intestine, where it is absorbed into the blood and then passes to the bone marrow.

(b) Explain why cancer patients are at risk for folic acid anemia.

_____

_____

(c) Folic acid supplements are recommended for pregnant women to prevent _____ defects (NTDs).

B9. Choose the two answers that match a type of anemia with a description of a person at high risk for that anemia.

(a) Pernicious anemia: postgastrectomy or postileectomy patient

(b) Folic acid anemia: patient with long-term alcoholism

(c) Aplastic anemia: newborn baby

(d) Hemolytic anemia: postsplenectomy patient

C. POLYCYTHEMIA

C1. In the following list of ratios between hematocrit and Hb, circle the answer that best suggests polycythemia.

    (a) 42:14

    (b) 30:10

    (c) 12:4

    (d) 66:22

C2. Mr. Miller, age 58 years, has a diagnosis of polycythemia vera. Answer these questions related to his case.

    (a) Circle all of the following that are likely to increase:

        (1) Red blood cell count

        (2) Hematocrit

        (3) Hemoglobin

        (4) Platelet count

        (5) White blood cell count

        (6) Plasma

    (b) Circle all of the following that are likely to increase:

        (1) Blood volume

        (2) Blood viscosity

        (3) Blood pressure

        (4) Risk of thrombus formation

    (c) Mr. Miller's skin, fingernails, and gums are likely to have what sort of appearance:

        (1) Pale

        (2) Dusky or cyanotic

    (d) Circle all treatments likely to be effective for Mr. Miller's polycythemia:

        (1) Withholding fluids

        (2) Removal of red blood cells by periodic phlebotomy

        (3) Reduction of white blood cells and platelets by chemotherapy or radiation

        (4) Increasing fluid intake

C3. Identify whether the following forms of polycythemia are classified as *absolute primary, absolute secondary,* or *relative.*

    (a) Mr. Leon fell on the floor of his apartment in 102° weather three days ago; he has no air conditioning and has been too weak to get himself food or drink: _____

    (b) Ms. Martin has been a heavy smoker for 54 years; she has been diagnosed with both emphysema and chronic bronchitis: _____

    (c) Mr. Miller (see Question C2): _____

D. AGE-RELATED CHANGES IN RED BLOOD CELLS

D1. Circle the correct answers within each statement about Jarred and Cassandra, both 2 months old.

    (a) Jarred was full term and weighed 8 pounds at birth. From shortly after birth until about 2 months of age, Jarred's RBC count, hematocrit, and hemoglobin levels were likely to have *(elevated? declined?)*. His body is increasing the production of *(HbF? HbA?),* which has a great capacity for giving up oxygen to tissues.

    (b) Cassandra weighed 4 pounds when she was born at 32 weeks' gestation. Her mother had smoked two packs of cigarettes per day throughout the pregnancy. Cassandra's blood is likely to have *(more? less?)* HbA (and more HbF) than Jarred's. Protein supplements *(are? are not?)* likely to help Cassandra raise her HbA levels. Cassandra had jaundice at birth; this condition is *(rare? common?)* among preterm infants.

D2. Fill in the blanks or circle the correct answer within each statement about hemolytic disease of the newborn (HDN).

    (a) HDN is more likely to occur in the *(first? second or third?)* Rh-positive baby delivered of an Rh-_____ mother.

    (b) As the baby's RBCs are destroyed by the mother's anti-Rh antibodies, the newborn's blood level of bilirubin is likely to be *(higher? lower?)* than usual. The condition known as _____ may occur, in which bilirubin deposits injure the _____, especially the basal ganglia. List several signs of severe injury to this area.

_____

_____

_____

(c) Treatment typically includes _____therapy, which is exposure of skin to _____. Bilirubin in skin is broken down to a chemical that can be excreted by the_____ and _____ systems.

(d) If this baby needs a transfusion, (s)he should receive Type O Rh-_____ blood. The baby will still be Rh-positive, but the Rh-neg blood (not vulnerable to the mother's anti-Rh antibodies) will help the child survive until its mother's anti-Rh antibodies are diluted from the baby's blood.

(e) Future HDN can be prevented by injection of Rh *(antigens? antibodies?)* to the Rh-negative mother during and following pregnancy with an Rh-positive baby.

D3. Hemoglobin levels typically *(increase? decrease?)* slightly with aging. Which type of anemia is most common among elderly people? _____

List three or more age-related factors that seem to contribute to increased risk for anemia.

_____

_____

_____

CHAPTER 12

Mechanisms of Infectious Disease

■ Review Questions

A. TERMINOLOGY

A1. Select terms from the following list that complete the exercise below. Use each term once.

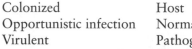

Colonized   Host
Opportunistic infection   Normal microflora
Virulent   Pathogenic

(a) Matthew, a newborn, has not yet established a _____ in his large intestine. After he ingests nutrients, bacteria will take up residence in his GI tract and produce vitamin K.

(b) Shawn has pneumonia. She is serving as _____ to a highly _____ strain of bacteria that have _____ her lungs.

(c) Peter has an infection caused by *Pneumocystis carinii* microbes that are not typically _____ in healthy persons. But in Peter's immunocompromised state, because he has AIDS, these microbes establish an _____ .

B. INFECTIOUS DISEASE

B1. Select the type of infectious agent that matches each description. Answers may be used more than once.

Bacteria   Chlamydiae
Fungi   Mycoplasma
Parasites   Prions
Rickettsiae   Viruses

(a) Some are oncogenic; some cause illnesses such as chickenpox, shingles, genital herpes, or AIDS: _____

(b) Contain no DNA or RNA, only proteins (PrpC); cause Creutzfeld-Jakob disease in humans and BSE ("mad cow disease") in animals: _____

(c) RNA or DNA core surrounded by a protein envelope derived from the membrane of the host cell; may remain latent in human cells for years and then become activated; incapable of replicating outside of living cells: _____

(d) Classified as prokaryocytes because they lack a true nucleus and organized organelles; they do contain DNA and RNA and can reproduce outside of human cells: _____

(e) The rigid cell wall (composed of peptidoglycan) of these microbes makes them vulnerable to antibiotics such as penicillin that attack this wall, but the antibiotic does not injure human cells because they lack this wall: _____

(f) Considerably smaller than bacteria, these microbes lack the rigid cell wall, so are resistant to penicillin; known to cause some pneumonias and genital infections: _____

(g) Include yeasts such as *Candida* and molds; cause athlete's foot, jock itch, and ringworm; produce a cell wall that is not made of peptidoglycan, so that the organism is not vulnerable to penicillin: _____

(h) Manifest characteristics of viruses (can reproduce only within a living cell) and of bacteria (have rigid peptidoglycan cell wall); depend on a vector such as a tick for transmission; cause Rocky Mountain spotted fever: _____

(i) Cause common genital infections; may cause blindness (trachoma) if the eyes of a baby are exposed to this microbe within the birth canal: _____

(j) Include protozoans (such as water-borne *Giardia lamblia*), worms (such as tapeworms), and arthropods (such as head or pubic lice, fleas, mites, and chiggers): _____

(k) Form a biofilm that favors survival of these microbes: _____

(l) An example is *Borrelia burgdorferi,* carried by deer ticks and infectious agent of Lyme disease: _____

B2. Circle the correct answers or fill in the blank in each statement about bacteria.

(a) Spherical bacteria are classified as (*bacilli? cocci? spirochetes?*). The bacteria that cause syphilis, *Treponema pallidum,* are classified as (*bacilli? cocci? spirochetes?*).

(b) *Staphylococci* are bacteria arranged in (*clusters? single lines? pairs?*), whereas diplococci are arranged in _____. In the name *Staphylococcus aureus, "aureus"* is the (*genus? species?*) name.

(c) Some bacteria form spores that (*increase? decrease?*) their resistance in unfavorable environments. *Mycobacterium tuberculosis* bacteria that cause tuberculosis are distinctive because of how they respond to an _____ stain.

(d) Bacteria that cannot survive in the presence of oxygen are called _____.
 (1) Aerobes
 (2) Anaerobes
 (3) Facultative anaerobes

(e) Gram-positive bacteria take a ___ stain with the Gram stain procedure.
 (1) Red (safranin)
 (2) Purple (crystal violet)

B3. Answer these questions about fungal infections.

(a) Paul's dermatophyte infections, commonly known as athlete's foot and jock itch, are caused by (*superficial? deep?*) pathogens that require relatively (*cool? warm?*) temperatures.

(b) Melissa just completed intensive antibiotic therapy for a respiratory infection; now she has a "yeast infection" (*Candida*) of her urethral and vaginal mucous membranes. Explain the connection.

_____

_____

B4. Complete this exercise about parasitic infections.

(a) Amebic dysentery is a GI infection caused by (*protozoa? worms? arthropods?*). List three mechanisms by which protozoan infections can be transmitted.

_____

_____

_____

(b) List three categories of worms that can infect humans.

_____

_____

_____

Such infections are a health problem primarily in (*the United States? developing nations?*).

(c) Mites, chiggers, lice, and fleas are all called _____-parasites because they infest the body through external surfaces, such as skin. Clothing, bedding, combs, or brushes are common modes of transmission for fleas and _____.

C. MECHANISMS OF INFECTION

C1. Ms. Leonard is a nurse-specialist in epidemiology for the Public Health Department. Write an appropriate job description for this position.

_____

_____

_____

C2. Select the term that best fits each description. Choose from these terms:

Endemic   Epidemic
Incidence   Pandemic
Prevalence

(a) Number of new cases of influenza in Detroit over a period of 3 winter months: _____

(b) Sudden outbreak of dysentery in a county in western Kentucky such that the prevalence exceeds normal rates for that county: _____

(c) Goiter was considered _____ to the Midwest before the general availability of fresh fish or iodized salt.

C3. Identify the mode of transmission in the following cases. Choose from these answers:

Direct contact   Ingestion
Inhalation   Penetration

(a) Jill, who was born with cystic fibrosis, currently has viral pneumonia:

_____

(b) Manuelo eats pork that is not fully cooked; he develops a tapeworm infection:

_____

(c) Patrick comes down with a case of *Shigella* infection after eating a salad prepared by a worker whose hands had fecal contamination: _____

(d) Raphael receives a tetanus infection after stepping on the sharp edge of a piece of farm equipment coated with soil containing *Clostridium tetani:* _____

(e) Sandra contracts genital herpes after unprotected sex: _____

(f) Mary Sue develops Lyme disease after she is bitten by an infected tick: _____

C4. List three examples of vertical transmission of infection (from mother to child).

_____

_____

_____

C5. Cite examples of factors that normally protect against infection of the:

(a) Respiratory tract

_____

(b) GI tract

_____

(c) Skin

_____

C6. Select the source of infections that fits the related description.

Endogenous agents   Fomites
Nosocomial   Zoonoses

(a) Shared brushes or hats (as vectors for lice eggs); improperly washed spoons or forks:

_____

(b) Rabies, Rocky Mountain spotted fever from a tick bite, or saliva from a cat bite:

_____

(c) An impetigo infection contracted during Danny's stay in the pediatric department of the hospital: _____

C7. Arrange the following stages in the course of a disease from first to last.

Acute   Convalescence and recovery

Incubation   Prodromal

_____ → _____ → _____ →

_____

Now identify the stage that fits each description:

(a) Microbes are actively replicating in the host, but no signs or symptoms are present:

_____

(b) A general feeling of malaise (slight fever, headaches, muscle aches, and fatigue) appears, but not signs highly specific to this disease: _____

(c) Following the period of maximal impact of the disease, resolution occurs:

_____

(d) This phase is prolonged in an insidious disease: _____

C8. Circle the correct answer within each statement about each disease.

(a) Celeste has a viremia which refers to a viral disease in (*blood? urine?*).

(b) Mrs. Jefferson's (*diverticulosis? diverticulitis?*) is a condition that involves inflammation.

(c) A disease with an abrupt onset is a(n) (*fulminant? insidious?*) illness.

(d) *Helicobacter pylori* is associated specifically with Nancy's (*gastric ulcers? foot abscesses?*).

C9. Complete this exercise about factors that increase virulence of microbes. Choose from the following answers:

Adhesive factors   Evasive factors
Invasive factors   Toxins

(a) Capsules or enzymes that cause clot formation are both mechanisms that protect microbes from WBCs: _____

(b) C toxins produced by microbes destroy WBCs: _____ _____

(c) Enzymes (*e.g.,* phospholipases) enable microbes to break through cell membranes:

_____

(d) Ligands (or adhesins) on microorganisms bind to specific receptors on target host cells: _____

(e) Examples are chemicals produced by the bacteria that cause diphtheria, pertussis, and tetanus (DPT), as well as traveler's diarrhea and many forms of food poisoning:

_____

D. DIAGNOSIS AND TREATMENT OF INFECTIOUS DISEASES

D1. Write the two requirements for diagnosis of an infectious disease:

(a) Finding of a specific _____

(b) Presence of _____

and _____

consistent with the specific diagnosis

D2. Match the diagnostic technique with the related description. Select from these answers:

Antigen detection   Culture
Genome sequences   Serology

(a) Checking antibody (IgG or IgM) titer from Naomi's blood to verify her suspected case of hepatitis B: _____

(b) Collection of microbes in Tom's sputum for growth on agar, followed by staining and microscopic examination: _____

(c) Use of DNA probes; polymerase chain reactions (PCR) to quantify the amount of HIV virus (viral load) in Barry's blood: _____

(d) Use of fluorescent antibodies that identify the specific pathogen causing Jerry's meningitis: _____

D3. List three major categories of treatments for infectious diseases.

_____

_____

_____

D4. Explain how ideal antimicrobial medications work.

_____

_____

_____

D5. Select the antibiotic that fits each description.

Aminoglycosides   Cephalosporins
Sulfonamides

(a) Broad-spectrum antibiotics that work by disrupting the bacterial cell wall:

_____

(b) Interfere with bacterial protein synthesis; may have nephrotoxic or ototoxic side effects: _____

(c) Interfere with normal metabolism of bacteria; may cause allergic effects:

_____

D6. List several mechanisms by which bacteria develop resistance to antibiotics.

_____

_____

_____

D7. Select the antimicrobial medication that fits each description.

Antibiotic   Antifungal
Antiparasitic   Antiviral

(a) Penicillin that targets the cell wall of bacteria: _____

(b) Reverse transcriptase inhibitors and protease inhibitors: _____

(c) Antimicrobials needed especially in poor, developing nations: _____

(d) Targets membrane lipid ergosterol, an essential component of cell membranes of certain microbes: _____

(e) A relatively new class of medications (echinocandins) that inhibit synthesis of β-1,3-glycan, a major cell wall polysaccharide in *Candida albicans, Pneumocystis carinii,* and *Aspergillus:* _____

D8. Fill in the blanks about immunotherapy treatment for infections. (See also Chapter 15.)

(a) Vaccines are used as _____ against many preventable infections such as MMR and DPT.

(b) Cytokines are chemicals produced by human _____ blood cells. These stimulate body defenses against infections; for example, _____.

(c) Interferons (IFNs) and interleukins (ILs) are examples of _____ made by WBCs.

(d) IVIG is an acronym for _____ and consists of anti-_____ that can boost immune capabilities of an infected host

D9. Identify the appropriate surgical intervention or condition requiring surgery.

Appendectomy   Debridement
Gas gangrene   Infected heart valve

(a) Infection of second- and third-degree burns required removal and cleaning of sections of Jimmie's skin: _____

(b) Mrs. Romanowski's hysterectomy led to ischemia of abdominal organs and infection that required removal of sections of her intestine and urinary bladder: _____

(c) Susannah's streptococcal infection as a child resulted in endocarditis that caused heart murmurs and related surgery: _____

(d) Billy required surgery to prevent organ rupture and possible peritonitis: _____

E. BIOTERRORISM AND EMERGING GLOBAL INFECTIOUS DISEASES

E1. Define bioterrorism.

_____

_____

Discuss the incident of bioterrorism in the United States in the fall of 2001 by filling in blanks and circling correct answers.

(a) Name the microorganism that causes anthrax: _____. This microbe more typically affects (*humans? plant-eating animals?*) and it is a (*common? rare?*) disease in the United States.

(b) List three systems that can serve as portals of entry for anthrax bacteria: _____, _____, and _____. State the specific mechanism of anthrax contamination in the outbreak of fall 2001: _____.

(c) What preparations have been implemented to defend against future bioterrorist attacks?

_____

E2. Circle the level of microorganism that poses the greatest risk of biothreat, based on risk of use, transmissibility, invasiveness, and mortality rate. Category (*A? B? C?*) Now identify the biothreat category of each of the following microorganisms.

(a) *Mycobacterium tuberculosis:* ___

(b) Yellow-fever virus: ___

(c) Food and water-borne agents, *Salmonella, Shigella,* and *E. coli 0157:H7:* ___

(d) *Staphylococcus aureus* toxin: ___

(e) Ebola virus that causes hemorrhagic fever: ___

(f) *Bacillus anthracis, Yersinia pestis* (cause of the plague), and smallpox virus: ___

E3. List four categories of individuals considered most critical to receive doses of the limited supply of smallpox vaccine to prevent a widespread outbreak of smallpox: _____, _____, _____, _____

E4. Identify the recent global disease that fits each description below. Choose from these answers:

MV (Monkeypox virus)
SARS (Severe acute respiratory syndrome)
WNV (West Nile virus)

(a) Outbreak in May 2003 in the Midwest, following possible infection of small mammals by a rat imported from Ghana; manifestations included fever, swollen lymph glands, and a rash:

_____

(b) A respiratory infection first reported in China in early 2003; it spread to 29 countries but was halted by summer 2003:

_____

(c) Mosquito-borne disease transmitted by birds or horses that can lead to meningo-encephalitis; caused more than 200 deaths in the United States during 2002:

_____

CHAPTER 13

The Immune Response

■ Review Questions

A. THE IMMUNE SYSTEM

A1. Write a paragraph explaining how the immune system is essential for survival. Include these terms: *disease, cancer, nonself,* and *recall.*

_____

_____

A2. Contrast the two major categories of the human body's defenses by writing *innate* or *adaptive* next to related descriptions or components of these defense systems below.

  (a) Immediate (or "early") responses that prevent or control an infection; responses are similar regardless of the type of infection: _____

  (b) Intact skin that serves as a barrier against microbial infection: _____

  (c) Natural killer cells, neutrophils and macrophages, mediators of inflammation such as complement, and cytokines:

  _____

  (d) Also known as acquired or specific immunity; responses distinguish between different microbes and molecules and "remember" previously encountered pathogens: _____

  (e) Lymphocytes and their products that are responsible for both humoral and cell-mediated immunity: _____

A3. Toll-like receptors are located on _____ cells of the innate immune system. These bind with molecules found on *(only specific microbes? a variety of pathogens?)*, for example, carbohydrates found in cell _____ of bacteria. Toll-like receptors are nicknamed the "_____ of the innate immune system" because they help phagocytes to recognize and then attack nonhuman cells.

A4. Circle the correct answers or fill in the blanks to answer these questions about immunity.

  (a) *(Antigens? Antibodies?)* are foreign to the host, and they *(stimulate? inhibit?)* an immune response. Antigens are also known as *(immunogens? immunoglobulins?)*.

  (b) Circle the antigens in the following list.

Bacteria	Bee venom
Fungi	Penicillin
Pollen	Protozoans
T lymphocytes	Transplanted organs
Viruses	

  (c) A site on an antigen that is recognized by a specifically shaped lymphocyte or antibody is called an antigenic determinant or an _____.

  (d) A single bacterium is likely to present *(only one? three? hundreds of?)* antigenic determinant(s) to human immune cells.

  (e) Penicillin is a(n) *(antigen? hapten?)*. Explain how Christopher can be allergic to penicillin. _____

A5. Match the three principal types of cells of the immune system with related descriptions below.

Antigen-presenting   Effector   Lymphocytes
  cells (APCs)   cells

  (a) Macrophages and dendritic cells that process antigens: _____

  (b) B cells that lead to antibody production are in this category: _____

  (c) Activated T lymphocytes, mononuclear phagocytes, and neutrophils that are responsible for the destruction of the antigens: _____

A6. Circle all answers that match a type of immune cell with a correct description.

  (a) Lymphocytes: normally make up about 99% of all leukocytes

(b) T lymphocytes: make up about 10% to 20% of all lymphocytes

(c) B lymphocytes: associated with antibody-mediated immunity

(d) T lymphocytes: associated with cell-mediated immunity

A7. Circle the correct answer or fill in the blanks within each statement about activation of immune cells.

(a) The trigger for activation of both B and T lymphocytes is recognition of an epitope on an anti_____ by B- or T-cell receptors.

   (1) B-cell antigen receptors consist of *(MHCs? immunoglobulins [antibodies]?)* bound to the B-cell membrane.

   (2) T-cell receptors recognize antigens only when they are bound to _____.

(b) Antigens are presented to lymphocytes by APCs (a_____ p_____ cells). List two examples of APCs: _____ _____

(c) Further activation of lymphocytes with chemicals known as cyto_____ causes B or T cells to _____.

(d) Activated B cells produce effector cells known as _____ cells that secrete antibodies (Igs) that bind to the intruding antigen and ensure its removal. Antibody-mediated immunity (or AMI) is also known as *(cytotoxic? humoral?)* immunity because antibodies are small and suspended in blood (a "humor").

(e) T cells are involved in _____-mediated immunity (or CMI), which is also known as *(cytotoxic? humoral?)* immunity because T cells exert toxic effects directly on antigens.

A8. Circle the correct answer or fill in the blank about "CDs."

(a) What is the meaning of CD in CD4+ or CD8+? _____

(b) Cytotoxic cells are known as *(CD4+? CD8+?)* cells, whereas *(CD4+? CD8+?)* cells are involved in humoral immunity.

(c) *(CD4+? CD8+?)* cells are destroyed by the HIV virus.

A9. Circle the correct answers or fill in the blanks within each statement about Kate's MHC molecules.

(a) MHC stands for m_____ h_____ complex molecules. "Histo-" (as in histology) refers to ____ of the body. These chemicals are coded for by DNA on Kate's chromosome _____. Because Kate's cells have unique MHC molecules, a kidney transplanted from Kate's friend Susan to Kate is likely to be recognized as *(self? nonself?)* because Susan's MHC molecules differ from Kate's. Because MHC molecules do play a role in transplant rejection, these chemicals are classified as anti*(gens? bodies?)*.

(b) Kate's MHC molecules should allow her immune system to recognize her own cells as "self," not "nonself." Errors in such recognition lead to _____ diseases (e.g., some forms of arthritis or diabetes) in which Kate's immune system would *(destroy? tolerate?)* her own cells. (See Chapter 15.)

(c) Write one sentence that describes the overall function of Kate's MHCs:

   _____

   _____

A10. Circle the correct answers or fill in the blanks within each statement about the two categories of MHC molecules.

(a) MHC I molecules are found on *(nearly every cell of the body? APCs and B cells?)*. As a result, they can flag the immune system if the body cell is altered by cancer or by viral invasion of human cells. The virus or cancer cell is degraded, and portions of it (antigens) complex with MHC I molecules. This complex is then recognized by *(helper? cytotoxic?)* T (CD8+) cells as an "intruder" that must be destroyed.

(b) MHC II molecules are found on _____, _____, and _____ cells. MHC IIs bind to antigens from microbes that have been phagocytosed and digested within macrophages. *(CD4+ helper? CD8+ cytotoxic?)* T cells recognize antigens complexed with MHC II complexes.

A11. Circle the correct answer or fill in the blanks within each statement.

(a) Human MHC proteins are also known as HLA (_____ _____ antigens) because they were first detected on

CHAPTER 13 ■ **The Immune Response**   **73**

_____ blood cells. MHC I molecules are divided into subtypes HLA-A, _____, and _____. MHC II are *(also? not?)* divided into subtypes. (See Table 13-1 in *Essentials of Pathophysiology.*)

(b) The combination of genes that determines a person's HLA type usually is inherited from each parent as a _____. Because of the diversity in MHC molecules, it *(is? is not?)* likely that each person's MHC (or HLA) antigens will be unique. For transplant compatibility, it is critical that donor and recipient MHC (or HLA) antigens be *(very similar? dissimilar?)*.

A12. Circle the correct answers or fill in the blank within each statement about macrophages.

(a) Macrophages develop from cells that produce *(neutrophils? monocytes?)* that are *(red? white?)* blood cells. Monocytes move from marrow into tissues where they mature into cells such as Kupffer cells, which are macrophages in the *(liver? lungs?)*, or microglial cells, which are macrophages in the _____.

(b) Macrophages take part in *(only innate? only adaptive? both innate and adaptive?)* immune responses. As part of the *(innate? adaptive?)* response, toll-like receptors on phagocytes bind to antigens of a variety of gram-positive or gram-negative bacteria. (See Question A3.)

(c) These phagocytic cells also secrete _____ such as TNF and IL-1 that will *(stimulate? inhibit?)* the inflammatory response.

(d) A role of macrophages in adaptive immunity is to serve as _____ that present antigen–MHC II complexes to *(CD4+? CD8+?)* cells.

A13. What function do dendritic cells share with macrophages?

_____

Dendritic cells are found in _____ tissue and also in skin, where they are known as _____ cells.

A14. Complete these statements about T lymphocytes by circling the correct answers or filling in the blanks. (See Questions A7 and A10.)

(a) T cells are more associated with control of *(bacteria? viral?)* infections. They do this by *(direct killing action? causing production of antibodies?)*, which is *(cell-mediated or CMI? humoral or AMI?)* immunity. T cells also activate other _____ cells and also _____ cells.

(b) T cells form in *(bone marrow? lymph tissue?)* and mature in the *(thymus? thyroid?)*, where helper T cells develop CD4 receptors and cytotoxic T cells develop ____ receptors.

(c) Helper T (CD__) cells activated by recognition of an antigen complexed with MHC *(I? II?)* molecules play key regulatory roles in immunity. Helper T cells secrete _____, such as interleukins (ILs), that activate most other types of immune cells (for example, attracting more _____ cells to the infected area).

(d) Cytotoxic T (CD__) cells are activated by MHC *(I? II?)* molecules complexed with cells infected with viruses or cancer (antigens); this process ensures that neighboring cells with MHC I but *not* infected with antigen will be spared from attack by CD8+ cells. List several mechanisms by which cytotoxic T cells destroy infected cells.

_____

_____

A15. Answer the following questions about B lymphocytes.

(a) B cells develop and mature in *(bone marrow? bloodstream? thymus?)*. During this process, they develop receptors that are _____. This process *(does? does not?)* require the presence of an antigen.

(b) List several functions of these immunoglobulins on B cells.

_____

(c) The mature B cells *(stay in bone marrow? migrate to peripheral lymphoid tissue?)*. Here, B cells that encounter complementary antigens and T-cell/cytokine stimulation will transform into _____ cells (and produce antibodies that bind to and remove specific antigens) or long-lived _____ cells that will

Copyright © 2007. Lippincott Williams & Wilkins. *Study Guide to Accompany Porth's Essentials of Pathophysiology: Concepts of Altered Health States 2e*, by Kathleen Schmidt Prezbindowski.

respond to future antigen exposure (see Question A7).

(d) B cells are more associated with destruction of *(bacteria and their toxins? fungi, protozoans, and viruses?).* They do this by *(direct killing action? causing production of antibodies?),* which is *(cytotoxic? humoral?)* immunity.

(e) B lymphocytes *(can? cannot?)* serve as APCs. Explain how B cells and T cells function in allergic reactions to penicillin

_____

_____

A16. Answer these questions about significant components of antibodies. Circle the correct answers or fill in the blanks within each statement.

(a) Antibodies or immunoglobulins are *(lipids? proteins?)* with *(1? 2? 4?)* polypeptide chains (2 light, 2 heavy) with at least ___ antigen-binding sites.

(b) Three classes of antibodies have shapes that resemble the letter Y. These are Ig__, Ig__, and Ig__.

(c) The function of the antibody is to bind to a(n) _____. These binding sites are found at the ends of the *(forked? tail?)* portion of the antibody; this region is known as the Fab or _____-binding fragment. This Fab end is *(constant? variable?)* in shape because this portion of all antibodies must conform to diverse antigens. The tail end (Fc fragment) is *(constant? variable?)* for the particular class of immunoglobulin (such as IgD or IgG).

A17. Identify the type of antibody likely to be secreted in each case.

IgA   IgD   IgE   IgG   IgM

(a) These antibodies are detected in baby Cleo's blood. Because these are the first antibodies to be secreted in response to an antigen and because they do not cross the placenta, it is determined that Cleo must have the related antigens (and infection that caused them): ___

(b) Baby Leo received these immunoglobulins from his mother because this type does cross the placenta and provide Leo with at least temporary immunity against many bacterial and viral infections; these Igs typically make up three quarters of all

circulating antibodies. There are four subsets of this class of Igs: ___

(c) Paul has conjunctivitis, which is normally prevented with the help of antibodies in tears in the eyes; these antibodies are also found in other secretions, such as saliva and the mucus of airways, GI tract, and vagina. They help to prevent adhesion of bacteria to epithelial linings: ___

(d) Dorothy has allergies to pollen and several foods that are mediated by antibodies that trigger release of histamine from her mast cells and basophils: ___

(e) Found on B lymphocytes as antigen receptors required for triggering differentiation of B cells: ___

A18. Circle the correct answers or fill in blanks within each statement about NK cells.

(a) NK (n_____-k_____) cells *(are? are not?)* lymphocytes. They destroy cancer cells or virus-infected cells *(directly? by releasing antibodies?).* They differ from T cells in that NK cells *(do? do not?)* need to be activated by the specific antigen. How do NK cells know not to kill normal human cells?

_____

(b) NK cells' mechanisms of destroying invaders mimic those of *(B? T?)* lymphocytes in that they produce cytotoxic chemicals such as _____ .

A19. Hussein is 20 years old and in excellent health. Circle the correct answers or fill in the blanks in these questions about his lymphoid organs.

(a) Circle all of his central lymphoid organs.

Bone marrow	Lymph nodes
MALT tissues lining	Peyer patches in
passageways into	GI organs
the body	Spleen
Thymus	Tonsils

(b) Hussein's thymus is likely to be located in his *(neck? thorax, anterior to his heart?).* His thymus is likely to be *(larger? smaller?)* now than it was when he was 10 years old.

(c) Normally, T cells mature within the thymus under the influence of _____ and _____ hormones. Most of these cells *(do? do not?)* leave the thymus.

(d) Normally, only T cells that can distinguish _____ antigens are selected to leave the thymus. This process is known as _____ selection. After about two days, mature cells leave the thymus and travel through the bloodstream to settle in _____.

(e) Most of Hussein's lymph nodes are likely to be located in his *(hands and feet? trunk and proximal ends of his extremities?)*. Refer to Figure 13-9 in *Essentials of Pathophysiology*. Maturing *(B? T? both B and T?)* cells are located in the lymph nodes. What other function do lymph nodes serve?

_____

(f) Hussein's spleen is likely to be located just posterior to his *(liver? stomach?)* on the upper *(right? left?)* of his abdomen. Old red blood cells are destroyed within *(red? white?)* pulp. White pulp serves as another location of _____ and _____ cells.

(g) Microbes inhaled into Hussein's airways will be greeted (and attacked) by immune cells in two sites, namely _____ and _____.

A20. Answer these questions about cytokines.

(a) Cytokines *(are made by? act on?)* immune cells, primarily *(B? T?)* lymphocytes and macrophages. These chemicals act on cells *(distant from? nearby?)* the cells that produce them, where they bind to specific _____. Most cytokines affect *(only one? more than one?)* type of cell and may lead to cascade effects.

(b) Name several cytokines that mediate inflammation by producing fever and mobilizing neutrophils. _____

(c) Name several cytokines that stimulate hematopoiesis.

_____

(d) Name an interleukin and its receptor that are critical for sustained T-cell proliferation. Drugs used to prevent rejection of transplanted kidneys, liver, or heart function by inhibition of this IL.

_____

(e) Explain how interferons (IFNs) help protect the body.

_____

_____

_____

_____

(f) Name a cytokine that is responsible for tissue wasting in "wasting diseases" such as chronic inflammations. _____

A21. Write *A* (active) or *P* (passive) to indicate the type of acquired immunity in each example.

(a) Immunization with injection of antigens to which the body develops immunity: ___

(b) Infection with a specific microbe (and its antigens): ___

(c) A dose of gamma globulin: ___

(d) Transfer of IgG antibodies from mother to baby across the placenta: ___

(e) Produces short-term protection that lasts only weeks to months: ___

A22. Production of antibodies in humoral immunity depends more directly on *(B? T?)* lymphocytes. List several mechanisms by which antibodies are able to combat infection.

_____

_____

_____

A23. Anastasia receives her DPT immunization and somewhat later receives a "booster." To which dose is she likely to mount a greater immune response (produce more antibodies)?

_____

A24. Answer the following questions about cell-mediated immunity.

(a) Name three types of antigens against which cell-mediated immunity offers protection.

_____

(b) Cell-mediated immunity depends more directly on *(B? T?)* lymphocytes and macrophages. *(Helper? Cytotoxic?)* T cells play a critical role in producing IL-2, which then stimulates killing activity by *(helper? cytotoxic?)* T cells and macrophages.

A25. Circle the correct answers or fill in the blanks within each statement about the complement system.

(a) The complement system consists of *(lipids? proteins?)* in blood and—similar to the process of blood coagulation—acts via a *(single reaction? cascade of reactions?)* to mediate *(cytotoxic? humoral?)* immunity.

(b) Name the three parallel pathways in the complement system: _____, _____, and _____-mediated pathway. All three result in reactions that successively cleave complement proteins. Where are these protein fragments then placed? _____

(c) Which of the three pathways can be initiated by antibodies (such as IgG or IgM) bound to antigens on the surface of microbes? _____ This pathway (the first studied) consists of proteins C1 to ____ plus other factors that enhance inflammation and destruction of microbes.

(d) Activation of complement leads to release of chemicals from mast cells and basophils, causing blood vessels to (constrict? dilate?) and have (increased? decreased?) permeability. This process, called _____, brings more phagocytic cells to the infected area.

(e) Coating of microbes that makes them more inviting to phagocytes is a process called _____; as a result, phagocytes are more attracted to these "tasty morsels," a process called _____.

(f) The late phase of the complement cascade triggers formation of the MAC (membrane _____ complex) that causes lysis of bacteria and cells, including _____.

A26. List two factors that exert checks and balances (self-regulation) on the immune system.

_____

_____

_____

B. DEVELOPMENTAL ASPECTS OF THE IMMUNE SYSTEM

B1. Arrange in correct sequence from first to last the following events in the development of the immune system. ____, ____, ____

(a) Development of spleen, lymph nodes, and tonsils

(b) Blood formation begins

(c) Development of the thymus and bone marrow

B2. Circle the correct answer or fill in the blank within each statement about immunity in infants.

(a) Sara, a full-term newborn, has antibodies in her blood that protect her from a number of diseases for several months. These are (IgAs? IgGs? IgMs?).

(b) Annie, born prematurely at 7 months, is likely to have (normal? deficient?) immunity. Explain why. _____

_____

_____

(c) Celia, a newborn whose mother has the HIV virus, (will? might? will not?) have IgGs against the HIV virus in her blood. Is Celia infected with HIV? _____

_____

_____

(d) IgM antibodies (can? cannot?) cross the placenta. What does the presence of IgM antibodies in 2-week-old Jill's blood indicate? _____

_____

(e) IgA antibodies are transferred from mother to baby Miji (across the placenta? through breast milk?). How can these antibodies help Miji?

_____

B3. Circle those factors that are likely to be decreased in elderly persons.

Incidence of autoimmune disease

Cell-mediated immunity

Antibody-mediated immunity

T-cell count

Infections

Cancers

Range of antibodies that can be recognized

IL-2 cytokine production

CHAPTER 14

Inflammation, Tissue Repair, and Fever

■ Review Questions

A. THE INFLAMMATORY RESPONSE

A1. Describe the "good news" and "bad news" of inflammation.

_____

_____

A2. Which part of the term *pericarditis* indicates that this condition is an inflammation? *(Peri-? Card-? -Itis?)*

A3. List five or more factors that can trigger an inflammatory response.

_____

_____

_____

A4. Explain the mechanisms that lead to the following cardinal signs and symptoms of an acute inflammation:

(a) Redness and warmth

_____

(b) Swelling (edema)

_____

(c) Pain and loss of function

_____

_____

A5. Acute inflammation involves two major stages. The first is the *(cellular? vascular?)* stage that accounts for redness, warmth, and edema. Which type of vascular response is a sunburn likely to cause?

(1) Immediate transient

(2) Immediate sustained

(3) Delayed hemodynamic

A6. Circle the correct answers or fill in the blanks within each statement about the cellular stage of inflammation. (See also Chapter 13.)

(a) The first cells to arrive on the scene are *(monocytes? neutrophils?)*. These cells produce chemicals known as _____ molecules that cause them to slow down and stick to the inner walls of vessels, a process known as _____. Neutrophils are likely to arrive at the injured area within *(1.5? 5?)* hours of the injury.

(b) Neutrophils move out of a dilated blood vessel by the process of _____. The cytoplasmic granules in these cells contain _____ that destroy the phagocytosed particles. White blood cells are attracted to the site of inflammation by the process of _____.

(c) To make sufficient neutrophils available during inflammation, the white blood cell count *(increases? decreases?)*; this process is called leuko*(cytosis? penia?)*. As a result, immature neutrophils known as *(segs? bands?)* may appear in circulating blood.

(d) Two other types of leukocytes known as _____phils and _____phils increase during allergic reactions or parasitic infections. *(Basophils? Eosinophils?)* release histamine that *(constricts? dilutes?)* vessels during acute inflammation.

(e) _____cytes are leukocytes that play important roles in chronic infection. Their lifespans are considerably *(longer? shorter?)* than those of neutrophils. Monocytes mature into cells known as _____. These may migrate to _____, where they act as APCs.

A7. List several chemicals that attract leukocytes to infected or inflamed areas.

_____

_____

A8. Arrange in correct sequence the stages of phagocytosis that follow chemotaxis:

Adherence/opsonization → Engulfment → Intracellular killing

_____ → _____ →
_____

A9. Choose from this list of chemicals to fill in the blanks within each statement.

Bradykinin   Histamine
Leukotrienes   Platelet-activating factor
Prostaglandin   Arachidonic acid
Complement   Cytokines
Serotonin

(a) Aspirin reduces inflammation and pain by inhibiting production of _____.

(b) _____ increase(s) capillary permeability, causing edema and pain.

(c) _____ cause(s) a wheal-and-flare reaction that accompanies some allergic reactions.

(d) _____ and _____ contribute to bronchial asthma.

(e) Found in platelets, basophils, and mast cells, _____ is released early in inflammation, causing vasodilation and increased permeability of vessels.

(f) _____ is found in platelets and has actions similar to those of histamine.

(g) _____ consists of a set of proteins that enhance adherence of phagocytes to bacteria.

(h) _____ is a 20-carbon fatty acid found in phospholipids of cell membranes; it leads to production of prostaglandins and leukotrienes.

(i) _____ include colony-stimulating factors, interleukins, interferons, and tissue necrosis factors.

A10. Virtually all chemicals listed for answers to Question A9 are vaso(_constrictors? dilators?_). Almost all these chemicals are (_cell? plasma?_)-derived mediators. Name two that are plasma derived: _____ and _____.

A11. Serous exudates are (_viscous? watery?_) fluids resulting from inflammation, whereas hemorrhagic exudates contain _____. Purulent exudates contain pus, which consists of _____.

A12. Contrast an _abscess_ with an _ulceration_.

_____

_____

A13. Indicate whether each of the following factors _increases_ or _decreases_ during acute-phase responses to inflammation.

(a) Plasma proteins such as fibrinogen or C-reactive protein (CRP) made by the liver: _____

(b) Body temperature in response to release of cytokines such as IL-1 and IL-6: _____

(c) Erythrocyte-sedimentation rate (ESR): _____

(d) Breakdown of skeletal muscle with release of amino acids from muscle proteins: _____

(e) Energy level: _____

A14. Circle the correct answers or fill in the blank within each statement about additional systemic inflammatory responses.

(a) In most severe infections, total white blood cell count is likely to (_increase? decrease?_). Write a typical count during such infections: _____/μL.

(b) The life span of white blood cells is typically about 10 (_hours? days? months?_). Rapid replacement with immature white blood cells is known as a "shift to the _____."

(c) In which condition(s) is/are the neutrophil count likely to increase?

Allergic reaction   Bacterial infection
Cancer   Parasitic infection
Viral infection

(d) In which condition(s) is/are the CD4$^+$ T-lymphocyte count likely to decrease?

Allergic reaction   Bacterial infection
Cancer   Parasitic infection
Viral infection

(e) In which condition(s) is/are the eosinophil count likely to increase?

Allergic reaction   Bacterial infection
Cancer   Parasitic infection
Viral infection

(f) Enlarged but painful lymph nodes more often accompany (_inflammation? cancer?_),

whereas enlarged but painless lymph nodes are more likely to be signs of
_____.

A15. Circle the correct answers or fill in the blanks within each statement about chronic inflammation.

(a) Chronic inflammation is more likely to involve rapid infiltration of affected tissue by *(neutrophils? monocytes?)*, which then develop into _____. In addition, _____ cells proliferate and lead to scarring and deformity.

(b) A *(nonspecific? granulomatous?)* inflammation occurs in response to presence of foreign bodies such as splinters, sutures, or asbestos. Tuberculosis is an example of a *(nonspecific? granulomatous?)* inflammation in which the center of the granuloma is *(cheesy? coagulated and hard?)*.

B. TISSUE REPAIR AND WOUND HEALING

B1. Arrange in correct sequence the degree to which these types of cells can regenerate, from most to least.

Labile   Permanent   Stable

_____, _____ , _____

Identify which of the above categories of cells fits each of the following descriptions of tissues.

(a) Mature skeletal muscle, cardiac muscle, and neurons that will never regenerate:

_____

(b) Cells that have a daily turnover, such as skin, linings of the mouth, GI tract, much of the genitourinary tract, and blood-forming cells in bone marrow:

_____

(c) Cells such as those in the liver that will grow if stimulated and if they have a supportive framework (stroma):

_____

B2. Circle the two true statements. (Pay particular attention to whether the **bold-faced** word or phrase makes the statement true or false.)

(a) Connective tissue that serves as a scaffolding for functional cells is known as **parenchymal tissue.**

(b) Cirrhosis is **more** likely than hepatitis to result in permanent liver damage.

(c) Healing by second intention is likely to occur **faster** and with **better** results than healing by first intention.

(d) Inflammation **is** considered **essential** to the normal wound-healing process.

B3. Complete these exercises about wound healing. First, arrange in correct sequence the phases of wound healing, from first to last.

(a) Proliferative Inflammatory Remodeling

_____ → _____ →

_____

(b) Next, arrange in correct sequence the following events that occur in the inflammatory phase, by number, from first to last. _____ , _____ , _____ ,

_____.

(1) Migration of neutrophils or polymorphonuclear cells (PMNs) to the scene of the injury or infection

(2) Arrival of monocytes that will develop into powerful macrophages

(3) Constriction of injured blood vessels due to release of vasoconstrictor chemicals

(4) Dilation and increased permeability of capillaries

B4. Describe the function of each of these cells or chemicals in the inflammatory and proliferative phases of wound healing:

(a) Macrophages

_____

_____

(b) Tissue-angiogenesis factor (TAF)

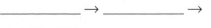

_____

(c) PMNs

_____

_____

(d) Fibroblasts

_____

_____

(e) Endothelial cells

_____

_____

B5. Determine whether each of the following is, in general, *G* (relatively good) or *B* (relatively bad):

(a) Granulation tissue and proud flesh: ____

(b) Keloid: ____

B6. Circle the two true statements about wound healing. (Pay particular attention to whether the **bold-faced** word or phrase makes the statement true or false.)

(a) During the remodeling phase of healing, **both** formation and lysis of collagen fibers occur.

(b) In general, large wounds heal from the **outside** toward the **inside.**

(c) At the point when sutures are removed (about a week after the injury), wound strength is at about **70%** of prewound strength.

(d) Usually wounds **do** ultimately heal to be 100% as strong as the prewound tissue.

B7. Match the vitamin with the related description.

Vitamin A   Vitamin B
Vitamin C   Vitamin K

(a) Most are water soluble so must be replaced daily to serve as cofactors for enzymes needed for healing: _____

(b) Facilitates formation of blood vessels: _____

(c) Needed for synthesis of the protein collagen: _____

(d) Helps to prevent bleeding that would slow the healing process: _____

B8. Circle the two true statements. (Pay particular attention to whether the **bold-faced** word or phrase makes the statement true or false.)

(a) Ischemic tissue is **more** likely to become infected during healing than tissue that is well supplied with blood.

(b) **Intrinsic** phagocytic disorders are those in which phagocytic cells **lack** the enzymes needed to do their jobs.

(c) Hyperglycemia, for example, in diabetics, **increases** the effectiveness of phagocytes.

(d) Corticosteroids **enhance** inflammation and **accelerate** the healing process.

(e) **Dehiscence** refers to excessive binding together of two sides of a wound.

B9. Ms. Alsop is receiving hyperbaric treatment for an infection that has resisted healing. List three mechanisms by which this type of treatment decreases infection and promotes healing.

_____, _____, _____

B10. Defend or dispute this statement: "Sutures enhance healing and help prevent infection."

_____

_____

_____

C. TEMPERATURE REGULATION AND FEVER

C1. Circle the two true statements. (Pay particular attention to whether the **bold-faced** word or phrase makes the statement true or false.)

(a) Core body temperature is normally about **42°C.**

(b) Body temperature is typically highest in the **morning.**

(c) The temperature control center is located in the **hypothalamus.**

(d) The thermoregulatory center regulates **core** (rather than surface) temperature.

(e) Because fat conducts heat **poorly,** adipose tissue is a **poor** insulator.

C2. Write *L* next to mechanisms by which the body loses heat, and write *P* next to mechanisms related to heat production (or heat gain).

(a) Release of catecholamines such as epinephrine produced during stress: ____

(b) Shivering: ____

(c) Strenuous exercise: ____

(d) Sweating: ____

(e) Use of a cooling blanket: ____

(f) Development of "goose bumps": ____

(g) Diuresis (for example, by use of diuretics): ____

C3. Match the heat loss mechanism with the related description.

Conduction   Convection
Evaporation   Radiation

(a) George feels a chill as a breeze from an open window reaches him while he is taking a shower: _____

(b) The backs of Julia's thighs feel cool as she sits on a metal bench in her running shorts: _____

(c) Emilio runs a 10K race on a 105°F day: _____

(d) This mechanism is likely to account for most of Lucy's heat loss as she sits outside on a 60°F day: _____

C4. Circle the correct answers or fill in the blanks within each statement about fever.

(a) Fever is caused by *(resetting the temperature set point in the hypothalamus? ineffectual temperature-regulating mechanisms?)*.

(b) The human temperature set point typically has an upper limit of ____°C (or ____°F). List two factors that might cause the core body temperature to exceed this.

_____ _____

(c) Fever is also known as _____. Antipyretic agents *(increase? decrease?)* body temperature by *(causing vasodilation? resetting the temperature set point?)*.

(d) Bacteria that cause fever release chemicals called *(endo? exo?)*genous pyrogens. These chemicals stimulate body cells to release _____genous pyrogens, such as _____-1, which, in turn, work through _____ E_2.

(e) List two mechanisms that the hypothalamus will initiate to increase core body temperature to the new set point.

_____ _____

(f) What causes the anorexia, malaise, and increased white blood count that are likely to accompany fever? _____

C5. Suggest a likely cause of fever in each of the following cases. (None of these patients has an infection.)

(a) Mrs. Graham has had a myocardial infarction (heart attack).

_____

_____

(b) Mr. Giovanni has Hodgkin disease.

_____

_____

(c) Infant Jeremy has increased intracranial pressure (ICP) following head trauma. He is not responding to antipyretic therapy.

_____

C6. Defend or dispute this statement: "Fever is beneficial."

_____

_____

_____

C7. Choose the class of fever for each.

Intermittent Relapsing Remittent Sustained

(a) Billy had a fever for 3 days, then a normal temperature for 2 days, and then the cycle repeated: _____

(b) Cicely's temperature has varied between 101°F and 104°F for 5 days: _____

C8. During a fever, heart rate and metabolic rate are both likely to *(increase? decrease?)*. As a result, the person has a(n) *(increased? decreased?)* need for hydration.

C9. Arrange these phases of a fever in correct sequence from first to last:

Chill Defervescence Flush Prodrome

_____ → _____

→ _____ → _____

Choose from the above list to match the fever phase with the related description.

(a) Shivering and goose bumps signal an attempt by the body to conserve heat to meet the body's new temperature set point: _____

(b) Stages that decrease body temperature back toward normal (two answers): _____, _____

C10. Lawrence has a history of herpes simplex type I (HSV-I). He breaks out with a fever blister now that he has a fever. Explain.

_____

_____

C11. Ms. Johnson's chart indicates that she has an "FUO." Define FUO and list several possible causes.

_____

_____

_____

C12. Body temperature is _(better? more poorly?)_ regulated in infants than in adults. Fever in children under the age of 3 years is defined as a temperature greater than _____°C (or _____°F).

C13. During a history and physical examination, Mr. Baker, age 87, reports to the nurse that he takes medicine for "my Parkinson disease and a water pill for my heart." The nurse records his oral temperature at 100.2°F. Explain why his temperature should be further monitored.

_____

_____

_____

_____

_____

CHAPTER 15

Alterations in the Immune Response

■ Review Questions

A. HYPERSENSITIVITY DISORDERS

A1. List three major categories of functions of the immune system.

_____

_____

_____

A2. List four major categories of dysfunction of the immune system.

_____

_____

_____

A3. Allergens are defined as any foreign substance that can _____.

List four ways allergens can enter the body.

_____

_____

A4. Refer to Table 15-1 in *Essentials of Pathophysiology* and circle the correct answers or fill in the blanks in this overview of the four classes of hypersensitivity responses.

(a) Antibodies (Igs) are involved in *(I? II? III? IV?)* class(es). These responses all involve *(B? T?)* lymphocytes. Which type involves IgE? _____ Which types involve IgG and IgM? _____

(b) In which class are T cells, not antibodies, involved? _____ The T cells directly destroy the antigen or secrete _____ that do the deed. These are *(immediate? delayed?)* hypersensitivity reactions because they occur 1 to 3 *(minutes? hours? days?)* after exposure to the antigen.

(c) Which classes involve complement? _____ and _____

(d) Which class involves formation of immune complexes (utilizing IgG) that can lead to vasculitis and edema with localized necrosis and severe organ damage? _____ List several examples of organs damaged by such antigen-antibody complexes:

_____

_____

_____

A5. Brenda has allergies to ragweed pollen. Circle the correct answers or fill in the blanks within each statement about her experience.

(a) When Brenda breathes in air containing the pollen, the _____ cells (with _____ attached) in the walls of her airways are exposed to the environmental antigens, in this case _____.

(b) The antigens then trigger release of allergy-producing mediators from granules in her mast cells, leading to an _____ response. Name several of these mediators.

_____

(c) Which type of hypersensitivity reaction is Brenda experiencing? *(I? II? III? IV?)* This is a(n) *(immediate? delayed?)*-type of hypersensitivity, which usually occurs within 5 to 30 *(minutes? hours? days?)* of exposure to the allergen.

(d) Brenda has a runny nose and watery eyes, signs of _____. Because her allergies occur annually in the same 2 months of the year, she has *(perennial? seasonal?)* allergies.

Explain causes of these manifestations.

_____

(e) Brenda states that she has periods during which she "just can't breathe." Explain.

_____

(f) State three roles of CD4$^+$ (type T$_H$2) cells in Brenda's allergy.

_____

_____

_____

(g) Like Brenda, several of her family members have allergies to ragweed pollen and several other allergens. Their allergies are likely to be *(atopic? nonatopic?)*. Brenda and family members with similar allergies probably have *(high? low?)* levels of basophils, mast cells, and IgEs.

A6. April, age 10, has a number of food allergies. She has gone into anaphylactic shock after eating cake containing egg and nuts. Circle the correct answer or fill in the blanks within each statement about April's condition.

(a) She is allergic to milk, eggs, and several types of nuts and fish. These foods are primarily *(proteins? carbohydrates?)*. The foods interact with Ig___ bound to cells lining the digestive tract, making this a type ___ allergic response.

(b) Food allergies more commonly manifest in *(adults? children?)*. List several types of manifestations of food allergies.

_____

_____

(c) The two major aspects of anaphylaxis that are potentially dangerous to April are:

(c1) Drop in blood pressure due to

_____

(c2) Airway obstruction and difficulty breathing related to effects of those chemical mediators:

_____

(d) Explain why April receives an injection of epinephrine: _____

(e) Suggest how April might best manage her allergies: _____

(f) Unlike food allergies and hay fever, some type I, IgE-mediated hypersensitivity responses are helpful. Give one example:

_____

A7. Sondra, a newborn, is Rh positive; she has a 2-year-old brother, Jason, who is also Rh positive. Their mother is Rh negative. Sondra has HDN,

an abbreviation for _____ disease of the _____. In this type ___ hypersensitivity reaction, her mother's *(Rh-positive RBCs? Rh antibodies?)* crossed the placenta to enter Sondra's blood. Specifically, these are Ig___ antibodies that can bind to and destroy Sondra's RBCs, leading to conditions such as

_____.

A8. Bob, a student nurse, is being tested to see whether he has tuberculosis. A dose of PPD (or _____ _____ _____) is injected *(intravenously? subcutaneously?)* at 2 PM on Tuesday. By 2 PM on Thursday, Bob has a small (less than 0.2 cm) reddened area at the site of the injection, indicating that Bob *(has tuberculosis? has enough sensitized T cells to cause a hypersensitivity reaction?)*. This is an example of a type ___ hypersensitivity reaction.

A9. Contact dermatitis is a type ___ hypersensitivity.

(a) List three or more examples of causes of contact dermatitis.

_____

_____

(b) Suggest how you might determine exactly what did cause the contact dermatitis.

_____

(c) The affected area typically becomes *(pale and cool? swollen, red, and warm?)*. What treatments would you suggest?

_____

_____

B. AUTOIMMUNE DISORDERS

B1. Answer the following questions about self-tolerance.

(a) Briefly define *self-tolerance*.

_____

_____

_____

(b) Describe the key to developing self-tolerance.

_____

_____

_____

(c) Explain how self-reactive (or autoreactive) lymphocytes are normally eliminated.

_____

_____

_____

B2. List several examples of autoimmune diseases.

_____

_____

_____

B3. Explain how each of the following factors plays a role in the development of autoimmune disease.

(a) Heredity

_____

_____

_____

(b) Trigger factors such as a chemical substance or virus

_____

_____

_____

(c) Gender

_____

_____

_____

(d) Decreased level of suppressor T cells

_____

_____

_____

B4. Wolfgang Amadeus Mozart may have died from heart failure associated with rheumatic fever. Circle the correct answer or fill in the blanks within each statement about his illness.

(a) Mozart may have suffered a group A beta-hemolytic _____coccal infection. A protein in the cell wall of these bacteria plays a very similar role to that of antigens in the endocardial lining of the _____, which forms heart valves.

(b) The streptococcal infection caused production of antibodies that should have been directed to _____ bacteria but,

in a case of "mistaken identity" or molecular _____, were instead directed to the antigens in Mozart's heart valves in association with his own specific _____. With the failure of the valves to direct blood properly, heart workload _(increased? decreased?)_, leading to heart _____. (See more in Chapter 19.)

B5. Blood (or serum) testing for diagnosis of an autoimmune disease involves identification of auto-_____ against a person's own tissues or cells. One example of such a test is the ELISA test, which refers to: _____-_____ _____ assay.

C. TRANSPLANTATION IMMUNOPATHOLOGY

C1. Phoebe, age 20, has received a kidney transplant. (See Question D1[d].) Answer these questions related to Phoebe's case.

(a) Phoebe's new kidney came from a female accident victim, age 38, who was unrelated to Phoebe. This is an example of a(n) _____ cadaver graft. (Select the answer from the following choices.)

(1) Allogeneic

(2) Autologous

(3) Syngeneic

(b) Over the past decade, the 1-year survival rate for kidney transplants has reached about _(15%? 45%? 70%? 95%?)_. The survival rate is highest when donor-host HLA antigens _(match closely? are unmatched?)_.

(c) Within 36 hours of the transplant surgery, Phoebe's immune system began to mount a response against the donor kidney tissues. This is known as _____ disease. (Select the answer from the following choices.)

(1) Graft-versus-host-disease (GVHD)

(2) Host-versus-graft-disease (HVGD)

(d) HVGD required activation of Phoebe's _(B? T?)_ lymphocytes, which then activated her ___ lymphocytes. As a result, Phoebe's antibodies initially attacked graft _(B or T cells? kidney tubule cells? blood vessels?)_, diminishing blood flow to the transplanted organ. This reaction is classified as a _(cellular? humoral?)_ rejection because Phoebe's antibodies destroyed donor kidney tissue.

C2. Arrange the types of transplant rejections in order of likelihood of occurrence, from most to least likely to occur.

Acute   Chronic   Hyperacute

_____ → _____ → _____

Phoebe's transplant rejection (in Question C1) is classified as _____.

C3. Circle the two true statements about graft-versus-host-disease (GVHD). (Pay particular attention to whether the **bold-faced** word or phrase makes the statement true or false.)

(a) GVHD **rarely** occurs in patients who have received bone marrow transplants.

(b) The risk of GVHD is greater if donor and host have very **different** HLA antigens.

(c) In GVHD, T cells within the donated tissue attack **recipient** (host) cells.

(d) The recipient's skin is **rarely** a target of GVHD.

C4. List typical signs and symptoms of GVHD as it affects these organs.

(a) Intestine

_____

(b) Liver

_____

(c) Skin

_____

C5. Identify treatments that are designed to prevent GVHD.

_____

_____

D. IMMUNODEFICIENCY DISORDERS

D1. Write *P* for primary (hereditary or congenital) immunodeficiencies or *S* for secondary (or acquired) immunodeficiencies next to each case. (The second lines are provided for answers to Question D2.)

(a) Tracy has frequent respiratory infections related to her radiation and chemotherapy treatments for cancer: _____ _____

(b) Peter has a shingles infection associated with his AIDS diagnosis: _____ _____

(c) Pete's thymus has failed to develop (DiGeorge syndrome caused by a defective gene on chromosome 22): _____ _____

(d) Phoebe, age 20, has received a kidney transplant. To reduce her risk for organ rejection, she will take immunosuppressant medications for the rest of her life: _____ _____

(e) Timmy, age 3 years, has repeated middle ear infections as a result of lack of maturation of B-lymphocyte stem cells and resulting IgG deficiency: _____ _____

D2. Classify the immunodeficiencies above according to the following categories. (Write these answers on the extra lines in the previous question.)

B-cell (humoral) deficiency
Combined B-cell and T-cell deficiencies
T-cell (cellular) deficiency

D3. Circle the two true statements in the following list. (Pay particular attention to whether the **bold-faced** word or phrase makes the statement true or false.)

(a) Genes that cause immunodeficiency are typically present on **autosomes,** and **few** are on **X chromosomes.**

(b) Maternal antibodies that protect the newborn from infections are **IgMs.**

(c) The **first** antibodies that infants produce are typically IgMs.

(d) By about the age of **2 years,** a child's antibody production level typically matches adult levels.

(e) Humoral immunodeficiencies are **more** likely to lead to fungal and protozoan infections than to bacterial infections.

D4. Circle the correct answers or fill in the blank within each statement.

(a) *(IgA? IgG? IgM?)* is the most common selective immunoglobulin deficiency. About *(10%? 25% 50%?)* of individuals with this type of deficiency have some form of allergy related to lack of these Igs in respiratory or digestive mucous membranes. Administration of IgA *(does? does not?)* help these individuals.

(b) There are four subclasses of *(IgA? IgG? IgM?)* antibodies. IgG2 antibodies are directed against *(protein? polysaccharide?)* antigens, for example, against microbes with capsules made of _____.

(c) Pat's nephrotic syndrome results in abnormal blood filtration with loss of IgA and IgG (but not IgM) antibodies in urine. Why not IgM?

_____

_____

D5. Most people with T-cell immunodeficiencies have *(primary? secondary?)* deficiencies. Explain why.

_____

_____

One example of a primary immunodeficiency is DiGeorge syndrome, which is an *(autosomal? X-linked)* disorder. Circle the signs and symptoms of this disorder:

Eyes set closely together
Large jaw (macrognathia)
Failure of thymus to develop
Failure of parathyroid gland to develop
Hypercalcemia
Heart defects
Increased risk of infections

D6. Answer the following questions about T-cell and B-cell immunodeficiencies.

(a) List several causes of such deficiencies:

_____

_____

_____

One sign of T-cell deficiencies is _____ infections, which are caused by normally harmless pathogens. Another sign is *anergy*. Describe this condition.

_____

_____

(b) What does the acronym SCIDS stand for?

_____

In this condition, *(B? T?)*-cell deficiency occurs. Without treatment, SCIDS patients are likely to die by the age of ___ years.

Treatments include _____ transplantation and _____ .

E. AIDS: TRANSMISSION OF HIV INFECTION

E1. Circle the two true statements. (Pay particular attention to whether the **bold-faced** word or phrase makes the statement true or false.)

(a) Most HIV infections are in the **United States.**

(b) AIDS is considered a **pandemic** disease.

(c) About **30 million people** with HIV infections live in Africa.

(d) Most new HIV infections occur among persons **over age 75.**

E2. Circle the three fluids that serve as "vectors" for almost all HIV transmission. Then underline the one other fluid that has been documented as a vector for HIV transmission.

Blood	Breast milk	Feces
Mosquito venom	Nasal secretions	Saliva
Semen	Sweat	Tears
Urine	Vaginal fluids	Vomitus (emesis)

E3. Explain how alcohol and cocaine use are related to HIV transmission.

_____

_____

E4. Circle the two true statements about HIV/AIDS. (Pay particular attention to whether the **bold-faced** word or phrase makes the statement true or false.)

(a) The "A" in the acronym AIDS stands for **autoimmune.**

(b) Since 1985, blood donations **have** routinely been tested for HIV.

(c) **Unprotected sex** is the most common means of HIV transmission.

(d) Occupational HIV infection by health-care workers is **common.**

E5. Circle the phrase that defines "seroconversion":

(a) Having a virus (or other antigen) in the bloodstream

(b) Having antibodies (developed against this antigen) in the bloodstream

E6. Circle the two true statements about HIV/AIDS. (Pay particular attention to whether the **bold-faced** word or phrase makes the statement true or false.)

(a) That Jonathan has a history of two STDs (genital herpes and chlamydia) **increases** his risk for having HIV infection.

(b) Although Gary has been infected with HIV, the fact that he has no signs or symptoms of HIV means that he **cannot** transmit the virus.

(c) On 2/1/06, Patrick had unprotected sex during which he was infected with HIV. On 3/15/06, he was **likely** to be in the "window period" for HIV seroconversion.

(d) HIV transmission **cannot** occur by oral sex.

F. PATHOPHYSIOLOGY OF AIDS

F1. How does AIDS kill? Primarily by destruction of (circle the correct answer):

(a) Many types of body cells, as in liver, kidneys, and lungs

(b) Immune cells, so that the body succumbs to infections and/or cancer

F2. Circle the two types of cells that are most commonly infected by the HIV virus.

B lymphocytes   CD4+ T cells
CD8+ T cytotoxic cells   Macrophages
Neutrophils

F3. Circle the three true statements. (Pay particular attention to whether the **bold-faced** word or phrase makes the statement true or false.)

(a) Most HIV infections worldwide are caused by the **HIV-2** virus.

(b) CD4+ T cells **do** have the role of recognizing foreign antigens.

(c) A retrovirus is one that carries its nucleic acid as **DNA.**

(d) The HIV virus carries its nucleic acid in the form of **DNA.**

(e) One normal function of CD4+ T cells is to **activate B lymphocytes** so that antibody production will occur.

(f) CD4+ cells **are** involved in regulating cytotoxic CD8+ T cells and NK cells.

F4. Arrange in correct sequence (from first to last) the steps in replication of HIV within human CD4+ T cells. (List the letters in the spaces that follow.)

(a) Assembly of protein-coated RNA leads to release of new HIV viruses.

(b) Attachment of HIV's gp120 and gp41 to a chemokine co-receptor on a CD4+ T cell occurs.

(c) Cleavage (with help of a protease) of the polyprotein into smaller viral proteins occurs.

(d) With the help of the enzyme integrase, viral-like DNA is integrated into the original DNA of the CD4+ cell.

(e) Reverse transcription occurs as viral RNA is copied to form viral-like DNA.

(f) Translation of viral-like mRNA forms a polyprotein.

(g) Transcription of the viral-like DNA results in formation of viral-like mRNA.

(h) Uncoating takes place as the protein coat is removed from the HIV virus.

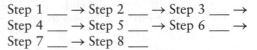

Step 1 ___ → Step 2 ___ → Step 3 ___ →
Step 4 ___ → Step 5 ___ → Step 6 ___ →
Step 7 ___ → Step 8 ___

F5. Describe the structure of the HIV virus by filling in the blanks.

(a) Name two glycoproteins found within the viral envelope: _____ and _____.

(b) HIV screening consists of a test for the presence of antibodies to the HIV core protein, named _____.

F6. Circle the correct answer(s) to complete this sentence: HIV-infected persons typically begin to show symptoms of HIV:

(a) As soon as the CD4+ T-cell level drops slightly

(b) Only when the CD4+ T-cell level drops dramatically

F7. Identify the CD4+ T-cell category (1 to 3) and the clinical category (A to C) of each patient listed in the following table. All three patients have experienced persistent swollen lymph nodes in neck or axillae, sore throat, and night sweats. The CD4+ counts listed are the patients' values before treatment.

Client	CD4+ Count	Category	Signs or Clinical Symptoms	Category
Carl	202 cells	____	Has had one AIDS-defining illness (PCP) and foot infections	____
Terry	512 cells	____	Headaches, malaise, and shingles	____
Kelsey	32 cells	____	Has had many AIDS-defining illnesses (esophageal candidiasis; recurrent pneumonia, including PCP and TB; CMV; invasive cervical cancer; HIV-wasting syndrome) and peripheral neuropathy	____

Determine which client(s) has/have AIDS, according to the CDC definition:

_____

F8. Match the typical phases of HIV infection with the descriptions that follow.

Primary (acute) infection phase
Latent period
Overt AIDS (or symptomatic)

(a) Phase in which viral load is high, approximately 2 to 4 weeks after infection:

_____

(b) Symptoms may mimic those of a flu: fatigue, fever, night sweats, lymphadenopathy, pharyngitis, GI problems, muscle and joint pain:

_____

(c) Viral load is down, CD4+ T-cell count is dropping, and the person has either no symptoms or only mild ones:

_____

(d) The CD4+ T-cell count may approach zero; signs and symptoms include opportunistic infections, cancers, and wasting syndrome:

_____

F9. Miguel was infected with HIV 16 years ago. Because he does not have overt AIDS at this point, he is classified as a *(rapid? slow? typical?)* progressor.

F10. Complete the table describing opportunistic infections (OIs) that are more likely to occur in AIDS patients than in persons with normal immune function. Fill in the blanks with one or more of the following **bold** abbreviations representing the systems commonly infected:

D-E = Digestive (esophageal)

D-I = Digestive (intestinal)

N-S = Nervous/Sensory

R = Respiratory

Name of Microbe	Class of Microbe	Commonly Infected Systems
Candida albicans	Fungus	D-E, N-S, and R
Cryptosporidium parvum	_____	_____
Cytomegalovirus (CMV)	_____	_____
Herpes simplex (HSV)	Virus	_____
Mycobacterium avian complex (MAC)	_____	_____
Mycobacterium tuberculosis	Bacterium	R
Pneumocystis carinii (PCP)	_____	_____
Toxoplasma gondii	_____	_____

F11. Identify the opportunistic infection (OI) from the table in Question F10 that matches each description.

(a) Common cause of diarrhea that may lead to serious dehydration and electrolyte imbalances: _____

(b) Cause of the yeast infection "thrush" of the esophagus (also of mouth, vagina): _____

(c) The most common presenting sign of AIDS during the 1980s; common once CD4+ T-cell levels drop below 200 cells/mL and rare in persons with normal immunity; diagnosis includes identification of the microbe in sputum or lavage specimens:

_____

(d) Leading cause of death from HIV globally; multidrug-resistant (MDR) forms pose special threats to persons with HIV:

_____

(e) Symptoms include painful swallowing:

_____

(f) OI of the brain involving headaches, lethargy, confusion, and seizures:

_____

F12. List three types of neurologic disorders for which persons with AIDS are at greater risk.

_____

_____

_____

F13. Name one type of opportunistic cancer that affects small blood vessels in the mouth, GI tract, and lungs and leads to violet lesions on skin; linked to a herpesvirus: _____

List two other types of cancers for which persons with AIDS are at increased risk:
_____, _____

F14. Bill has had AIDS-defining illnesses over the course of 7 years. His HAART regimen includes two reverse-transcriptase inhibitors, a protease inhibitor, and several prophylactic medications. Identify Bill's HIV-related disorders.

(a) Bill is 6′1″ tall. His weight has dropped from 182 lb before HIV was diagnosed to his current weight of 142: _____

(b) Although his weight is down and his face and extremities appear lean, Bill has a noticeable "belly." His cholesterol and triglyceride levels are elevated:

_____

F15. Circle the two true statements about HIV diagnosis. (Pay particular attention to whether the **bold-faced** word or phrase makes the statement true or false.)

(a) The Western blot test is the **first** test normally performed to detect HIV status.

(b) Both **ELISA** and Western blot test for HIV antibodies (not HIV antigens).

(c) PCR tests identify the presence of the HIV **virus** rather than the **antibody** to HIV.

(d) Newborns whose mothers have HIV infections can be better diagnosed for HIV infection by the **ELISA** and **Western blot tests** than by PCR.

(e) Home testing kits for HIV identify the presence of **the HIV virus** in blood or saliva.

F16. HAART refers to _____ _____ _____ therapy. HAART drugs include PIs and NRTIs. Refer to the eight phases of HIV identified in Question F4 and match the HIV phase to the following HAART drugs.

(a) Protease inhibitors (PIs) such as indinavir (IDV) or saquinavir (SAQ): ___

(b) NRTIs such as AZT, ddI, or ddC: ___

F17. Explain why vaccines and prophylactic medications are also taken by many AIDS patients.

_____

G. HIV INFECTION IN PREGNANCY AND IN INFANTS AND CHILDREN

G1. Circle the two true statements. (Pay particular attention to whether the **bold-faced** word or phrase makes the statement true or false.)

(a) Most infants who become infected with the HIV virus contract it **through blood transfusions.**

(b) If a newborn's mother is HIV-positive, the newborn **will also test positive** for the HIV antibody.

(c) If a newborn's mother is HIV-positive, the newborn **will also test positive** by PCR testing for HIV-like DNA.

(d) Administration of the RTI zidovudine (sometimes abbreviated AZT) does **decrease risk** of HIV transmission during pregnancy, labor, or delivery.

(e) The U.S. Public Health Department recommends HIV counseling and testing **only** if a pregnant woman is considered at "high risk" for HIV infection.

G2. Circle the factors that increase risk of perinatal transmission from an HIV-positive mother to her baby:

(a) A high maternal HIV viral load

(b) High maternal $CD4^+$ count

(c) Exposure of the fetus to a large amount of maternal blood during the birth process

(d) Short time from rupture of the amnion to delivery of the baby

(e) Breast-feeding by an HIV-positive mother

G3. Newborns infected with HIV are likely to demonstrate a pathogenesis that is *(similar to?*

different from?) that of adults with HIV. For example, PCP is likely to occur relatively *(early? late?)* in the course of the child's condition. HIV-infected babies typically weigh *(more? less?)* than their non-HIV counterparts and *(do? do not?)* experience failure to thrive (FTT) and developmental delays.

CHAPTER 16

Control of Cardiovascular Function

■ Review Questions

A. ORGANIZATION OF THE CIRCULATORY SYSTEM

A1. List the components of the circulatory system.

_____

_____

A2. Choose the two true statements. (Pay particular attention to whether the **bold-faced** word or phrase makes the statement true or false.)

(a) The aorta is a **systemic** artery.

(b) Blood moves **faster** and under **greater pressure** through the aorta than through the pulmonary artery.

(c) The right ventricle pumps blood into the **aorta.**

(d) The average (mean) arterial blood pressure (BP) is **greater** in pulmonary vessels than in systemic blood vessels.

A3. Arrange the following terms in correct sequence.

(a) Amount of blood (from greatest to least) at any given time.

Arteries and arterioles   Venules and veins   Heart

_____ → _____ → _____

(b) Blood pressure (from greatest to least):

Arteries   Veins   Capillaries

_____ → _____ → _____

(c) Pathway of blood (from first to last):

Pulmonary artery   Superior vena cava   Right side of the heart

_____ → _____ → _____

A4. Compared with the right side of the heart, the left side normally pumps _(more? less? the same amount of?)_ blood with each contraction. Blood moves through the heart and blood vessels from _(high to low? low to high?)_ pressure. The systemic circulation contains about _(seven times? the same? one seventh?)_ amount of blood as the pulmonary circulation.

B. PRINCIPLES OF BLOOD FLOW

B1. Circle the correct answers or fill in the blanks to answer the following questions about factors that determine blood flow through body tissues and maintain blood pressure (BP).

(a) According to Poiseuille's law, when a blood vessel is narrowed to half its original diameter, resistance to flow through that vessel increases _(2? 4? 8? 16? 32?)_ times. List three mechanisms by which blood vessels may become narrowed.

_____

_____

_____

(b) Blood flow through vessels is directly related to _(blood pressure? resistance?)_ in those vessels and inversely related to _(blood pressure? resistance?)_ in those vessels. This can be expressed by the equation $F = $ _____/_____.

(c) Dawn's hematocrit is 62, which is _(higher? lower?)_ than normal. As a result, Dawn's blood has a _(high? normal? low?)_ viscosity, which _(increases? decreases?)_ resistance to flow.

(d) Blood flows most rapidly (i.e., with greatest velocity) through _(the aorta? capillaries? veins?)_, and it flows most slowly through _____. Explain how these differences in velocity are advantageous to the human body.

_____

_____

(e) Blood flow is most rapid _(within the center? against the wall?)_ of a blood vessel. Smooth blood flow is known as _(laminar?_

turbulent?) flow. Turbulent flow (which increases risk of clot formation) is more likely to occur *(in curving or branching? at straightaway?)* sections of blood vessels.

(f) An aneurysm is a section of a vessel that has "ballooned out." Such an area has *(more? less?)* wall tension than a vessel of normal diameter. This factor *(increases? decreases?)* risk of rupture. Relationships between vessel diameter (or radius) and wall tension are described by the _____ law.

(g) *(Arteries? Capillaries? Veins?)* have greatest distensibility and compliance, meaning that these vessels can hold large amounts of blood with only slight changes in pressure.

C. THE HEART AS A PUMP

C1. Circle the correct answers within each statement about the heart.

(a) The *(left? right?)* side of the heart is more anterior in location.

(b) *(Atria? Ventricles?)* have thicker walls, which is consistent with their functions as *(pumps? reservoirs?)*. Atria serve primarily as *(pumps? reservoirs?)*.

(c) Most of the heart wall is formed of *(endo? myo? peri?)*cardium.

C2. Arrange the following structures of the heart in sequence from outermost to innermost.

Endocardium   Fibrous pericardium
Myocardium   Pericardial cavity
Parietal pericardium   Visceral pericardium

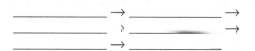

C3. Write *C* for cardiac muscle or *S* for skeletal muscle next to the following descriptions.

(a) Contractions are voluntary: ___

(b) Contractions are of longer duration: ___

(c) Muscle cells are separated from each other by intercalated disks that permit muscle cells to contract as a unit (or syncytium): ___

(d) Calcium channel blockers particularly inhibit this type of muscle, which stores less calcium in its cells: ___

(e) Measurement of troponin T and troponin I are used to measure the extent of infarction of this type of muscle: ___

C4. Describe the "fibrous skeleton" of the heart and state its importance.

_____

_____

_____

_____

C5. Match each valve with the related description.

Aortic   Bicuspid
Pulmonary   Tricuspid

(a) Located immediately inferior to the openings into the coronary arteries: _____

(b) Also known as the mitral valve: _____

(c) Prevent retrograde blood flow from the ventricles into the atria: _____ and _____

(d) Also known as semilunar valves: _____ and _____

(e) Anchored by chordae tendineae and papillary muscles that prevent these valves from everting: _____ and _____

C6. Circle the correct answers or fill in the blanks within each statement about the cardiac conduction system.

(a) Most myocardial cells *(can? cannot?)* initiate and conduct impulses. Specialized pacemaker and conduction tissues generate impulses at a *(faster? slower?)* rate than other heart tissues.

(b) Arrange in sequence from first to last these structures in the conduction pathway:

AV node   Bundle and bundle
Purkinje fibers   branches
SA node

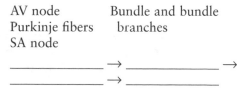

(c) Which structure in part (b), above, is the normal "pacemaker"? _____ It is located in the wall of the *(right? left?)* atrium.

(d) Conduction through the AV node and bundle is *(rapid? slow?)*. State an advantage of this.

_____

_____

(e) Which structure provides the only connection between conductile tissue of atria and ventricles? (Choose from the list in Question C6[b].) _____ State an advantage of this arrangement.

_____

_____

_____

(f) Where are the bundle branches located?

_____

(g) Purkinje fibers have *(rapid? slow?)* transmission. State an advantage of this.

_____

_____

C7. Circle the correct answers or fill in the blanks within each statement about the cardiac conduction system.

(a) Define an action potential.

_____

_____

(b) The inside of a resting cardiac muscle cell membrane typically has a charge of *(+90? –90?)* mV with many more *(Na+? K+?)* located inside the membrane and more *(Na+? K+?)* located outside of the cell membrane.

(c) A stimulus triggers entrance of *(Na+? K+?)* into the cell. Fast Na^+ channels open at a point known as the _____. Electrical potential then rises to a peak of about _____ mV. This period is known as phase *(0? 1?)* or _____ polarization.

(d) Repolarization starts with a(n) *(downward? upward?)* slope (phase 1) as the inside of the membrane develops a more *(positive? negative?)* potential.

(e) The slope flattens out in phase 2 (the _____ phase). What accounts for this plateau, and what is its impact?

_____

_____

(f) The phase 3 slope forms *(dramatically? gradually?)* as K^+ ions move *(into? out of?)* the cell and the influx of Na^+ and Ca^{2+} *(begins? ceases?)*.

(g) Phase 4 requires the Na^+/K^+ pump, which pumps Na^+ *(out of? into?)* the cell and pumps K^+ *(out of? into?)* the cell to return the cell to its original (resting) state.

C8. Circle the correct answers or fill in the blanks within each statement about other aspects of the conduction system.

(a) The *slow response* is initiated by the slow calcium-sodium channels found at the *(AV node? SA node? Purkinje fibers?)*. These are the sites where cardiac action potentials begin (the natural pacemaker or ____ node) or are *slowly* transmitted (____ node) from atria to ventricles.

(b) The *fast response,* which opens fast sodium channels, occurs in the normal myocardial cells of _____, _____, and Purkinje fibers.

(c) A hallmark of SA and AV nodes is slow inward leak of Na^+ through slow channels. This inward flow of Na^+ continues until the threshold is reached and then the SA or AV node spontaneously ___polarizes.

(d) A steep downward slope in phase 4 quickly readies the myocardium for another contraction (producing a rapid heart rate). Drugs such as epinephrine *(increase? decrease?)* heart rate because they increase this slope downward toward resting membrane potential, allowing another action potential and contraction to quickly begin. The vagus nerve is a *(sympathetic? parasympathetic?)* nerve because it *(increases? decreases?)* the slope, ____creasing heart rate.

C9. Circle the correct answers or fill in the blanks within each statement about the refractory period.

(a) The heart is unresponsive to any stimuli whatsoever during:

(1) Absolute refractory period

(2) Relative refractory period

(3) Supernormal excitatory period

As a result, a second myocardial contraction *(can? cannot?)* normally be superimposed over a first one.

(b) The heart can respond to a weak stimulus during the _____ period. In heart disease, ischemia can generate extra _____ beats during this period.

C10. Match the different forms of arrhythmias and conduction disorders with the related descriptions that follow.

Bradyarrhythmias
Complete heart block
Preventricular contractions (PVCs)
Supraventricular arrhythmias
Ventricular arrhythmias

(a) Atria and ventricles are likely to beat independently of each other: _____

(b) Ventricular fibrillation (a quivering heart) is an example of these most life-threatening conduction disorders: _____

(c) Any arrhythmia that originates in the SA node, atria, or AV node: _____

(d) Heart rate of 50 bpm: _____

(e) Occurs when an ectopic pacemaker initiates a beat: _____

C11. Mrs. Pohlmann is having a clinical ECG performed. Complete this exercise about her ECG.

(a) It is likely that ____ leads will be placed on her body. Draw a normal ECG in the margin at left.

(b) Select the part of Mrs. Pohlmann's ECG that best fits each description. Choose from these answers:

P wave   PR interval   QRS complex
RR interval   ST segment   T wave

(b1) Represents repolarization of ventricles: ____

(b2) Represents depolarization of ventricles: ____

(b3) Represents depolarization of the AV node, bundle of His, and Purkinje fibers: ____

(b4) A measure of the length of one cardiac cycle: ____

C12. Refer to Figure 16-15 in *Essentials of Pathophysiology* and answer these questions about the cardiac cycle.

(a) The ECG is a recording of *(electrical? contractile?)* activity of the heart. Recall

that the P wave is associated with impulses that lead to contraction of the *(atria? ventricles?)*, whereas the *(QRS complex? T wave?)* heralds ventricular contraction.

(b) Arrange the following events in the cardiac cycle in correct sequence from first to last, beginning with the QRS complex. (Order the letters in the spaces that follow.)

(A) AV valve closure as ventricular pressure surpasses atrial pressure

(B) Opening of semilunar valves as ventricular pressure surpasses pressure in the great arteries (pulmonary artery and aorta)

(C) Start of ventricular contraction

(D) Dramatic drop in ventricular pressure to less than atrial pressure causing AV valves to open; rapid ventricular filling follows

(E) Ejection period

(F) Semilunar valve closure as ventricular pressure drops below that in the great arteries

(G) T wave signaling the start of ventricular relaxation

(H) P wave signaling atria to give blood an "extra push" into ventricles

___ → ___ → ___ → ___ → ___ → ___ → ___ → ___

(c) Identify the events listed in Question C12(b) that are most closely associated with these heart sounds:

(c1) First heart sound ("lubb"): ___
(c2) Second heart sound ("dup"): ___
(c3) Third heart sound (if present): ___
(c4) Fourth heart sound (if present): ___

(d) Identify the event listed in Question C12(b) that causes the incisura (or notch) in the aortic pressure tracing: ____

(e) Which valves remain open during ventricular diastole (so ventricles can fill during this time)? *(AV? Semilunar?)* Which valves are open only during ventricular systole? *(AV? Semilunar?)*

(f) The two periods during which blood volume stays the same (isovolumetric) are just at the start and end of *(atrial? ventricular?)* systole. Ventricles pump out most of their blood volume *(early? late?)* in ventricular systole. The total volume of blood pumped out with each ventricular contraction is known as _____ volume (SV).

(g) At its highest level, ventricular pressure reaches the same level as pressure within the *(atria? great arteries?)*. In Figure 16-15 in *Essentials of Pathophysiology*, that value is ____ mm Hg.

(h) What factor determines pressure in the aorta during ventricular diastole? _____ Figure 16-15 in *Essentials of Pathophysiology* indicates that diastolic BP in the aorta is ___ mm Hg.

(i) Circle the correct answers. Write in normal values to validate your answers.

(i1) Stroke volume is calculated as:

A. SV = ESV − EDV

B. SV = EDV − ESV

SV = ____ mL − ____ mL = ____ mL/beat

(i2) Ejection fraction is calculated as:

A. SV/EDV

B. SV/ESV

C. ESV/EDV

EF = ____ mL/ ____ mL = ____ %

(j) Because Mrs. Lewis has a diagnosis of congestive heart failure, she is likely to have a(n) *(increase? decrease?)* in both stroke volume and ejection fraction, leading to a(n) *(increase? decrease?)* in EDV.

C13. Circle the correct answers within each statement about right atrial pressure (RAP).

(a) Suzanna's RAP is 0 mm Hg. This value is *(high? normal? low?)*.

(b) Mrs. Pope's RAP is 9 mm Hg, suggesting *(strong? weak?)* pumping of the right side of the heart. A sign of this RAP is likely to be *(bulging? sunken?)* veins in the neck.

C14. Circle the correct answers or fill in the blanks within each statement about heart function. Refer to the left side of Study Guide Figure 17-1.

(a) Determine the average cardiac output (CO) of a resting adult:

Cardiac output (CO) = stroke volume × heart rate

= _____ mL × ____ beats/min

= _____ mL/min = ____ L/min

(b) At rest, Tony has a cardiac output of 6 L/minute. During a strenuous cross-country run, his maximal cardiac output is 18 L/minute. Tony's cardiac reserve is _____.

(c) As he runs, Tony's muscles surrounding his leg veins squeeze *(more? less?)* blood back to his heart, therefore *(increasing? decreasing?)* his venous return and his end-diastolic volume (EDV) or preload. As a result, his myocardial fibers have stretched *(more? less?)*.

(d) Within limits, a stretched muscle (much like a stretched rubber band or balloon) contracts with *(greater? less?)* force as stretching causes maximal overlap of _____ and _____ filaments in the muscles. This is an example of the _____-Starling mechanism.

(e) List several reasons why venous return might be reduced, leading to decreased stretching of the heart, RAP, preload, stroke volume, and cardiac output.

_____

_____

_____

(f) Mr. Stinson has hypertension and aortic valve stenosis; both of these factors tend to *(increase? decrease?)* afterload and *(increase? decrease?)* stroke volume. Stroke volume is *(directly? inversely?)* related to afterload.

C15. Answer these questions about Mrs. Rosenthal, age 76.

(a) Mrs. Rosenthal's resting cardiac output is 1.2 L/minute, and her heart is "enlarged." Explain the connection.

_____

_____

_____

(b) She is taking digoxin, a drug with positive inotropic effects. Such a drug is designed to increase the heart's *(contractility? rate?)*.

(c) Mrs. Rosenthal's resting heart rate is 120 beats/minute. At this rate, the length of one cardiac cycle is ____ second(s). When Mrs. Rosenthal becomes anxious, her heart rate increases to 180 beats/minute, allowing only ___ second(s) for each cardiac cycle. Such rapid heart rates especially shorten the time allotted for ventricular *(systole? diastole?)*, which is the period when ventricles *(eject? fill?)*. This factor contributes to her *(high? low?)* cardiac output.

D. BLOOD VESSELS AND THE PERIPHERAL CIRCULATION; MICROCIRCULATION AND LOCAL CONTROL OF BLOOD FLOW

D1. Arrange the layers of the wall of an artery or vein in sequence from outermost to innermost.

Externa   Intima   Media

_____ → _____ →

_____

Which layer contains smooth muscle that permits constriction of the vessel? _____

D2. Describe the functions of these parts of blood vessels:

(a) Endothelial cells of the tunica intima.

_____

_____

(b) Smooth muscle of the tunica media that permits blood vessels to maintain a constant state of muscle tone and also to contract to return blood to the heart. Include the following terms: *sarcoplasmic reticulum, fast sodium channels, extracellular calcium, norepinephrine,* and *alpha-adrenergic receptors.*

_____

_____

_____

_____

_____

D3. Refer to Figure 16-2 in the text to answer the following questions.

(a) Define *pressure pulse.*

_____

_____

_____

(b) How is the concept of pressure pulse applied clinically?

_____

_____

_____

(c) Pressure pulse *(becomes greater? dissipates?)* as blood passes through arterioles, capillaries, venules, and veins. As a result, "a pulse" *(can? cannot?)* normally be palpated on these vessels.

D4. Match the type of vessel with the descriptions that follow.

Arterioles   Arteries   Capillaries
Lymphatic vessels   Veins   Venules

(a) Site of gas, nutrient, and waste exchange: _____

(b) Act as site of greatest resistance (and drop in blood pressure): _____

(c) Have thick, muscular walls that can withstand a high level of blood pressure: _____

(d) Connect capillaries with veins: _____

(e) Thin-walled, distensible vessels; most have valves to prevent backflow: _____

(f) These vessels return blood to the heart; they contain the lowest pressure, normally between 10 and 0 mm Hg: _____

(g) Carry fats absorbed from intestines toward major veins in the neck: _____

(h) Collectively known as microcirculation (three answers):

_____, _____, _____

D5. Identify the two locations on the body where all lymph fluid flows into blood plasma.

_____

_____

D6. Six years ago, Mrs. Reese had a right mastectomy in which 10 axillary lymph nodes were removed. She has since experienced several infections related to *Staphylococcus aureus* that were serious enough to require hospitalization. Her right arm is constantly swollen to about three times the size of her left arm. Explain.

_____

_____

_____

D7. Select from this list of terms the answer that best fits each of the following descriptions:

Fenestrations   Lymphatic vessels
Metarterioles   Nutrient flow
Non-nutrient flow   Precapillary sphincters

(a) Control blood flow into arterial ends of capillaries: _____

(b) Capillaries that involve exchange of gases and nutrients between blood and tissues: _____

(c) Vessels that link arterioles with capillaries: _____

(d) Remove fluid from interstitial spaces, as well as proteins and other particles that are too large to pass through capillary walls: _____

D8. Hyperemia refers to a(n) *(increase? decrease?)* in local blood flow. Blood flow to Ruth's arm is reduced by application of pressure on the skin of her arm. Once the pressure is relieved, blood flow returns to her arm. This phenomenon is known as _____ hyperemia.

D9. Classify the following chemicals as *vasoconstrictors* or *vasodilators* that regulate local blood flow.

(a) Nitric oxide (NO) derived from endothelial lining of blood vessels: _____

(b) Endothelin-1 _____

(c) Histamine, bradykinin, and prostaglandin E_2 released during inflammation: _____

(d) Serotonin that is associated with migraine headaches: _____

(e) Norepinephrine released by sympathetic nerves to blood vessels in skin, kidneys, and gastrointestinal tract: _____

D10. Dr. Sewell is having surgery to repair her right femoral artery, which was injured by her fractured right femur. Explain how her right lower extremity receives a blood supply before and during the surgery when blood flow through the injured vessel is cut off.

_____

_____

E. AUTONOMIC NERVOUS SYSTEM CONTROL OF CIRCULATORY FUNCTION

E1. You have just studied chemicals that dilate or constrict blood vessels in attempts to increase or decrease blood flow through specific tissues or organs. Complete this exercise about the more widespread effects of autonomic nerves on the regulation of circulation.

(a) Control centers for circulation and blood pressure are located in the *(cerebellum? medulla? pons?)* of the brain. Name two types of receptors that provide information to this part of the brain about the need for changes in circulation, for example, during stress, exercise, or sleep. _____, _____

(b) The right and left vagus nerves contain most of the *(sympathetic? parasympathetic?)* nerve fibers in the body. Circle the major effect(s) of the vagus nerves:

(1) Increase heart rate (pulse)
(2) Decrease heart rate (pulse)
(3) Increase force of cardiac contraction
(4) Vasoconstriction of blood vessels in skin, gastrointestinal tract, and kidneys
(5) Vasodilation of blood vessels in skin, gastrointestinal tract, and kidneys

(c) Sympathetic nerves exit from the *(brainstem in cranial nerves? spinal cord segments T1-L2? spinal cord segments S2-S4?)*. Identify (from the list in Question E1[b]) the major effect(s) of sympathetic nerves: _____

E2. Match the chemicals that are associated with the autonomic nervous system (ANS) with the related descriptions that follow.

Acetylcholine   Dopamine
Epinephrine   Norepinephrine

(a) Neurotransmitter released by all parasympathetic neurons: _____

(b) Neurotransmitter released by sympathetic neurons that stimulate the heart or blood vessels: _____

(c) Hormone produced by the adrenal medulla that stimulates sympathetic neurons: _____

CHAPTER 17

Disorders of Blood Flow and Blood Pressure

■ Review Questions

A. BLOOD VESSEL STRUCTURE AND FUNCTION

A1. Describe blood vessel structure by filling in the blanks within each statement. Choose from these answers (tunica): *externa, intima,* and *media.*

(a) Large vessels such as arteries and veins consist of three layers. Arrange layers in correct sequence from outermost to innermost: tunica _____ → tunica _____ → tunica _____.

(b) Endothelial cells form most of the tunica _____; even the smallest vessels (capillaries) contain this layer. Smooth muscle cells and elastic fibers make up most of the tunica _____.

A2. Discuss the roles of endothelial cells by filling in the blanks.

(a) List four or more normal functions of endothelial cells. _____

_____

(b) List five or more factors that can lead to *endothelial dysfunction.* _____

_____

A3. Describe function and dysfunction of smooth muscle cells by circling correct answers and filling in the blanks.

(a) Smooth muscle cells of blood vessels are supplied by *(sympathetic? parasympathetic?)* nerves. Release of the neurotransmitter *(acetylcholine? norepinephrine?)* leads to contraction of smooth muscle and vaso*(constriction? dilatation?).*

(b) Smooth muscle cells can migrate to the tunica intima and proliferate there as part of the blood vessel disorder known as _____. List several factors that promote atherosclerosis.

_____

B. DISORDERS OF THE ARTERIAL CIRCULATION

B1. Circle the correct answers or fill in the blanks within each statement about lipoproteins.

(a) *(HDL? LDL? VLDL?)* is the main carrier of cholesterol that is released into the bloodstream and settles in blood vessels. For this reason, these lipoproteins are called the *(good? bad?)* cholesterol. *(Low? High?)* blood levels of these lipoproteins are associated with atherosclerosis leading to heart disease. What does the abbreviation LDL stand for?

_____

(b) *(HDL? LDL? VLDL?)* consists of a relatively low concentration of cholesterol and a high level of phospholipids. These lipoproteins are called the *(good? bad?)* cholesterol because they transport cholesterol away from plaque lining the blood vessels and back to the liver for excretion. *(Low? High?)* blood levels tend to help prevent heart disease. Smoking and metabolic syndrome both tend to *(increase? decrease?)* HDLs.

(c) Which lipoproteins transport most triglycerides that are made in the body? _____

(d) The human body *(can? cannot?)* convert VLDLs into LDLs.

(e) The proteins that make up part of lipoproteins are known as _____ proteins. Explain their importance.

_____

B2. Choose the two true statements about high cholesterol. (Pay particular attention to whether the **bold-faced** word or phrase makes the statement true or false.)

(a) High blood cholesterol levels caused by complications of diabetes or obesity are examples of **primary** hypercholesterolemia.

(b) High-calorie diets, even if not high in fats, **do** increase LDL levels.

(c) Excessive dietary intake of triglycerides, cholesterol, and other saturated fats **suppresses** LDL receptor numbers or function.

(d) The National Cholesterol Education Program (NCEP) targets **triglycerides** as the primary target for lowering cholesterol.

B3. Answer the following questions about Amy, age 35, whose mother (but not father) has familial hypercholesterolemia (type 2A).

(a) Because this is an autosomal *(dominant? recessive?)* genetic disorder and one of her parents has the defective gene, Amy *(can? cannot?)* inherit this disorder. In fact, she has a *(0? 25? 50? 100?)%* chance of having this disorder. The incidence of this disorder is about ___ persons per 1,000.

(b) Amy's total cholesterol level is 298 mg/dL with an LDL of 170 mL/dL. These values are *(high? normal?)*. Her LDL level is related to the *(high? low?)* level of effective LDL receptors on her cells.

(c) Amy's physical examination by her cholesterol specialist includes palpation of her Achilles tendons. Explain why.

_____

_____

(d) The nutritionist suggests that Amy's management of her cholesterol disorder should include:

(d1) *(Increased? Decreased?)* exercise, which is likely to *(increase? decrease?)* her HDLs above her current level of 45 mg/dL.

(d2) Increased intake of foods such as

_____.

(d3) Decreased dietary intake of

_____ and _____, especially *(saturated? unsaturated?)* fats.

(e) Amy has a lipid-lowering medication prescribed. Match types of drugs with descriptions below. Select from these answers.

Ezetimibe   Fibric acid derivatives
Nicotinic acid   Statins

(e1) The cornerstone of LDL cholesterol-lowering drugs, these block synthesis of cholesterol in the liver; these

medications also decrease triglyceride levels: _____

(e2) Inhibits cholesterol absorption from foods: _____

B4. Sean is a 21-year-old whose mother died of a heart attack at age 42. Sean smokes two packs of cigarettes a day; has a cheeseburger, chips, and a shake for lunch and dinner almost daily; and has not exercised in a year. His cholesterol is 248 mg/dL and his blood pressure is 134/84 mm Hg.

(a) Identify Sean's risk factors for coronary heart disease that *can* be modified by change in his health behaviors.

_____

_____

_____

(b) Identify Sean's risk factors that are *not* modifiable.

_____

_____

(c) Which is Sean's strongest risk factor for atherosclerosis?

_____

(d) Is it likely that Sean's blood vessels would demonstrate any atherosclerotic changes at his current age?

_____

B5. Circle the correct answers or fill in the blanks within each statement about additional risk factors for atherosclerosis.

(a) Homocysteine is associated with *(increased? decreased?)* risk of blood clots as well as damage to the lining of _____. This chemical is derived from *(meats? vegetables?)*. Plasma levels of homocysteine may be lowered by intake of

_____

(b) CRP (or _____ _____ protein) is a sign of inflammation that may damage blood vessels and set the stage for atherosclerosis.

(c) Name several microbes that may be associated with atherosclerosis.

_____

_____

B6. Refer to Figure 17-8 in *Essentials of Pathophysiology* and list in sequence these events that appear to contribute to the development of atherosclerosis. (Arrange the letters in the spaces that follow.)

(A) Platelets adhere to injured, exposed areas of the vessel; platelets release growth factors

(B) Smooth muscle in vessel walls proliferates under the influence of growth factors

(C) Lipids released from foam cells accumulate to form the core of an atherosclerotic plaque covered by a cap of connective tissue and smooth muscle

(D) Damage to endothelium, for example, by smoking and/or mechanical stress of hypertension, with recruitment of inflammatory cells

(E) Formation of foam cells as macrophages in blood vessel walls ingest and oxidize excessive lipids and become foam cells; vessel lining is left with exposed areas

(F) The lesion encroaches upon the lumen, gradually narrowing the lumen of the vessel and reducing blood flow

____ → ____ → ____ →
____ → ____ → ____

B7. Match these possible effects of atherosclerosis with the related description:

Infarction   Ischemia
Occlusion   Thrombosis

(a) Thrombi that catch on damaged endothelium may lead to clot formation (_____), which is the most important complication of atherosclerosis.

(b) Reduction in diameter of the lumen of a blood vessel is known as _____.

(c) Reduction of blood flow to tissues is a condition known as _____.

(d) Death of tissue or organ due to inadequate blood flow is known as _____.

B8. The term *vasculitides* is plural for blood vessel inflammation and necrosis, or _____. Select from this list of etiologic categories the one that best matches each example of vasculitis:

Direct injury   Infectious agent
Immune process   Physical agent
Secondary to other disease

(a) One manifestation of Genevieve's lupus (SLE) is skin sensitivity to sunlight; she has a characteristic "butterfly rash" on her face: _____

(b) Peter has hives (urticaria), which is a group III hypersensitivity vasculitis: _____

(c) Ms. Alvino developed frostbite on toes of both feet after she was stranded in a snowstorm: _____

B9. Match the condition with the related description of patients seen by an emergency room nurse.

Acute arterial occlusion
Atherosclerotic occlusive disease
Giant cell temporal arteritis
Polyarteritis nodosa
Raynaud phenomenon
Thromboangiitis obliterans

(a) Anna-Maria, age 30, came to the ER after a hand injury in a restaurant kitchen where she works. Anna-Maria states her concern about recent episodes in which fingers of both hands developed numbness and tingling. At first pale, her fingers then turned deep red and began to throb. These attacks occurred especially when she was anxious and working in the "cold room" of the kitchen: _____

(b) Mr. Knight, age 60, presents with acute pain and paresthesia (numbness and tingling) in his left leg; the leg is pale and cool. He has a left femoral pulse, but left popliteal and dorsalis pedis pulses are absent. Mrs. Knight reports that her husband has a history of atrial fibrillation (with resulting stasis of blood in the left atrium that increases risk of embolus formation): _____

(c) Gilbert Scanlon, age 68, has a history of two strokes. Today, his BP is 180/106. His skin manifests a bluish mottling and he reports numbness. His serum creatinine level of 4.8 mg/dL indicates about 25% of normal kidney function. He is treated with steroids: _____

(d) Jack Whitehead, age 38, is a chain-smoker. Skin on his hands and feet appears thin and shiny with noticeable ulcer formation on his right foot. He has bilateral leg pain when he walks. (*Hint:* his condition is also known as Buerger disease.)

_____

(e) Mrs. Sonneborn, age 70, presents with severe pain and tenderness at her right temple and blurred vision. Her diagnostic testing included a biopsy of her right temporal artery: _____

(f) Mr. Vonnahme, age 74, was diagnosed with type 2 diabetes mellitus 10 years ago. All pulses in his lower extremities are diminished and bruits are noted over his femoral arteries. He reports calf pain "whenever I walk even out the driveway to the mailbox." With his feet on the floor, his legs appear red (dependent rubor); when his legs are raised above heart level they develop pallor. (*Hint:* this condition is also called arteriosclerosis obliterans.)

_____

B10. Name the four conditions listed in Question B9 that are called peripheral vascular diseases because they primarily affect circulation in the extremities.

_____, _____,

_____, _____

B11. Which patients in Question B9 have signs of intermittent claudication?

_____

B12. Explain why cigarette smoking is contraindicated for clients with arterial disease.

_____

_____

B13. Circle the three true statements about aneurysms. (Pay particular attention to whether the **bold-faced** word or phrase makes the statement true or false.)

(a) Most aneurysms involve abnormal **narrowing** of blood vessels.

(b) Abdominal aortic aneurysms (AAAs) are **more** common than thoracic aortic aneurysms.

(c) The greatest risk with AAAs is **rupture** of the aneurysm.

(d) Berry aneurysms most commonly occur in arteries that supply the **legs.**

(e) Atherosclerosis, hypertension, and congenital defects are **all** factors that can cause aneurysms.

(f) Clot formation is **less** likely to occur in aneurysms than in vessels with normal diameter.

B14. Mr. Fey experiences an intense, ripping pain, "like a sword slashed down my back." Within an hour, he faints (syncope), has pallor and poor capillary refill, and within 4 hours he dies. Mr. Fey had a history of hypertension. On autopsy, the site of the primary tear of Mr. Fey's aneurysm was located in the ascending aorta; the tear extended to 8 cm below the point where the aorta pierces the diaphragm. What type of aneurysm did Mr. Fey most likely experience?

_____

C. DISORDERS OF ARTERIAL BLOOD PRESSURE

C1. Choose the two true statements about blood pressure (BP). (Pay particular attention to whether the **bold-faced** word or phrase makes the statement true or false.)

(a) Systolic pressure occurs when the heart is **contracting.**

(b) Diastolic BP is **higher** than systolic BP.

(c) Mean arterial pressure (MAP) is a **good** indicator of tissue perfusion.

(d) Pulse pressure (MAP) is normally about **80** mm Hg.

C2. Refer to Figure 17-1 of the Study Guide. Name the two major factors that determine arterial blood pressure: _____ and _____. List three or more factors that contribute to development of PVR (peripheral vascular resistance).

_____

_____

_____

C3. As you progress through this chapter, fill in the blanks and complete the arrows in Figure 17-1 of the Study Guide to show how nervous, hormonal, and other factors increase blood pressure.

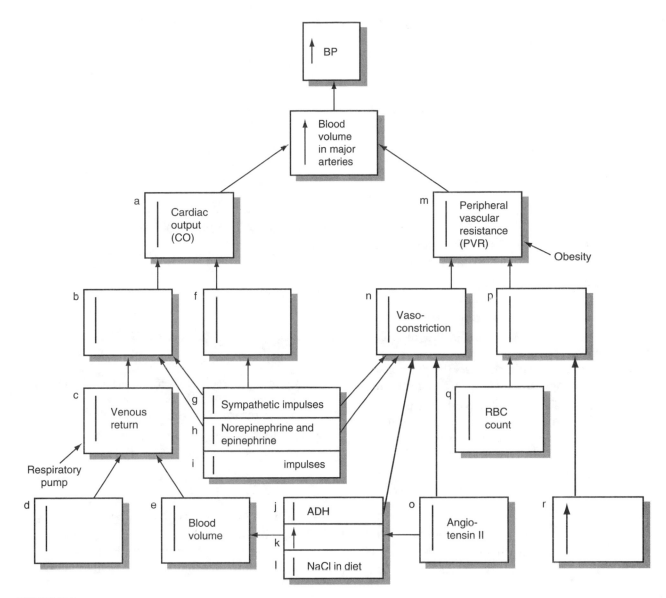

FIGURE 17-1

C4. Answer the following questions about blood pressure (BP).

(a) Circle the factors that are likely to increase diastolic BP.

(1) Vasoconstriction of small arteries and arterioles

(2) Sympathetic nerve impulses

(b) Most of the peripheral vascular resistance (PVR) that controls BP is built up in:

(1) Arterioles and small arteries

(2) Venules

(3) Capillaries

(c) Pulse pressure is likely to increase with:

(1) A rise in systolic BP

(2) Decreased diastolic BP

(3) Aortic valve regurgitation

C5. Classify the following factors as those involved in *L* (long-term) or *S* (short-term) regulation of BP and blood flow through tissues.

(a) Dr. Lang, age 83, has chronic hypertension. Her kidneys sense the high BP and attempt to lower it by eliminating more water (diuresis) and sodium (natriuresis) in urine: _____

(b) As Mrs. Lister stands up quickly, blood accumulates in her lower body. Baroceptors in her neck sense low BP there and signal the brainstem to raise her BP: _____

(c) During Juliet's 10-K run, lactic acid and other products of muscle metabolism build up in her legs: _____

(d) Release of aldosterone from Mr. Nunez's adrenal cortex causes his kidneys to retain sodium and water: _____

C6. The RAA (renin-angiotensin-aldosterone) mechanism *(increases? decreases?)* BP.

Fill in the blanks to arrange the following RAA events in correct sequence from first to last:

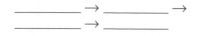

(a) The angiotensin-converting enzyme (ACE) made by the lungs converts angiotensin I to angiotensin II.

(b) The enzyme renin converts the plasma protein angiotensinogen into angiotensin I.

(c) Angiotensin II exerts two effects that raise BP: it stimulates aldosterone production and it increases peripheral vascular resistance (PVR) by vasoconstricting arterioles in skin, GI tract, and kidneys.

(d) Renin is released from kidneys in response to low BP in renal vessels.

C7. Classify the following chemicals as *constrictors* or *dilators* that regulate blood flow.

(a) ADH (vasopressin) released from the posterior pituitary: _____

(b) Angiotensin II (part of the renin-angiotensin-aldosterone mechanism): _____

(c) Epinephrine and norepinephrine: _____

C8. Compare and contrast chemoreceptors with baroreceptors.

_____

_____

_____

C9. Circle the correct answers or fill in the blanks to answer the following questions about Mrs. Lister's (Question C5[b]) sudden drop of BP when she stands up.

(a) If baroreceptors sense decreased BP, they send impulses to Mrs. Lister's *(cerebellum?*

cerebrum? medulla?), where neurons in her *(vasomotor? cardioinhibitory?)* center will initiate *(sympathetic? parasympathetic?)* impulses. These will then *(elevate? lower?)* her blood pressure by two mechanisms. Name them.

_____

_____

(b) If Mrs. Lister's BP-regulating reflexes do not respond quickly, she may become dizzy and fall as a result of _____ hypotension.

D. ESSENTIAL HYPERTENSION

D1. Circle the factor that carries a higher risk for hypertension.

(a) Being a 25-year-old *(woman? man?)*

(b) Being a *(35? 55?)*-year-old woman

(c) *(Higher? Lower?)* socioeconomic group

(d) *(African? European?)* American ancestry

D2. Circle the correct answers about Mrs. Shaw, age 58, who weighs 240 lb. Her blood pressure (BP) is recorded as 162/102 mm Hg.

(a) Mrs. Shaw's BP is categorized as:
  (1) High-normal
  (2) Prehypertensive
  (3) Stage 1 hypertensive
  (4) Stage 2 hypertensive

(b) The National Heart, Lung, and Blood Institute describes an ideal BP for adults age 18 and older as less than _____ mm Hg:
  (1) 160/100
  (2) 140/90
  (3) 130/85
  (4) 120/80

D3. Essential hypertension is chronic high blood pressure with *(a single? no?)* known cause. However, all forms of hypertension do involve a(n) *(increase? decrease?)* in cardiac output and/or a(n) *(increase? decrease?)* in peripheral vascular resistance (as shown in Study Guide Figure 17-1). Hypertension is also likely to involve an increase in *(sympathetic? parasympathetic?)* activity and a(n) *(increase? decrease?)* in the RAA mechanism, which results in sodium and water *(elimination? retention?)*.

D4. Circle the factors that have been shown to increase risk of high BP.

(a) "Pear" shape (fat in hips and thighs) rather than "apple" shape (fat in abdomen)

(b) Obesity

(c) Snacks of fruits or vegetables rather than chips or ice cream

(d) Cessation of use of oral contraceptives

(e) Family history of hypertension

(f) Physical inactivity

(g) Low stress level

(h) No alcohol intake

(i) Sleep apnea

D5. Answer the following questions about hypertension.

(a) Persons in early stages of hypertension are likely to have *(many? no?)* signs or symptoms.

(b) List organs that are usually "target organs" of chronic hypertension.

_____

(c) Risk of strokes is greater with *(systolic? diastolic?)* hypertension.

(d) The left ventricle must *(increase? decrease?)* its force when pumping into systemic vessels with hypertension. Explain how this change can lead to myocardial ischemia and heart attack and/or heart failure.

_____

_____

(e) Can hypertensive therapy reduce such left ventricular hypertrophy (LVH)?

_____

(f) Explain how the effects of high blood pressure on kidneys can exacerbate hypertension.

_____

_____

D6. Answer the following questions about Mrs. Shaw (Question D2), who has her blood pressure taken by the clinic nurse.

(a) The circumference of Mrs. Shaw's arm is 12". The width of the BP cuff should be at least:

(1) 3"

(2) 4.8"

(3) 7.2"

(4) 9.6"

If the cuff is too small for her arm, BP is likely to be *(over? under?)* estimated.

(b) Mrs. Shaw's diagnosis of stage 2 hypertension should be based on her BP of 162/102 recorded:

(1) In one measurement of BP

(2) In two or more measurements of BP during one clinic appointment

(3) In two or more measurements of BP during two or more appointments after her initial screening visit

D7. Mr. Lanter tries to adopt a lifestyle that will reduce his stage 1 hypertension. Answer the following questions related to his case.

(a) Mr. Lanter considers eating a soup with a label that lists 1,200 mg of sodium per serving. This serving would account for *(2%? 20%?)* of a sodium intake that he tries to limit to 6 g/day.

(b) Reduction of *(saturated? unsaturated?)* fats is recommended for cardiovascular health.

(c) Mr. Lanter would like to drink two 6-oz glasses of wine at dinner. This *(does? does not?)* exceed the daily limit recommended by the JNC-VI report.

(d) Which form of exercise would be more beneficial for Mr. Lanter? *(Brisk walk? Weight-lifting?)*

D8. Select the antihypertensive medication that fits each description by selecting from the list and filling in the blanks with your answers.

Angiotensin-converting enzyme inhibitors (or ACE-Is)
α_1-Receptor antagonists β-Blockers
Central adrenergic blockers   Diuretics
Calcium channel blockers

(a) Directly inhibit sympathetic nerves:

_____

(b) Dilators that decrease peripheral vascular resistance and workload of the heart:

_____ _____

(c) Selectively affect the heart, decreasing its rate and contractility: _____

(d) Directly reduce blood volume and cardiac output: _____

(e) Interfere with conversion of angiotensin I to angiotensin II: _____

D9. Mr. Lanter (Question D7) is still hypertensive after 4 months of attempts at lifestyle changes. Circle the correct answers or fill in the blanks to answer the following questions about him.

(a) Mr. Lanter's BP is currently 148/92. His essential hypertension is classified by JNC-VI guidelines as:

(1) Systolic

(2) Diastolic

(3) Systolic/diastolic

(b) Mr. Lanter's pulse pressure is ____ mm Hg. Typical of systolic hypertension, his pulse pressure is *(greater? less?)* than normal. Describe several effects of such a "widened pulse pressure."

_____

_____

_____

(c) Mr. Lanter is likely to be started on a *(low? high?)* dosage of medication and to build up *(rapidly? step-wise?)*. His compliance is likely to be greater with a prescription for *(one? three?)* dose(s) per day.

E. SECONDARY HYPERTENSION

E1. Choose the two true statements about secondary hypertension. (Pay particular attention to whether the **bold-faced** word or phrase makes the statement true or false.)

(a) **Almost all** hypertension is of this type.

(b) Many of the conditions causing secondary hypertension **can** be cured or corrected.

(c) Secondary hypertension is **rarely** seen in persons under age 30.

(d) A common cause of secondary hypertension is **kidney** disease.

E2. Answer the following questions about several types of secondary hypertension.

(a) Define renovascular hypertension.

_____

(b) Reduced renal flow associated with hypertension can initiate release of _____ from kidneys. This chemical

triggers the renin-angiotensin-aldosterone (RAA) mechanism, which further increases BP. Angiotensin II is a powerful vaso*(constrictor? dilator?)* that increases PVR. Angiotensin II also stimulates release of the hormone _____ that causes kidneys to *(eliminate? retain?)* Na$^+$ and H$_2$O. Aldosterone also leads to *(hyper? hypo?)*kalemia.

(c) Besides the RAA mechanism, aldosterone levels can be increased by:

(1) Addison disease

(2) Primary hyperaldosteronism

(3) Cushing disease

(d) Epinephrine and norepinephrine are the two major hormones produced by the adrenal *(cortex? medulla?)*. These chemicals are classified as _____. A tumor of cells that make these hormones is known as a _____oma. These tumors can also arise in *(sympathetic? parasympathetic?)* ganglia, sites of nerve cells that release catecholamines. The most common symptom is _____. Circle other signs of this type of tumor:

(1) Decreased sweat

(2) Palpitations

(3) Pallor

(4) Weight gain

(e) Coarctation of the aorta is a *(dilation? narrowing?)* of the vessel. Affected persons are likely to have high BP in the *(arms? legs?)*.

E3. Choose the two true statements about malignant hypertension. (Pay particular attention to whether the **bold-faced** word or phrase makes the statement true or false.)

(a) Malignant hypertension is caused by chemicals released by **cancer** cells.

(b) For a diagnosis of this type of hypertension, diastolic pressure must be greater than **160** mm Hg.

(c) Associated spasms of cerebral vessels can lead to **encephalopathy.**

(d) **Papilledema** is assessed by observation of the optic nerve for swelling.

(e) Malignant hypertension can usually be treated **gradually at home.**

E4. Circle the three true statements about hypertension in pregnancy. (Pay particular attention to whether the **bold-faced** word or phrase makes the statement true or false.)

(a) Incidence of hypertension in pregnancy is **greater** among African American women than among white women.

(b) Incidence of hypertension in pregnancy is **greater** among younger mothers than among older mothers.

(c) Persistent headache and visual problems **are** signs of preeclampsia/eclampsia.

(d) **Decreased** liver enzymes such as ALT and AST are signs of preeclampsia/eclampsia.

(e) Pregnancy-induced hypertension is thought to involve **decreased** placental blood flow and release of toxic chemicals that alter endothelial cells lining blood vessels.

E5. Circle the correct answer and then explain: Edema *(never? sometimes? always?)* accompanies pregnancy-induced hypertension (PIH) or preeclampsia.

_____

_____

E6. Circle the factors that increase risk for preeclampsia.

(a) Single (rather than multiple) fetuses

(b) Women with a history of chronic hypertension

(c) Presence of a hydatidiform mole (cystic, pathologic ovum)

(d) Diabetes mellitus

(e) Proteinuria early in pregnancy

E7. Describe the HELLP syndrome associated with high mortality pregnancy-induced hypertension.

_____

E8. Contrast preeclampsia with eclampsia.

_____

_____

E9. Identify the type of hypertension in each of the following pregnancies. Fill in the blanks using terms in the following list.

Chronic hypertension
Gestational hypertension
Preeclampsia-eclampsia

(a) A normal level of protein in a 24-hour urine is less than 300 mg. Faith's 24-hour urine protein level is 650 mg. Her BP at 24 weeks of gestation has elevated dramatically to 162/98 mm Hg. This is her first pregnancy: _____

(b) Betty Sue, 17, has no history of hypertension, but her BP now (at 24 weeks' gestation) is 142/84 mm Hg. Results of tests for protein in her urine are negative. If her BP returns to normal by about 3 months postpartum, this will confirm her diagnosis: _____

(c) Mrs. Swedeland, 39, has a history of stage 1 hypertension. Her BP actually decreased during her first trimester. Now at 30 weeks' gestation, her BP is 160/102 mm Hg: _____

E10. Circle the helpful interventions for PIH or preeclampsia.

(a) Avoidance of alcohol and tobacco use

(b) Bed rest

(c) Birth of the fetus

(d) ACE-inhibitors

(e) Dietary salt restriction

F. HYPERTENSION IN CHILDREN AND THE ELDERLY

F1. Circle the correct answers within each statement.

(a) That Donnie's parents both are hypertensive places Donnie at *(higher? lower?)* risk for high BP.

(b) In infancy or early childhood, hypertension is more likely to be *(essential? secondary?)*, with the most common cause being *(coarctation of the aorta? kidney disorders?)*.

(c) At age 3, Donnie is in the 95th percentile for height and his BP is over 113/67 mm Hg on three occasions. This indicates that his BP is in the *(25th? 75th? 95th?)* percentile for his age, which classifies his BP as *(normal? high normal? stage 1 hypertensive? stage 2 hypertensive?)*. Donnie *(need not? should?)* be evaluated and treated.

F2. List three factors that can cause adolescents to develop high blood pressure.

_____

_____

F3. Circle the two true statements. (Pay particular attention to whether the **bold-faced** word or phrase makes the statement true or false.)

(a) Prevalence of hypertension among older adults is about **25%** for persons in their sixties and **35%** for those 70 years and older.

(b) In the most common type of hypertension among elderly, **diastolic but not systolic** BP is elevated.

(c) With aging, baroreceptor sensitivity is likely to **decrease.**

(d) With aging, walls of the aorta and other large arteries are likely to become **stiffer.**

F4. List several factors that can help ensure accurate measurement of BP in the elderly.

_____

_____

F5. Briefly describe guidelines for treatment of hypertension in the elderly.

_____

_____

G. ORTHOSTATIC HYPOTENSION

G1. Answer the following questions about the mechanism that normally regulates BP when a person stands up.

(a) On standing, blood shifts to _(upper? lower?)_ parts of the body. As a result, BP _(increases? decreases?)_ in the upper body.

(b) State the normal locations of baroreceptors: _____ and _____. When these sense a drop in BP, the following responses are typically initiated: an _(increase? decrease?)_ in heart rate and vaso_____. Contraction of leg muscles to support the standing position also _(increase? decrease?)_ venous return (review Study Guide Figure 17-1).

G2. Define orthostatic hypotension.

_____

Answer the following questions about factors that can lead to orthostatic hypotension.

(a) List several mechanisms by which circulating blood volume might be reduced.

_____

_____

(b) List examples of medications that can lead to orthostatic hypotension.

_____

(c) Explain how diabetes or stroke can contribute to orthostatic hypotension.

_____

G3. Gladys, age 85, has been in bed with a severe respiratory infection for most of the past 4 days. Today Gladys has gotten out of bed three times. Each time she feels weak and dizzy just after she stands up. Answer the following questions about her.

(a) Explain the probable causes of her dizziness.

_____

_____

_____

(b) List several interventions that can help reduce risk of falls for Gladys.

_____

_____

H. DISORDERS OF THE VENOUS CIRCULATION

H1. List two factors that normally assist veins with the job of returning blood from the lower extremities to the heart.

_____

_____

H2. Answer the following questions about three types of veins in the lower extremities.

(a) List the three types of veins in the lower extremities, from most superficial to deepest.

_____

(b) Explain how blood in deep veins is normally prevented from moving to superficial ones when calf muscles contract.

_____

_____

CHAPTER 17 ■ **Disorders of Blood Flow and Blood Pressure** 109

(c) More than 80% of blood normally flows through _____ veins. When deep veins are blocked, blood is forced out into superficial veins, leading to *(primary? secondary?)* varicose veins. The most common cause of this type of varicose veins is DVT (_____ _____ _____).

H3. Circle all the factors that are likely to increase risk of varicose veins.

Male gender   Pregnancy
Obesity   Age over 50 years
A family history of   Working in a job
     varicose veins   that involves long-term standing or heavy lifting

H4. *(Deep? Superficial?)* veins are more likely to become varicose. Circle the correct answer and explain why.

_____

_____

H5. List several behaviors that can help prevent the harmful effects of varicose veins.

_____

_____

H6. Circle the correct answers within each statement.

(a) The saphenous vein is a *(deep? superficial?)* vein in the *(upper? lower?)* extremity.

(b) Edema is a major sign of chronic *(arterial? venous?)* insufficiency, whereas ischemia is a major sign of chronic *(arterial? venous?)* insufficiency.

(c) A thrombus that is in the posterior tibial vein is more likely to pass directly to the *(liver? lung?)*.

H7. Match the vascular condition with the most likely signs and symptoms.

Chronic venous   Deep venous
     insufficiency   thrombosis
Peripheral arterial   Varicose veins
     disease

(a) Unsightly appearance, aching, and possibly edema that subsides when legs are elevated:

_____

(b) Ischemia: _____

(c) Often asymptomatic, but may manifest pain, swelling, and other signs of inflammation, such as fever, malaise, and high white blood cell count; may lead to pulmonary embolism:

_____

(d) Stasis dermatitis, edema, necrosis of subcutaneous tissue, skin atrophy, and possibly ulcers of tissues covering the inner ankle: _____

H8. The three major factors, first described by Virchow, that lead to venous thromboses are listed here. Identify which factor is involved in each of the following cases of thromboses.

Hypercoagulability   Vessel injury   Venous stasis

(a) Congestive heart failure or heart attack:

_____

(b) Pregnancy or limited mobility postpartum:

_____

(c) Hip surgery:

_____

(d) Indwelling venous catheter:

_____

(e) A smoker taking oral contraceptives:

_____

(f) Sitting on a plane ride from Boston to Los Angeles and drinking only one glass of water: _____

H9. Swelling, deep muscle tenderness, and pain (as in a positive Homans sign) *(always? often? never?)* accompany DVT. Name a serious potential outcome of a DVT. _____

H10. List several effective treatments for DVT.

_____

_____

_____

CHAPTER 18

Disorders of Cardiac Function

■ Review Questions

A. DISORDERS OF THE PERICARDIUM

A1. Fill in the blanks to answer the following questions about the pericardial cavity.

(a) The pericardial cavity is located between the _____ and the _____. (Choose from the following options.)

Fibrous pericardium   Myocardium
Parietal pericardium   Visceral pericardium

(b) State the major concern about pericardial disorders.

_____

_____

A2. Mrs. Barrett has pulsus paradoxus. Circle the correct answers or fill in the blank within each statement about her condition.

(a) During inspiration, lung volume normally *(increases? decreases?)* and pressure within lungs *(increases? decreases?)*, "inviting" increased venous return to the heart. As the right side of the heart fills and exerts pressure on the septum, the volume of the left side of the heart *(increases? decreases?)*. As a result, stroke volume normally *(increases? decreases?)* by about _____ mm Hg during inspiration.

(b) Mrs. Barrett's systolic blood pressure decreases by about 10 mm Hg during her inspiration. This alteration leads to *(more? less?)* than normal stroke volume during inspiration. This *(is? is not?)* an indicator of pulsus paradoxus, which can indicate cardiac tamponade. Explain.

_____

_____

A3. Select pericardial disorders that fit the following descriptions.
Acute pericarditis   Cardiac tamponade
Constrictive pericarditis   Pericardial effusions

(a) Scar tissue binding visceral and parietal layers of the pericardium that interferes with cardiac filling: _____

(b) Life-threatening condition in which the heart cannot fill adequately because it is compressed by excessive pericardial fluid:

_____

(c) Characterized by this triad of signs and symptoms: chest pain, "leathery" pericardial friction rub, and ECG changes:

_____

(d) Exudate within the pericardial cavity; especially dangerous if volume is large or when it accumulates rapidly:

_____

(e) Inflammation in which pericardial capillaries dilate and become more permeable: _____

A4. Choose the two answers in which a term is matched with a correct description. (Pay particular attention to whether the **bold-faced** word or phrase makes the description correct or incorrect.)

(a) Pain due to acute pericarditis is best described as a **suffocating pressure.**

(b) A **purulent** exudate is one that contains "**pus**" (consisting of WBCs and microbes).

(c) Constrictive pericarditis **can** occur from pericardial effusions that lead to pericardial scarring.

(d) In cardiac tamponade, excessive fluid **expands the chambers of the heart.**

(e) Pericardiocentesis refers to **excessive fluid in the pericardial cavity.**

B. CORONARY HEART DISEASE

B1. Circle the correct answer within each statement.

(a) The circumflex artery is a branch of the *(left? right?)* coronary artery.

(b) In most persons, the posterior portion of the interventricular septum is supplied with blood by the *(right? left?)* coronary artery.

(c) There are anastomoses between the *(large? small?)* branches of coronary arteries.

B2. Identify which of the major categories of factors controlling coronary blood flow are used in descriptions below.

Metabolic   Neural   Endothelial   Physical chemicals

(a) Sympathetic nerves supplying smooth muscle of coronary arteries: _____

(b) Left ventricular contractions that determine blood pressure of the aorta:

_____

(c) Adenosine and other dilator chemicals produced by working myocardial cells:

_____

(d) Nitric oxide and endothelins produced by cells lining coronaries; serve as vasodilators and anticoagulants: _____

B3. Circle the correct answers within each statement.

(a) Coronary heart disease (CHD) *(is? is not?)* closely associated with atherosclerosis.

(b) Atherosclerotic lesions occur most often in *(proximal? distal?)* areas of coronary arteries.

(c) *(Stable? Unstable?)* "fixed" atherosclerotic plaque narrows blood vessels and leads to occlusion and chronic *(stable? unstable?)* angina.

(d) Unstable or "vulnerable" plaque can rupture, resulting in *(grayish-white? red?)* thrombus formation and *(stable? unstable?)* angina and myocardial infarction.

B4. Mr. Adilifu has a pulse of 160 beats/minute and a blood pressure of 120/50 mm Hg. As a result, his coronary artery perfusion (blood supply) is likely to be *(higher? lower?)* than normal. Explain.

_____
_____
_____

B5. Answer the following questions about chronic ischemic heart disease.

(a) Define ischemia.

_____

(b) Clot (thrombus) formation is one of the three main mechanisms by which chronic cardiac ischemia is likely to occur. List the other two.

_____
_____

(c) List several reasons why Mrs. Caruso, who has normal coronary blood flow, may have inadequate coronary perfusion to meet the needs of her heart muscle.

_____
_____
_____

B6. Mr. Clark, age 66, moderately overweight, and a two-pack-a-day smoker, reports to Dr. Sewell that over the past month he has been having "bouts of pain in my chest whenever I walk up to the top floor (two flights) to go to bed, but the pain stops just about as soon as I stop." He also reports, "I never have pain at rest, and the pain episodes have not gotten worse over the past month." Answer the following questions related to his case.

(a) Mr. Clark's symptoms suggest *(chronic ischemic heart disease? acute coronary syndrome with possible infarction)*. Which of these two conditions is likely to occur earlier in the progression of heart disease?

_____

(b) The consistency of Mr. Clark's chest pain on exercise suggests chronic *(stable? unstable?)* angina. Angina pectoris literally means _____. The pain is most likely *(sharp or stabbing? squeezing or suffocating chest pain?)*. Anginal pain *(never? sometimes?)* radiates.

(c) When Mr. Clark experiences angina, it is probably better that he *(sit? lie?)* down. Explain.

_____
_____

(d) List several interventions other than medications or surgery that may reduce Mr. Clark's frequency of angina.

_____
_____

(e) Dr. Sewell prescribes nitroglycerin pills. Mr. Clark is advised to *(swallow each pill? place the pill under his tongue but not swallow it?)*

(f) List other treatment methods for stable angina:

(f1) Medications

_____

(f2) Surgeries

_____

(g) Several months later, Mr. Clark experiences chest pain in bed at about midnight on a regular basis. This condition is most likely to be *(stable angina? variant angina? silent myocardial ischemia?)*. This condition is usually caused by *(thrombus formation? spasms?)* of coronary vessels. Which two classes of drugs listed in your answer to Question B6f(1) are most likely to reduce Mr. Clark's night pain?

_____

B7. Circle the correct answers or fill in the blanks to answer the following questions about myocardial ischemia and myocardial infarction (MI).

(a) Mrs. Holly, a diabetic, states that she "never exercises" and lives on the first floor of her house so does not need to "do steps." Over recent weeks, she has begun to experience angina for periods as long as a half hour as she sits and watches television at night. Her angina is classified as *(stable? unstable?)* angina.

(b) A coronary angiogram indicates that Mrs. Holly has significant coronary atherosclerosis, yet she states that she has "not had chest pain" until this month. Explain.

_____

_____

_____

(c) Mrs. Holly's unstable angina is probably caused by a *(fixed obstruction? disruption?)* of atherosclerotic plaque.

(d) Mr. Ravin has manifestations similar to those of Mrs. Holly except that he has elevated cardiac enzyme levels; an ECG reveals that his ST segment is not elevated. These findings indicate *(no? some?)* myocardial injury with a probable diagnosis of:

(1) Unstable angina

(2) Non–ST-segment elevation (non–Q-wave) MI (NSTEMI)

(3) ST-segment elevation (Q-wave) MI (STEMI)

(e) Arrange the diagnoses listed in Question B7(d) according to amount of myocardial damage likely, from most to least damage: ___, ___, ___

(f) Which diagnosis in Question B7(d) is commonly known as *heart attack* or *acute myocardial infarction* (AMI)? _____

(g) An AMI with ST-segment elevation is more serious if a Q wave is *(absent? present?)* as a(n) *(elevation? dip?)* in the ECG tracing. (*Hint:* Refer to Figure 18-8 in *Essentials of Pathophysiology*.)

B8. Serum cardiac markers are helpful in diagnosis of MIs because these chemicals, which are normally found in *(intact myocardial cells? blood serum?)*, are released as a result of damage or death of heart cells. The level of these "markers" in blood is *(directly? inversely?)* related to the extent of myocardial injury. Serum levels of most of these markers rise and then decline to almost normal levels within about 3 to 10 *(hours? days? weeks?)* of onset of the MI. Select markers from this list that fit the following descriptions:

Total creatine kinase (CK)   Myoglobin
Troponin

(a) A low molecular weight molecule, it is the first of these chemicals to be released post-MI: _____

(b) TnI and TnT; help regulate myocardial contractions; useful for diagnosing MIs in which CK-MB levels are too low to detect: _____

(c) Name an enzyme that helps provide ATP to cardiac cells: _____. Explain why assessment of MB isoenzyme is performed.

_____

B9. Choose the two true statements about myocardial infarctions (MIs). (Pay particular attention to whether the **bold-faced** word or phrase makes the statement true or false.)

(a) Variant (or Prinzmetal) angina is related to presence of **thrombi** and typically occurs during **maximal exercise** and at **mid-afternoon**.

(b) The onset of an MI is **abrupt** and typically involves **severe, crushing, often radiating pain.**

(c) Pain of an MI **is** typically relieved by nitroglycerin.

(d) Early hospitalization after onset of symptoms of an MI **does** reduce the risk of sudden death from the MI.

B10. Circle the manifestations that may accompany a heart attack that are due to sympathetic nerve activity:

(a) Nausea and vomiting

(b) Tachycardia and pale, cool, moist skin

B11. Circle the correct answers within each statement about heart attacks and manifestations.

(a) About *(5% to 10%? 10% to 20%? 30% to 50%? 70% to 80%?)* of persons with AMI die of ventricular fibrillation within the first few hours of symptoms. *(Subendocardial? Transmural?)* infarcts involve the full thickness of the myocardial wall and are *(ST-AMIs? non-ST-AMIs?)*. Which type of AMI is more common? *(Subendocardial? Transmural?)*

(b) Early reperfusion by thrombolytic therapy, within *(20? 60? 180?)* minutes of the onset of ischemia can prevent cell death. The reperfused and recovering area of myocardium is known as *(necrotic? stunned?)* myocardium. It *(will? may? will not?)* regain full function.

B12. Circle the correct answers or fill in the blanks to answer the following questions about treatment modalities for AMI patients.

(a) *(None? Some?)* of the interventions for MI is/are similar to those for angina (Question B6), such as nitroglycerin which *(vasoconstricts? vasodilates?)* both coronary arteries as well as veins to *(increase? decrease?)* workload of the heart.

(b) _____ should be administered by nasal prongs.

(c) Morphine is often given *(by mouth? intramuscularly? intravenously?)* for rapid pain and anxiety control that reduces workload of the heart.

(d) AMI patients *(should? should not?)* have ECG monitoring, and thrombolytic

therapy should be continued (see Question B11[b]).

(e) Fill in the blanks to complete the descriptions of other revascularization procedures.

(1) PTCA is an acronym for

_____, also known as a "_____ angioplasty," with or without stent (see Figure 18-10 in *Essentials of Pathophysiology*). PTCA with or without a stent is an example of a PCI or _____ _____ _____ , meaning interventions involving access to coronary arteries by an incision made through

_____ .

(2) Brachytherapy uses _____ within coronary arteries.

(3) CABG is an acronym for _____ _____ _____ _____ . Vessels used to reperfuse the heart usually include the _____ vein and/or the _____ artery. (See Figure 18-11 in *Essentials of Pathophysiology*.)

B13. Circle the correct answers or fill in the blanks within each statement about recovery after a myocardial infarction.

(a) Which portion of an infarcted heart is most severely damaged? *(Injured? Ischemic? Necrotic?)* myocardium

(b) Post-MI inflammation of the necrotic tissue along with newly formed granulation tissue leads to *(soft? scar?)* tissue within a *(day? week?)* after the MI. This soft tissue is at greater risk for _____ compared with healthy heart muscle. The inflammation also leads to *(hypothermia? fever?)* and *(increase? decrease?)* in white blood cell count and sedimentation rate.

(c) Necrotic myocardial tissue is usually completely replaced with scar tissue by 2 *(months? years?)* after the MI. This tissue *(is? is not?)* likely to conduct impulses and contract normally. The extent of damage determines heart function and can be detected by changes in the _____ . This scar tissue is at risk for a potentially fatal outpouching known as a ventricular _____ .

(d) A sharp chest pain within 1 day to several weeks after the MI may indicate the complication of (endo? peri?)carditis.

C. MYOCARDIAL AND ENDOCARDIAL DISEASE

C1. Differentiate myocarditis and cardiomyopathies from MI.

_____

_____

C2. Circle the two true statements about myocarditis. (Pay particular attention to whether the **bold-faced** word or phrase makes the statement true or false.)

(a) Myocarditis is most often caused by **viral infection.**

(b) ECG changes and elevated cardiac marker levels **are** used to diagnose myocarditis.

(c) Most cases of myocarditis are **fatal.**

(d) Treatment focuses on **active exercise** immediately after diagnosis.

C3. What is the major cause of primary cardiomyopathies? _____. Select the type of cardiomyopathy from this list that fits each related description below:

Dilated   Restrictive   Hypertrophic   Peripartum

(a) Ventricular muscle walls thicken and stiffen, resulting in decreased volume for diastolic filling; microscopic examination of heart muscle tissue indicates abnormal organization of muscle fibers: _____

(b) As shown in Figure 18-14 in _Essentials of Pathophysiology,_ this cardiomyopathy involves the greatest ventricular radius or diameter: _____

(c) Ventricle walls become rigid, limiting their filling and stroke volume; may involve amyloid infiltration; form of cardiomyopathy endemic to parts of Asia, Africa, and South America but uncommon in the United States: _____

(d) The most common cause of sudden death in young persons; idiopathic, but may be genetic: _____

(e) Occurring during pregnancy or in months following childbirth: _____

(f) Likely to involve dyspnea, decreased stroke volume and ejection fraction, and possibly heart failure: _____

C4. Circle the correct answers or fill in the blanks to complete this exercise about Lucy, age 16, who has infective endocarditis as a complication of a serious infection from _Staphylococcus aureus._ She has no known history of heart problems or IV drug abuse.

(a) Most cases of infective endocarditis are caused by (bacteria? fungi? viruses?). Most persons who develop this condition (do? do not?) have a history of previous valve disorders, valve replacement, or congenital heart defects. Because Lucy does not have such a history, she is likely to have (acute? subacute?) bacterial endocarditis.

(b) This condition requires two independent factors, which are a damaged _____ and a _____.

(c) Vegetative lesions on heart valves are composed of _____.

(d) Arrange in correct sequence (from first to last) the events likely to occur in the course of bacterial endocarditis:

(1) Initiation of immune responses to bacteria that can cause systemic injury

(2) Formation of vegetative lesions that damage heart valves

(3) Release of emboli containing microbes from free edges of valve surfaces

___ → ___ → ___

(e) Lucy's acute bacterial endocarditis (is? is not?) likely to be accompanied by a spiking fever and chills. List other signs and symptoms that Lucy is likely to have.

_____

_____

_____

(f) Name the most definitive diagnostic procedure for infective endocarditis.

_____

What technique can detect sites of vegetative lesions?

_____

C5. Circle the correct answers or fill in the blanks to complete this exercise about Antonio, age 9, who has been diagnosed with rheumatic fever (RF) almost a month after a "strep sore throat" with headache, swollen neck glands, and fever.

(a) RF follows a GAS infection, which refers to _____ A _____; it *(can? cannot?)* be prevented by antibiotics for streptococcal infections. This condition is more likely to occur in persons with *(poor? excellent?)* health care.

(b) This condition *(affects only heart valves? is systemic?)*. Circle the organs of the body other than the heart that are most likely to be affected:

Central nervous system   Joints
Kidneys   Liver   Skin

(c) Select the organ (from C5[b]) that fits the sign or symptom of RF:

  (c1) Erythema marginatum and subcutaneous nodules: _____

  (c2) Sydenham chorea: _____

  (c3) Polyarthritis that responds to aspirin therapy: _____

  (c4) Aschoff bodies, lesions that consist of necrosed tissue surrounded by immune cells: _____

(d) The manifestations described in C5(c) are likely to be *(permanent? temporary?)* effects of RF.

(e) If Antonio moves into a chronic phase of RF, it is likely to involve *(temporary? permanent?)* valve damage that occurs *(within the next month? decades?)* after the triggering event. Circle the valve that most often stenoses as a result: *(aortic? mitral? pulmonary? tricuspid?)*.

(f) If valve disease persists, Antonio should have prophylactic therapy with the antibiotic _____ before _____ (or other) procedures in which GAS bacteria might access Antonio's bloodstream.

D. VALVULAR HEART DISEASE

D1. Answer the following questions about heart valve disorders.

(a) Write two or more causes of heart valve disorders: _____

(b) State the major problem resulting from heart valve disorders.

_____

_____

(c) Stenosis is a problem with *(opening? closing?)* a valve, whereas regurgitation is a problem with *(opening? closing?)* the valve. Valve incompetence is an alternative term for valvular *(regurgitation? stenosis?)*.

(d) Explain how diseased valves produce heart murmurs.

_____

D2. Refer to Figure 18-18 in your text and identify the valve disorders that fit the related descriptions.

Aortic valve regurgitation
Aortic valve stenosis
Mitral valve prolapse
Mitral valve regurgitation
Mitral valve stenosis

(a) The left atrium enlarges as blood accumulates there and increases risk for mural (wall) clot and embolus formation; anticoagulation therapy is used:

_____

(b) Most likely to lead to dyspnea related to pulmonary congestion and edema and possible pulmonary hypertension and right-sided heart failure: _____

(c) Because the valve acts as a swinging door, blood sloshes back and forth between the left atrium and left ventricle; may result in no symptoms for decades but can eventually lead to left atrial overload and pulmonary congestion: _____

(d) Also known as floppy mitral valve syndrome; more common in women, and usually asymptomatic; avoidance of caffeine, alcohol, and tobacco can control symptoms that do occur:

_____

(e) The left ventricle hypertrophies as it works to pump out blood; this may lead to heart failure; slower pulse because left ventricular systole takes longer: _____

(f) Because coronary arteries perfuse during ventricular diastole, perfusion of these vessels decreases as diastolic pressure drops in this condition: _____

(g) Pulse pressure widens as diastolic pressure decreases when the aortic valve allows blood to flow back into the left ventricle during diastole; stroke volume and systolic pressure increase as the left ventricle pumps out that same blood repeatedly:

_____

D3. List several techniques used to diagnose valve disorders.

_____

_____

_____

_____

E. HEART DISEASE IN INFANTS AND CHILDREN

E1. Circle the correct answers or fill in the blank within each statement about normal and defective heart development.

(a) About *(4,000? 40,000?)* babies are born in the U.S. each year with congenital heart defects. Presence of congenital heart defects in parents or siblings *(does? does not?)* increase risk for such defects in a developing fetus.

(b) Most heart development occurs between the fourth and eighth *(weeks? months?)* of prenatal development. Most congenital heart defects develop *(during? after?)* this period of time.

(c) Endocardial cushions form *(AV? semilunar?)* valves as well as parts of the atrial and ventricular _____.

(d) The septum primum and septum secundum contribute to formation of the *(atrial? ventricular?)* septum in the fetus. An opening between these two septa that allows fetal blood to pass from right atrium directly to left atrium is known as the foramen _____.

E2. Select the structure in fetal circulation that fits each description.

Ductus arteriosus	Ductus venosus
Foramen ovale	Placenta
Umbilical arteries	Umbilical vein

(a) Carry/ies "blue" blood (high in CO_2, low in O_2) from fetal internal iliac arteries to placenta: _____

(b) Carries blood from umbilical vein to inferior vena cava: _____

(c) Two structures that allow fetal blood to bypass the deoxygenated lungs; normally close within days after birth:

_____ , _____

E3. A red blood cell (RBC) is in the fetal descending aorta. Arrange in correct sequence (from first to last) the structures that the RBC will pass through in the most direct route to the fetal brain. Use answers from the list in Question E2. (One structure will not be used.)

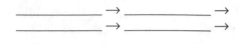

E4. Circle the correct answers or fill in the blank within each statement about fetal and postnatal circulation.

(a) Fetal PO_2 and O_2 saturation are typically *(higher? lower?)* in fetal life than postnatally.

(b) During fetal life, the lungs are filled with *(air? fluid?)* and are *(well oxygenated? hypoxic?)*. As a result, pulmonary vessels vaso*(constrict? dilate?)*, causing fetal lungs to present *(high? low?)* resistance to flow. For this reason, most blood in the fetal pulmonary artery flows into lower pressure *(lungs? ductus arteriosus?)*.

(c) At birth, the baby's first breath causes lung volume to *(increase? decrease?)* and pressure there to *(increase? decrease?)*. This *(raises? lowers?)* pulmonary resistance and *(increases? decreases?)* pulmonary blood flow, which contributes to closure of both the ductus arteriosus and the _____. Premature babies whose lungs do not inflate well are more likely to have these fetal structures *(close early? remain open?)*.

(d) List a second reason for decrease in pulmonary vascular resistance and pulmonary blood after birth:_____

_____

_____

E5. Circle the correct answers or fill in the blanks to answer the following questions about types of shunts resulting from congenital heart defects.

(a) Which type of shunt leads to right ventricular hypertrophy (RVH) with possible RV failure?

(1) Left-to-right shunt

(2) Right-to-left shunt

(b) Which type of congenital heart defect is classified as "with cyanosis"?

(1) Left-to-right shunt

(2) Right-to-left shunt
Explain your answer.

_____

(c) Describe how cyanosis can be assessed in infants.

_____

E6. Explain why infants with congenital heart defects are at risk for "failure to thrive."

_____

_____

_____

E7. Select the types of congenital heart defects listed here that fit the following descriptions.

Atrial septal defect
Coarctation of the aorta
Endocardial cushion defects
Patent ductus arteriosus
Pulmonary stenosis
Tetralogy of Fallot
Transposition of the great vessels
Ventricular septal defect

(a) Which of these defects lead to cyanosis ("blue babies")? _____

(b) This defect allows blood to flow from left atrium to right atrium, leading to right ventricular and pulmonary artery overload: _____

(c) Involves four defects: pulmonary stenosis, aortic shifting to the right, ventricular septal defect, and right ventricular hypertrophy; may require surgical creation of an aorta-to-pulmonary artery shunt to increase pulmonary blood flow:

_____

(d) Narrowing of the aorta, almost always distal to the ductus arteriosus; as a result, blood pressure is considerably higher in the brachial artery than in the femoral artery, leading to systemic hypertension:

_____

(e) The aorta and the pulmonary artery have their locations and roles "switched"; may be corrected by an "arterial switch" surgery: _____

(f) In this defect, some of the neonate's aortic blood flows back into the pulmonary artery, overloading the lungs, possibly causing left-sided failure; may be caused

by excessive prostaglandin production because these are vasodilators:

_____

(g) The most common congenital heart defect (20% to 30% of all congenital heart defects); symptoms depend on the size of the defect; large defects with severe left-to-right shunts can lead to pulmonary hypertension and pulmonary congestion; as pulmonary vascular resistance increases, a right-to-left shunt develops: _____

(h) Common heart defect in children with Down syndrome; likely to affect tricuspid or mitral valve: _____

(i) Because blood flow to lungs is limited, treatment may include use of prostaglandin E to maintain patency of the ductus arteriosus (two answers):

_____,

_____

E8. Describe causes and symptoms of "tet" spells in infants with tetralogy of Fallot.

_____

_____

_____

E9. Circle the correct answer or fill in the blank within each statement about Kawasaki disease.

(a) Kawasaki disease is a *(rare? common?)* form of acquired heart disease in young children.

(b) Kawasaki disease is an inflammation of the *(heart? blood vessels?)* that *(is? is not?)* thought to be of immune origin.

(c) This disorder affects *(only the cardiovascular system? many systems?)*. Its most important effect is on the

_____.

E10. Circle each of the following that is a sign or symptom of the *acute* phase of Kawasaki disease.

(a) Spiking a fever of 104°F over the course of 5 days

(b) Itchy skin rash

(c) Conjunctivitis with yellowish discharge

(d) Swollen, red palms and soles

(e) Red throat and strawberry tongue

(f) Peeling of skin on fingers and toes

CHAPTER 19

Heart Failure and Circulatory Shock

■ Review Questions

A. HEART FAILURE

A1. Review the concepts listed here by returning to Study Guide Chapter 16 (Questions C12–C15) and Chapter 17 (Questions C1–C4, D3, D8). See also factors that regulate cardiac output and peripheral vascular resistance in Study Guide Figure 17-1.

Cardiac output	Cardiac reserve
Stroke volume	Venous return
Frank-Starling mechanism	Afterload
End-diastolic volume (EDV) or preload	Ejection fraction Inotropic effects
Cardiac contractility	Peripheral vascular resistance (PVR)

A2. Complete this overview of heart failure by filling in the blanks about the two major categories of factors that lead to heart failure.

(a) Failure of the _____ as a pump. List several possible causes for heart failure in each subcategory:

(a1) Cardiac disorders such as

_____

(a2) Excessive workload of the heart related to _____

(b) Compensatory (_____) mechanisms in three subcategories:

(b1) Excess preload related to

_____

(b2) Excess afterload related to

_____

(b3) Cardiac contractility related to

_____

A3. Circle all adaptations (among your answers to Question A2[b]) that occur within minutes or hours (rather than weeks or months) of decreased output and may temporarily improve cardiac performance.

A4. Test your understanding of preload and afterload by circling the correct answers or filling in the blanks within each statement.

(a) Indicate whether end-diastolic volume (EDV) and preload are likely to *increase* or *decrease* in each case.

(a1) When venous return increases during active exercise: _____

(a2) When stroke volume is reduced, as in heart failure or aortic valve regurgitation: _____

(a3) With fluid retention, as in renal failure: _____

(b) Afterload increases when systemic vessels vaso*(constrict? dilate?)*, causing an increase in peripheral vascular resistance (PVR). Afterload also increases in *(hyper? hypo?)*tension and in aortic *(stenosis? regurgitation?)* because the heart must do more work if any of these factors are present.

(c) *Inotropic* refers to _____ of the heart. Circle all factors that have positive inotropic effects on the heart.

Digitalis	Epinephrine
Myocardial infarction or ischemia	Sympathetic nerve impulses
Vagus nerve impulses	

A5. Answer the following questions about alterations associated with heart failure.

(a) In heart failure, the heart is likely to be *(overstretched? not stretched adequately?)*, so that the diameter of the heart *(increases? decreases?)*. Contractility of the heart then *(increases? decreases?)* as actin and myosin filaments are *(better? inadequately?)* juxtaposed.

(b) Circle the factors that are likely to decrease in heart failure.

Afterload	Cardiac output
Ejection fraction	Ventricular wall
End-diastolic volume	tension
Stroke volume	Cardiac reserve

(c) Circle each of the following that is likely to be a compensatory mechanism that the body will carry out to try to "fix" heart failure.

   (1) Vasodilation

   (2) Increased sympathetic nerve impulses

   (3) Increased heart rate

   (4) Release of renin and aldosterone

   (5) Hypertrophy of the ventricular wall

   (6) Increased blood flow to kidneys

(d) Explain the pros and cons of an increase in sympathetic nerve impulses as a compensatory mechanism in persons with heart failure.

   (d1) Pros

   _____

   _____

   (d2) Cons

   _____

   _____

(e) Circle the correct answers or fill in the blanks within each statement about how the RAA (renin-angiotensin-aldosterone) mechanism affects heart failure.

   (e1) Angiotensin II is a powerful vaso *(constrictor? dilator?)*. One of its effects is to *(increase? decrease?)* renal perfusion, which *(increases? decreases?)* urine output and *(increases? decreases?)* blood volume. This *(improves? exacerbates?)* heart failure.

   (e2) Angiotensin II stimulates release of _____ from the adrenal *(medulla? cortex?)*. This hormone causes kidneys to retain _____ and _____.

   (e3) ADH serves as a vaso *(constrictor? dilator?)* and causes kidneys to *(retain? eliminate?)* H_2O.

   (e4) The combined effects of angiotensin II, aldosterone, and ADH cause a(n) *(increase? decrease?)* in preload and afterload.

   (e5) _____ is a class of hormone that increases urinary output of both Na^+ and H_2O and therefore *(mimics? opposes?)* ADH, angiotensin, and aldosterone. List three organs in which these chemicals are found.

   _____ _____ _____

(e6) Name three chemicals discussed in this exercise that lead to hypertrophy of the myocardium by stimulating growth of myocytes (see Question A2[b3]): _____ _____ _____

A6. Write *ICF* next to causes of heart failure that result from impaired cardiac function, and write *EWD* next to those related to excess work demands of the heart. (Refer to Question A2[a])

   (a) Excessive production of thyroid hormone: _____

   (b) IV fluid overload: _____

   (c) High blood pressure: _____

   (d) Tetralogy of Fallot: _____

   (e) Heart attack: _____

   (f) Valvular heart disease: _____

A7. Most forms of CHF are *(high? low?)* output. Give examples of causes of CHF in which output is normal but still inadequate for body needs.

   _____

   _____

   _____

A8. Circle the correct answers or fill in the blanks within each statement about systolic and diastolic heart failure.

   (a) Systolic failure is also known as *(backward? forward?)* failure in which the heart has a problem with *(ejection? filling?)*. As a result, ventricular wall tension *(increases? decreases?)* and end-diastolic volume *(increases? decreases?)*. Major symptoms are related to *(edema? ischemia?)*.

   (b) Diastolic failure is also known as *(backward? forward?)* failure in which the heart has an impaired *(ejection? filling?)*. Diastolic failure is often related to ventricular hypertrophy, in which the volume of ventricular chambers is diminished. Signs and symptoms all involve *(edema? ischemia?)*.

   (c) Write *D* for diastolic failure and *S* for systolic failure next to each disorder to indicate likely effects on the heart.

   (c1) Mitral stenosis: ____

   (c2) Hypertension: ____

(c3) Aortic valve regurgitation: _____

(c4) Tachycardia (e.g., during the stress of exercise of a diseased heart): _____

A9. Fill in the blanks with selections from this list to indicate manifestations of each type of CHF.

AA: Abdominal discomfort and anorexia
APE: Acute pulmonary edema
Asc: Ascites
DN: Dyspnea at night
F: Fatigue
HS: Hepatomegaly and splenomegaly
ICP-P: Increased capillary pressure in pulmonary capillaries
ICP-S: Increased capillary pressure in systemic capillaries
JVD: Jugular vein distention
SA: Swollen ankles
PSOB: Perceived shortness of breath

(a) Left-sided CHF: _____, _____, _____, _____, _____

(b) Right-sided CHF: _____, _____, _____, _____, _____, _____

A10. Define each of these terms and explain why they are frequent signs of CHF.

(a) Orthopnea

_____

_____

(b) Diaphoresis

_____

_____

(c) Cool, clammy skin

_____

_____

(d) Nocturia

_____

_____

(e) Cheyne-Stokes breathing

_____

_____

(f) Exertional dyspnea

_____

_____

A11. Indicate which type of heart failure each of the following conditions is more likely to cause. Write *R* for right-sided and *L* for left-sided.

(a) Aortic stenosis: _____

(b) AMI resulting from occlusion of the circumflex branch of the left coronary artery: _____

(c) Cor pulmonale secondary to chronic bronchitis related to 40 years of cigarette smoking: _____

(d) Congenital heart defect of pulmonary stenosis: _____

(e) Chronic systemic hypertension: _____

A12. Mrs. Griffin was diagnosed with left-sided heart failure 8 years ago related to decades of uncontrolled hypertension. She is in skilled nursing care on oxygen by nasal cannula 24 hours a day. Mrs. Griffin remains in bed or in a wheelchair because she has episodes of angina and dyspnea even at rest. Her weight has dropped from 160 lb to 93 lb over the past 2 years. Recently she had a "PEG" (percutaneous esophageal gastrostomy) feeding tube inserted. Circle the correct answer or fill in the blanks within each statement related to her case.

(a) Mrs. Griffin's condition is categorized as Class *(I? II? III? IV?)* heart failure according to the New York Heart Association Functional Classification.

(b) Explain how her weight loss is related to heart failure.

_____

_____

(c) Explain what a sudden gain of 2 lb may mean.

_____

_____

(d) She manifests signs of both left-sided and right-sided heart failure. Explain.

_____

_____

(e) Mrs. Griffin's ejection fraction is 19%. Write a value for a normal ejection fraction. _____

A13. Match the technique used for diagnosis of heart failure with the related description.

BNP   Chest x-ray
Echocardiography   History and physical
                        examination

(a) Provides information about the size and shape of the heart: _____

(b) Demonstrates motion of ventricles and valve function during the cardiac cycle: _____

(c) Elevated levels confirms the diagnosis of heart failure (see Questions A5[e5]): _____

(d) Identifies presence of dyspnea, enlarged liver, ascites, and peripheral edema: _____

A14. Select the treatments for heart failure that fit the following descriptions.

ACE inhibitors   Dietary modifications
Digitalis   Diuretics

(a) Restriction of sodium and fat intake: _____

(b) Interrupts part of the renin-angiotensin-aldosterone (RAA) pathway: _____

(c) Slows conduction through the heart, reducing heart rate in a tachycardic heart; may improve cardiac contractility: _____

(d) Decreases preload: _____

A15. Circle the signs and symptoms that are likely to accompany acute pulmonary edema:

(a) Air hunger
(b) Bradycardia (slow heart rate)
(c) Calm demeanor
(d) Dyspnea
(e) Dry skin
(f) Crackles heard upon auscultation
(g) Pink, frothy sputum
(h) Confusion and lethargy

A16. Mrs. Griffin (Question A12) has an episode of acute pulmonary edema. Her blood pressure is 98/48 mm Hg. Answer the following questions related to her case.

(a) This condition is the most dramatic effect of *(right? left?)*-sided heart failure.

(b) Why might lipstick or nail polish on Mrs. Griffin interfere with assessment of this condition? _____

(c) Describe a simple measure that can relieve some of her orthopnea. _____

(d) What effect would a powerful diuretic such as furosemide (Lasix) be likely to have on her? _____

(e) How can morphine sulfate help Mrs. Griffin? _____

A17. Cardiogenic shock is shock that results from a _____ problem. Circle the three true statements about cardiogenic shock. (Pay particular attention to whether the **bold-faced** word or phrase makes the statement true or false.)

(a) The most common cause of this type of shock is **thyrotoxicosis.**

(b) In **all** cases of cardiogenic shock, cardiac output is **inadequate.**

(c) In cardiogenic shock, both end-systolic pressure and end-diastolic pressure are likely to **increase.**

(d) Lips and nailbeds are likely to appear **cyanotic.**

A18. Answer the following questions about treatments for cardiogenic shock.

(a) Nitroprusside and nitroglycerin are vaso*(constrictors? dilators?)* that will *(increase? decrease?)* venous return as blood pools in abdominal organs, skin, and kidneys. Therefore these drugs *(increase? decrease?)* preload and *(increase? decrease?)* peripheral vascular resistance (PVR).

(b) Catecholamines such as epinephrine may be helpful because they *(increase? decrease?)* cardiac contractility; however, they are also vaso*(constrictors? dilators?)* that will *(increase? decrease?)* PVR.

(c) *(A ventricular assist device [VAD]? An intra-aortic balloon pump?)* increases diastolic blood pressure, which *(increases? decreases?)* coronary perfusion.

(d) Define refractory heart failure. _____

Name two techniques used in attempts to prolong survival of refractory heart patients. _____

B. CIRCULATORY FAILURE (SHOCK)

B1. Shock can be defined as

_____

(a) List four factors required for adequate oxygenation of tissues.

_____

_____

(b) Cardiogenic shock was just discussed as a failure of the heart as a pump. Now list three major categories of circulatory shock.

_____

_____

(c) As you progress through the sections of your text on shock, identify the category of shock in each of the following cases. Select from your answers to Question B1(b).

(c1) Loss of body fluid by second- and third-degree burns with third-spacing: _____

(c2) Hemorrhage: _____

(c3) Vomiting over the course of a week: _____

(c4) Pulmonary embolism: _____

(c5) Anaphylactic shock resulting from an allergic reaction to a bee sting: _____

(c6) Septic shock in a trauma victim: _____

B2. Review Study Guide Figure 17-1 and circle the correct answers or fill in the blanks to answer the following questions about compensatory mechanisms the body uses to reverse shock by increasing cardiac output and blood pressure.

(a) Sympathetic nerve activity *(increases? decreases?)*. Effects include *(brady? tachy?)*cardia and *(increased? decreased?)* strength of contraction (dependent on current cardiac ability).

(b) Vaso*(constriction? dilation?)* of veins and venules occurs, which is helpful because veins store *(much? little?)* of the body's blood volume. As a result, venous return *(increases? decreases?)*, which (according to the _____-Starling mechanism) should *(increase? decrease?)* stroke volume and cardiac output.

(c) Circle vessels that are typically constricted by sympathetic nerve activity.

(1) Cerebral

(2) Coronary

(3) Vessels to skin, kidneys, and abdominal organs

(d) Another sympathetic effect is *(increased? decreased?)* sweat production, which together with vasoconstriction leads to *(warm, flushed? cool, clammy?)* skin in most forms of shock.

(e) Fill in the blanks within each statement about two mechanisms that are physiologic attempts to restore blood volume and increase cardiac output and blood pressure.

(e1) Hypothalamic responses include _____ as well as release of the hormone _____.

(e2) Renal retention of fluid is caused by renal vasoconstriction related to _____ nerves and the chemicals _____ and _____, and is also caused by hormones _____ and _____.

(f) These compensatory mechanisms for shock tend to *(increase? decrease?)* preload and *(increase? decrease?)* afterload; if prolonged, they are likely to cause more harm than good.

B3. Circle the correct answer or fill in the blanks to answer the following questions about Donald, age 24, who has lost about 1,500 mL (about 3 pints) of blood in a motorcycle accident that occurred 2 hours earlier.

(a) Donald's hypovolemic shock is due to *(hemorrhage? third-spacing?)*. His total blood volume is reduced by _____%.

(b) Which drops at a slower pace in hypovolemic shock? Donald's *(cardiac output? mean arterial pressure [MAP]?)*. Explain.

_____

(c) Circle treatments that are likely to be helpful for Donald.

(1) Administration of IV fluids

(2) Oxygen

(3) Vasodilators such as dopamine

(4) Supine position with elevated legs

(d) Donald's shock is worsening; however, treatments appear to be helping somewhat. His diagnosis is most likely to be *(nonprogressive? progressive? irreversible?)* hypovolemic shock.

(e) At first Donald is restless and then apathetic. The following day he moves into a stupor and then into a comatose state. Blood tests indicate that his kidneys are failing (see Question B8). Explain how these manifestations occur in severe and prolonged shock.

_____

B4. In distributive shock, total blood volume is *(increased? decreased? normal?)*, but venous return *(increases? decreases?)* as blood vessels *(constrict? dilate?)* excessively. This type of shock results from *(increased? decreased?)* sympathetic nerve activity or from release of vaso*(constrictor? dilator?)* chemicals.

Circle the types of shock that are forms of distributive shock.

Anaphylactic	Cardiogenic
Hypovolemic	Neurogenic
Obstructive	Septic

B5. Ms. Fern is a nurse who has developed hypersensitivity to latex. Answer the following questions related to her case.

(a) Exposure to latex causes her cells to release the chemical _____, which is a vasodilator. It also *(increases? decreases?)* permeability of blood vessels. As a result, her blood pressure *(increases? decreases?)* and blotchy red spots appear on her skin. These are _____.

(b) Ms. Fern experiences bronchospasm and dyspnea. Explain.

_____

(c) Epinephrine is administered quickly. How does this help?

_____

B6. Identify the type of shock in each of the following cases. Choose from the list of answers to Question B4.

(a) Brain injury that injures sympathetic nerves:
_____

(b) The most common form of distributive shock, it has a mortality rate of about 40%:
_____

(c) MI leading to congestive heart failure (CHF): _____

(d) Cardiac tamponade: _____

(e) Low blood glucose (hypoglycemia) resulting from an insulin reaction: _____

B7. Mr. Chabot, age 92, has sepsis involving gram-negative bacteria probably introduced to his bloodstream through an infection from his indwelling catheter. The microbes trigger release of cytokines from his immune system, including _____ and _____.

Circle all of the signs or symptoms that are likely to be seen in Mr. Chabot.

(a) Temperature of 96.0°F

(b) Skin pallor

(c) Cool, clammy skin

(d) Inappropriate behavior

(e) Hypotension

(f) Blood cultures positive for bacteria

(g) Hyperventilation

B8. Betsy, age 32, has irreversible hypovolemic shock resulting from severe burns suffered in a house fire 10 days ago. Answer the following questions about her complications of shock.

(a) Ischemia of kidneys for _____ is known to destroy renal function.

(1) 1 to 2 minutes

(2) 15 to 20 minutes

(3) 12 to 18 hours

(4) 3 to 4 days

Explain why acute renal failure often accompanies shock.

_____
_____
_____

How can Betsy's renal function be assessed?

_____
_____

(b) Betsy has developed a bleeding peptic ulcer. Explain.

_____
_____

(c) ARDS is an acronym for _____
_____ _____ _____.
Typically, signs of ARDS begin about 1 to 2 *(hours? days? weeks?)* after the original trauma. ARDS damage to Betsy's lungs makes them *(stiffer? more compliant?)*.

(d) Betsy is at increased risk for DIC (disseminated intravascular coagulation), which occurs in about _____% of septic clients. (See Study Guide Chapter 10, Question C6, on DIC.)

B9. MODS is an acronym for _____ _____ _____ _____. This condition is most likely to occur in the state of *(compensated? decompensated?)* shock. Mortality due to MODS *(is? is not?)* directly related to number of organs affected. List several factors associated with shock that lead to MODS.

_____

_____

_____

C. CIRCULATORY FAILURE IN CHILDREN AND THE ELDERLY

C1. Ashley, age 2 months, has right-sided heart failure resulting from a ventricular septal defect (VSD). Currently, she has no respiratory infection.

  (a) Circle the signs and symptoms likely to be present in Ashley.

    (1) Ascites
    (2) Bradycardia
    (3) Ankle edema
    (4) Dyspnea
    (5) Oliguria
    (6) Fatigue
    (7) Diaphoresis
    (8) Use of her accessory muscles while breathing
    (9) Jugular vein distention
    (10) Grunt on inspiration
    (11) Warm hands and feet
    (12) Slow feeding
    (13) Hepatomegaly
    (14) Rapid respiratory rate

  (b) Ashley is weighed daily. Explain why.

_____

_____

  (c) Circle treatments that are likely to be used to treat Ashley.

    Digitalis   Dilators
    Diuretics   Oxygen
    Small, frequent meals by tube feeding
    Supine (lying flat, face up) positioning

C2. Choose the two true statements. (Pay particular attention to whether the **bold-faced** word or phrase makes the statement true or false.)

  (a) Congenital heart defects are the **most common** cause of congestive heart failure (CHF) in children.

  (b) Congestive heart failure is a **rare** cause of disability in elderly.

  (c) With aging, blood vessels tend to become **stiffer,** which **increases** afterload.

  (d) **Complete bed rest** is usually advised for elderly persons with CHF.

  (e) Nocturia is a **late** manifestation of heart failure in elderly persons.

CHAPTER 20

Control of Respiratory Function

■ Review Questions

A. STRUCTURAL ORGANIZATION OF THE RESPIRATORY SYSTEM

A1. Arrange in correct sequence the structures through which air normally passes when you inhale.

Alveolar ducts   Alveolar sacs
Bronchi   Bronchioles
Larynx   Nose or Mouth
Pharynx   Trachea

_____ → _____ →
_____ → _____ →
_____ → _____ →
_____ → _____

A2. Alan smokes 2.5 packs a day (ppd). List two or more effects of cigarette smoke on Alan's airways.

_____

_____

A3. Which structure listed in Question A1 is common to both the respiratory system and the digestive system? Explain the significance of this anatomical arrangement.

_____

_____

A4. Which structure listed in Question A1 functions both in speech and as the "watchdog of the lungs?" _____ The space between the vocal folds is known as the *(glottis? epiglottis?)*. The *(cricoid? epiglottis? thyroid?)* cartilage is a leaf-shaped structure that normally prevents food or liquids from entering airways during swallowing.

A5. Dr. Kirkland has a tracheostomy tube through which air enters his trachea. What functions of his upper airways must mechanical equipment replace for Dr. Kirkland?

_____

A6. The walls of bronchioles *(do? do not?)* have cartilage rings. How is this fact significant during an asthma attack?

_____

A7. Choose the two true statements about respiratory structures. (Pay particular attention to whether the **bold-faced** word or phrase makes the statement true or false.)

(a) Vocal cords are located in the **pharynx.**

(b) In the tracheobronchial tree there are typically **23** levels of branching.

(c) The **base** of each lung lies on the diaphragm.

(d) Lungs produce angiotensin-converting enzyme (ACE) that helps **raise** blood pressure.

(e) **Type I** alveolar cells produce surfactant that tends to cause alveoli to **collapse.**

(f) Lungs contain a total of about **300** alveoli.

A8. *(Bronchial? Pulmonary?)* arteries supply lungs with blood that is high in O_2 and low in CO_2.

A9. Ms. Espada has a diagnosis of "pleural effusions." This means that she has an abnormal amount of fluid in her:

Pleural cavity   Parietal pleura
Visceral pleura

Arrange the three answers above from most superficial to deepest:

_____ → _____ → _____

B. EXCHANGE OF GASES BETWEEN THE ATMOSPHERE AND THE LUNGS

B1. Circle the correct answer or fill in the blanks within each statement about gases.

(a) The atmosphere around you contains enough molecules of gases to exert pressure on a column of mercury (Hg) to make it rise _____ inches.

(b) Air is almost 80% nitrogen and about 20% _____. Calculate the PO_2 in the atmosphere: 760 mm Hg × 0.20 = _____ mm Hg. To what does the "P" in PO_2 refer? _____

(c) Heidi is placed on 60% oxygen to help her get adequate oxygen while she has pneumonia. She will now breathe *(2? 3? 5?)* times the amount of oxygen in environmental air, or a pressure of _____ mm Hg.

(d) Besides nitrogen and oxygen, 47 mm Hg worth of _____ and a negligible amount of CO_2 are the other gases that normally comprise a major amount of alveolar air. Jillian is sitting outside on a hot, humid day. The air has 90% humidity. Which is likely to have a higher humidity? *(The atmosphere? Alveoli in Jillian's lungs?)*

B2. Answer these questions about pressure by filling in the blank with *Intrapleural* or *Intrapulmonary (or alveolar)*.

(a) Which pressure is inside of airways and alveoli? _____

(b) Which pressure is found between the parietal and visceral pleurae? _____ This value is normally always *(positive? negative?)*. Explain why.

_____

_____

_____

(c) Which pressure is likely to be the higher value? _____

(d) Which pressures increase during forced expiration such as in a Valsalva maneuver? _____

B3. Circle the correct answers or fill in the blanks to answer the following questions about ventilation.

(a) The chest cavity is a(n) *(open? closed?)* cavity. Name the structures that form it.

_____

Normally the one opening into this cavity is the _____.

(b) What is (are) the principal muscle(s) involved in ventilation? *(Diaphragm? Intercostals?)* The nerve supply to this muscle mass consists of the *(phrenic? intercostal?)* nerves, which are derived from the mid*(cervical? thoracic?)* portion of the spinal cord. Contraction of this muscle causes the diaphragm to move *(superiorly? inferiorly? laterally?)* with each normal inspiration.

(c) As these muscles contract, the volume of the thorax and lungs *(increases? decreases?)*, whereas the pressure within these closed spaces *(increases? decreases?)*. As a result, air is *(pushed out of? sucked into?)* lungs; this process is ___piration.

(d) Expiration is a(n) *(active? passive?)* process in which the diaphragm *(contracts? relaxes?)* and moves *(down? up?)*, causing pressures within the chest to *(increase? decrease?)*, and air is *(pushed out of? sucked into?)* lungs. This process is normally assisted by elastic _____ of lungs.

(e) *(External? Internal?)* intercostal muscles aid in *(ex? ins?)*piration because they help to *(lift? lower?)* ribs. ___ternal intercostals have the opposite effect during ___piration.

B4. Mrs. Villella has advanced emphysema. She sits on the side of her bed, with arms braced on a bedside table, breathing with pursed lips, and using her accessory muscles to help her exhale. Name the accessory muscles that aid expiration.

_____

_____

B5. Answer the following questions about lung compliance.

(a) Compliance means *(ease of? resistance to?)* inflation. Which type of balloon has more compliance? A balloon that:

(1) Is new and has never been inflated

(2) Has been inflated 50 times

(b) Explain why lungs are likely to be less compliant than normal in the following persons.

(b1) Baby Anastasia is born at 27 weeks' gestation rather than the normal 38 to 40 weeks: _____

_____

Anastasia's condition is known as

_____.

(b2) Mr. Wzolek, a coal miner for 35 years, has "black lung" with carbon particles and fibers in his lung interstitium.

_____

B6. Choose the two true statements about surfactant in lungs. (Pay particular attention to whether the **bold-faced** word or phrase makes the statement true or false.)

(a) Surfactant **lowers** surface tension and **increases** lung compliance.

(b) Surfactant is made primarily of **carbohydrates.**

(c) Surfactant has hydrophilic ends pointing toward the **inside** of alveoli.

(d) Surfactant causes alveoli to be **wetter.**

(e) Without surfactant, alveoli with the **smallest** diameter would collapse sooner than larger alveoli.

B7. Circle the correct answers or fill in the blank about air flow within lungs.

(a) Resistance to air flow is greater in *(small? large?)* airways. This is a statement of the *(Laplace? Poiseuille?)* law.

(b) Resistance to air flow is normally greater during *(ins? ex?)*piration; it is also greater if airways are partially blocked by mucus. For these reasons, asthmatics typically have more difficulty during ___piration.

(c) Airways collapse when *(compressing? distending?)* pressure is excessively high.

B8. Choose the term from this list that best fits each description. (The second blank line will be used for Question B9).

Expiratory reserve volume	Inspiratory reserve volume
Functional residual capacity	Minute volume
	Residual volume
Total lung capacity	Tidal volume
Vital capacity	

(a) A normal breath at rest: _____; <u>500</u> mL

(b) The maximal amount of air that a healthy adult can exhale after taking in the largest possible breath (IRV + TV + ERV): _____; _____ mL

(c) The volume of air remaining in the lungs at the end of a normal exhalation that can be used to oxygenate blood prior to the next inhalation: _____; _____ mL

(d) Tidal volume × respiratory rate: _____; _____ mL

B9. Fill in the normal volumes for each answer in B8. Follow the completed example in Part (a).

B10. Choose the two true statements. (Pay particular attention to whether the **bold-faced** word or phrase makes the statement true or false.)

(a) A **spirometer** is used primarily to measure **heart rate.**

(b) $FEV_{1.0}$ is measured in **seconds** (or fractions of seconds) rather than in **volume** (mL or liters).

(c) An emphysemic (who has difficulty with exhalation) is likely to have a **decreased** $FEV_{1.0}$.

(d) Persons with stiff, noncompliant lungs tend to breathe at a **faster** rate, taking more **shallow** breaths.

C. EXCHANGE AND TRANSPORT OF GASES

C1. List the three steps in the process of respiration.
_____ _____ _____

Answer the following questions about ventilation and perfusion.

(a) As you sit in a chair, which part of each of your lungs is likely to ventilate better? *(Apex? Base?)* Explain.

_____
_____
_____
_____

(b) If you lie on your back, which parts of your lungs will inflate better? *(Posterior or dependent? Anterior or nondependent?)* Explain.

_____

(c) Perfusion refers to *(air? blood?)* flow through a capillary bed. Based on gravity, which part of the lungs is likely to perfuse better? *(Apex? Base?)*

(d) Which vessels contain higher levels of O_2 and lower levels of CO_2? Pulmonary *(artery? veins?)*

C2. When lung tissue is hypoxic, pulmonary blood vessels vaso*(constrict? dilate?)*. Describe the "good news" and "bad news" of this response.

(a) Good news

_____

_____

(b) Bad news

_____

_____

C3. Match the clinical cases below with one of the listed factors that affect diffusion across the alveolar-capillary membrane.

Diffusion distance
Partial pressure of gases
Surface area for gas exchange
Solubility and molecular weight of gases

(a) Mrs. Westerfield was diagnosed with emphysema 6 years ago:

_____

(b) Mr. Frederick has interstitial viral pneumonia: _____

(c) Nina is hiking at 10,000 feet:

_____

(d) Senator Reider has left-sided heart failure causing pulmonary edema. Her arterial PO_2 is greatly decreased, but her PCO_2 is only slightly elevated: _____

C4. In a normal breath, Jules, a healthy 19-year-old, inspires 500 mL; this is a normal _____ volume. Typically, about *(150? 350?)* mL will reach his alveoli (alveolar ventilation). The remaining _____ mL, known as _____ dead space, never gets into his conducting airways.

C5. Identify which type of mismatch occurs in each of these disorders: *atelectasis* and *pulmonary embolism*. Select the correct term and write it on the line.

(a) Ventilation without perfusion (air without blood): _____

(b) Perfusion without ventilation (blood without air): _____

C6. Nina's newborn has the congenital heart defect known as tetralogy of Fallot. The baby is a "blue baby" because blood is passing from right to left ventricle through a defect in the ventricular septum without passing through pulmonary vessels. This baby has *(ventilation without perfusion? perfusion without ventilation?)*. The baby's congenital heart defect is an example of a(n) *(anatomic? physiologic?)* shunt.

C7. Answer the following questions about gas transport within blood.

(a) By the time blood leaves the pulmonary capillary bed to enter pulmonary veins, the left side of the heart, the aorta, and then other large arteries, the levels of PO_2 and PCO_2 are *(higher than? lower than? about the same as?)* levels of those gases in alveoli.

(b) When Jeremy has arterial blood gases (ABG) checked, his arterial PO_2 is 50 mm Hg, and his PCO_2 is 48 mm Hg. Are these typical values for a healthy adult? _____

(c) Normally, more than ____% of O_2 is carried in blood attached to hemoglobin (Hb) in red blood cells. Each Hb has four sites where O_2 can bind. If all Hbs had three of the four Hbs "saturated" with O_2, then the O_2 saturation (SO_2) would be ____%. This is a normal SO_2 for *(arterial? venous?)* blood. SO_2 for arterial blood is typically ___%.

(d) Only about 1% of O_2 is dissolved in _____. This amount can be increased when a person is exposed to a _____ chamber, for example, when Hb is permanently bound to CO (_____).

(e) Visualize your muscles when you are actively exercising. List several changes in active muscle tissue that will cause O_2 to detach from Hb, enter plasma, and soon reach your active muscles. Refer to Figure 20-18 in *Essentials of Pathophysiology*.

_____

_____

(f) In exercising muscles, the O_2-Hb dissociation curve shifts to the *(left? right?)*, indicating that *(more? less?)* O_2 is detaching from Hb and oxygenating tissues at any given level of PO_2.

(g) Figure 20-18 in *Essentials of Pathophysiology* points out that *(PO_2? SO_2?)* may reach lower levels that are still compatible with life than are possible for *(PO_2? SO_2?)*. Which value can reach levels greater than 100? *(PO_2? SO_2?)*

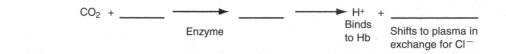

FIGURE 20-1

C8. Answer the following questions about transport of carbon dioxide (CO_2).

   (a) Most CO_2 is typically carried in blood:

      (1) As dissolved CO_2

      (2) As bicarbonate

      (3) On hemoglobin (Hb)

   (b) Write the chemical formulas for:

      (b1) Carbonic acid: _____

      (b2) Bicarbonate: _____

   (c) Show how bicarbonate is formed in blood by filling in the blanks in Study Guide Figure 20-1.

   (d) What is the role of the enzyme carbonic anhydrase in the reaction shown in that figure?

   _____

   _____

   (e) The reactions in that figure demonstrate that the increase in CO_2 in the body (as in most respiratory disorders) will tend to cause a(n) *(increase? decrease?)* in acid (H^+) in the body.

   (f) What percentage of CO_2 is carried in blood as carbaminohemoglobin (Hb-CO_2)? ___ %

D. CONTROL OF BREATHING

D1. Circle the primary location of the respiratory control.

   (a) Basal ganglia

   (b) Brainstem

   (c) Cerebral cortex

   (d) Limbic system

D2. Choose the two true statements. (Pay particular attention to whether the **bold-faced** word or phrase makes the statement true or false.)

   (a) The **pneumotaxic** center stimulates inspiration and tends to cause prolonged inspirations.

   (b) Hypoxia serves as the **main** stimulus of respiration in normal, healthy persons.

   (c) Chemoreceptors that sense elevation in CO_2 are **central** (rather than **peripheral**) receptors.

   (d) Chemoreceptors that sense hypoxia are those that are in the **aortic** and **carotid bodies.**

D3. Mr. Friday has chronic obstructive pulmonary disease (COPD). His chart indicates that his oxygen should be administered at 1 to 2 L/minute. Why not administer oxygen at 5 L/minute so that Mr. Friday will feel better faster?

   _____

D4. Circle the correct answers or fill in the blank within each statement about reflexes involving the respiratory system.

   (a) As you take a deep breath, visualize the *(irritant? J? stretch?)* receptors in your airways that are being stimulated. These will inhibit *(ins? ex?)*piration and promote *(ins? ex?)*piration. This is called the _____ reflex.

   (b) The cough reflex is triggered by receptors in the *(alveoli? pharynx? trachea and bronchi?)* Irritating substances there initiate nerve impulses along the _____ nerves to the cough center located in the *(hypothalamus? medulla? midbrain?)*.

D5. List several reasons that might account for absence of a cough reflex.

   _____

   _____

CHAPTER 21

Respiratory Tract Infections, Neoplasia, and Childhood Disorders

■ Review Questions

A. RESPIRATORY TRACT INFECTIONS

A1. Circle the correct answers in this exercise.

(a) *(Bacteria? Viruses?)* are the most common cause of respiratory tract infections.

(b) *(The common cold? Influenza or "flu"?)* is the most common viral infection of the respiratory tract. Most adults have *(2–4? 8–10?)* colds per year.

(c) The common cold is known to be caused by *(one specific virus? more than 100 types of viruses?)*. In persons 5 to 40 years of age, the *(adeno? corona? rhino?)*virus most commonly causes colds.

(d) Cold viruses *(can? cannot?)* live on hard surfaces. Colds are spread primarily by *(coughing or sneezing? infected fingers?)*.

(e) Effective vaccines for the common cold *(have? have not?)* been developed. Explain.

_____

_____

A2. Explain the importance of hand washing in preventing colds in yourself.

_____

_____

_____

A3. Circle the single best treatment for the common cold.

(a) Antibiotics

(b) Antihistamines

(c) Vitamin C

(d) Decongestants

(e) Rest and drugs that reduce fever

A4. Mrs. Kelley has right maxillary rhinosinusitis. Complete this exercise about her condition.

(a) Arrange sinuses according to location from most superior to most inferior:

Ethmoid and sphenoid
Frontal
Maxillary

_____, _____, _____

(b) All of these sinuses are known as _____ sinuses; they drain into the _____ . Explain how nasal polyps can interfere with drainage.

_____

_____

(c) These sinuses are lined with _____ membranes that *(do? do not?)* have cilia.

(d) Mrs. Kelley has had her bacterial rhinosinusitis for 2 weeks; her condition is classified as *(acute? subacute? chronic?)* sinusitis. At this point, she *(is? is not?)* likely to experience irreversible changes of the lining of her sinuses.

(e) Circle the manifestations Mrs. Kelley is likely to exhibit.

(1) Pain in her right cheek

(2) Pain in her upper right teeth

(3) Pain in the right side of her forehead

(4) Increased headache when she bends forward

(5) A sense of fullness in the ears

(f) Circle the three most likely treatments for Mrs. Kelley at this point.

(1) Antibiotics

(2) Antihistamines

(3) Decongestants

(4) Surgery

(5) Guaifenesin (mucolytic)

A5. Ms. Drach, age 69, lives in her own home. She was infected with the flu on March 1 during a visit from her brother who had the flu. Answer the following questions related to her case.

(a) The virus is most likely to incubate until March ___, when symptoms begin *(rapidly? insidiously?)*. Ms. Drach probably will be contagious from about March ___ until March ___.

(b) List several symptoms of the flu.

_____

_____

_____

(c) Ms. Drach's symptoms are likely to peak on about March ____ and disappear by about March ____.

(d) She is more likely to develop viral pneumonia if the infection begins by:

(1) Large droplet spray in the nose or throat, or infection from fingers

(2) Small droplets that directly infect lungs before immune defenses can be built up

(e) Circle appropriate treatments for Ms. Drach beginning on March 4.

(1) Antibiotics

(2) Rest

(3) Cooling the body

(4) Drinking fluids

(f) It *(is? is not?)* advisable for Ms. Drach to get a flu shot. Once she does, she should get another flu shot *(each fall? in 5 years?)*.

(g) Flu is more commonly caused by influenza virus *(A? B?)*. Typically, viral infection is *(more? less?)* contagious than bacterial respiratory infections.

A6. Circle the correct answers or fill in the blanks to answer the following questions about pneumonias.

(a) Circle the structures that are infected in pneumonia:

Alveoli   Bronchioles   Bronchi
Larynx   Pharynx (throat)

(b) Pneumonia *(is? is not?)* a common cause of death in the United States. Among infectious diseases, pneumonia is the *(leading? sixth leading?)* cause of death in the United States.

(c) Typical pneumonias are caused by *(bacteria? viruses?)*. *(Typical? Atypical?)*

pneumonias are likely to have less striking symptoms.

(d) List two causes of pneumonia other than infection.

_____

_____

A7. Ms. Drach (Question A5) developed a secondary bacterial infection superimposed on her flu. Answer the following questions related to her case.

(a) She is admitted to the medical unit with pneumonia on March 9 because her brother is concerned that "she just isn't acting right—she seems a little incoherent and she hasn't had a thing to eat in 2 days." She has *(community? hospital?)*-acquired pneumonia.

(b) The most likely bacteria to cause her pneumonia are *(Streptococcus? Klebsiella?) pneumoniae*. These microbes also are known as _____cocci. These are gram-*(positive? negative?)* bacteria with virulence based largely on the presence of a polysaccharide _____.

(c) It is likely that her oxygen saturation of hemoglobin is *(increased? decreased?)* and her respiratory rate is *(increased? decreased?)*.

(d) Explain why sputum or bronchoscopy samples are likely to be obtained.

_____

(e) To what does the "23-valent" pneumococcal vaccine refer?

_____

Is Ms. Drach in a category of persons who should receive this vaccine?

_____

A8. Mr. Lungren, age 75, was admitted July 21 with dyspnea related to cancer of the pleura (mesothelioma). He has chest tubes draining excessive pleural fluid. On July 28, he received a diagnosis of pneumonia. Answer the following questions related to his case.

(a) Based on the timing of its onset, Mr. Lungren has *(community? hospital?)*-acquired pneumonia. It also is called _____. Almost all of such pneumonias are *(bacterial? viral?)*, and they are likely to begin at least ____ hours after admission.

(b) The presence of bacteria in the lungs normally does not cause infection. List five or more reasons why acute bacterial infections may occur.

_____

_____

_____

_____

A9. Select from the list to identify the type of pneumonia likely to result in each of the following patients who have deficiencies of normal defenses against different types of microbes.

Bacteria (B)
Staph aureus, Aspergillus, Candida, or gram-negative bacilli (SACG)
Viral, fungal, mycoplasmal, or protozoan (VFMP)

(a) Franklin has neutropenia: ____

(b) Grace's antibody production is deficient: ____

(c) Erich has a T4 count of 148 as a result of his HIV infection: ____

A10. Tabatha, age 4 years, has a diagnosis of sickle cell anemia. Explain why she is at increased risk for pneumococcal pneumonia.

_____

_____

_____

A11. Answer the following questions about Legionnaires disease.

(a) This disorder is a *(common? rare?)* community-acquired pneumonia.

(b) The gram-*(positive? negative?)* microbe can be found *(only in the human body? in warm, standing water?).*

_____

(c) List four or more systems likely to be affected by this infection.

_____

_____

A12. List two or more categories of microorganisms that can cause atypical pneumonias.

_____

_____

A13. Circle the correct answers or fill in the blanks to answer the following questions about tuberculosis (TB) infection.

(a) TB is a *(rare? common?)* disorder globally. Its incidence is greater in *(crowded? sparsely populated?)* communities because this *(is? is not?)* an airborne infection.

(b) TB bacteria are resistant largely because of the waxy *(capsules? spores?)* that they form. This structure helps make these microbes identifiable by _____ staining.

(c) Which organs are most affected by *Mycobacterium tuberculosis hominis?* _____ TB in other organs is known as _____ TB.

(d) TB bacteria harm lungs by:

(1) Direct destruction of lung tissue

(2) Initiating hypersensitivity responses that lead to chronic granulomatous lung inflammation

A14. Arrange in correct sequence the events in a primary TB infection.

(a) Engulfment of TB bacilli by macrophages in which the microbes slowly grow for up to 3 months

(b) Embedding of TB bacilli in alveoli

(c) Inhalation of droplet nuclei containing the TB bacillus

(d) Presentation of TB bacilli antigens to T cells as part of a cell-mediated response

(e) Lesions known as Ghon foci form from TB bacilli, macrophages, and immune cells

(f) Caseous necrosis of Ghon foci and migration into lymph nodes leads to Ghon complexes.

___ → ___ → ___ → ___ → ___ → ___

A15. Answer the following questions about TB.

(a) Explain why immunosuppressed persons such as those with AIDS are more likely to develop active cases of tuberculosis.

_____

_____

_____

_____

(b) Describe how chest x-rays can reveal a history of TB.

_____

_____

(c) Contrast symptoms of primary TB to those of secondary TB.

_____

_____

(d) What does a positive tuberculin test indicate?

_____

(e) Immunodeficient persons who have been exposed to TB are likely to have false- *(positive? negative?)* reactions known as anergy.

(f) How can results from a false-negative reaction be verified?

_____

_____

_____

(g) What is isoniazid (INH)?

_____

TB drug therapy is typically *(long? short?)* term. Explain why multidrug regimens are used.

_____

A16. Manifestations of fungal infections *(are? are not?)* similar to those of tuberculosis. List several of these manifestations.

_____

Select the fungal infection that fits each description.

Blastomycosis Candidiasis
Coccidioidomycosis Histoplasmosis

(a) Distinctive among fungal infections by the fact that a skin test is not available; may spread to skin, bones, or prostate:

_____

(b) Common fungal infection in the Midwest, especially in river valleys; the fungus grows well in soil: _____

(c) Present in soil and dust; most prevalent in the southwest and Texas; known as "valley fever": _____

(d) Common opportunistic infection in immunosuppressed patients; caused by a yeast-like microbe: _____

B. CANCER OF THE LUNG

B1. Circle the correct answers or fill in the blanks to answer the following questions about Mr. Polk, age 62, who has lung cancer.

(a) He has the *(leading? fourth leading?)* cause of cancer deaths in the United States.

(b) Mr. Polk was an asbestos worker for 30 years; he smoked for 45 years and stopped smoking last year. Because of being a smoker in his profession, Mr. Polk's risk of developing lung cancer was *(greater than? the same as? less than?)* for nonsmoker asbestos workers.

(c) Sharp, severe chest pain *(is? is not?)* a typical early symptom of lung cancer. List several early manifestations that Mr. Polk is likely to experience.

_____

_____

(d) Mr. Polk's chart indicates that he exhibits these additional signs of lung cancer. Describe them.

(d1) Hemoptysis

_____

(d2) Hoarseness

_____

_____

(e) Mr. Polk's presenting symptoms were pain in his right hip and thigh, which led to evidence of metastasis in these bones. Explain the clinical significance.

_____

_____

_____

(f) Mr. Polk has high blood levels of ADH, PTH, and Ca^{2+}. Explain. _____

_____

_____

(g) Overall, the 5-year survival rate for individuals with lung cancer is about _____%.

B2. Match the types of lung cancer to the related descriptions.

Adenocarcinoma   Large cell carcinoma
Small cell carcinoma   Squamous cell carcinoma

(a) Mr. Polk's carcinoma is a type found commonly in male smokers; it started in his right bronchus, and carcinoma cells eventually were identified in his sputum: _____

(b) Highly anaplastic (poorly differentiated); this type of lung cancer metastasizes early and has a poor prognosis: _____

(c) Mrs. Jordan has this type of cancer, which is common in women; she was never a smoker. The cancer started in her smallest airways (bronchioles) and her alveoli: _____

(d) Which type of lung cancer is also called an "oat cell" tumor that spreads early and is not staged by the TNM method? _____

(e) Which two types of lung cancer are associated with the best prognosis because they are less likely to spread? _____, _____

(f) These three types of lung cancer are categorized as NSCLCs: _____ _____ _____

C. RESPIRATORY DISORDERS IN INFANTS AND CHILDREN

C1. Choose the two true statements about lung development. (Pay particular attention to whether the **bold-faced** word or phrase makes the statement true or false.)

(a) Lungs mature **faster** than most other organs of the body.

(b) Lungs typically **are** developed sufficiently so that they are capable of adequate respiration to permit survival by 25 to 28 weeks of gestation.

(c) **Type II** alveolar cells produce surfactant.

(d) Normally all 300 million alveoli are present in lungs by **the time of birth.**

C2. Circle the correct answers within each statement.

(a) A newborn's chest wall and lungs normally are *(compliant? stiff or rigid?)*. This factor typically makes the neonate's breathing *(easier? more difficult?)*.

(b) Chest retractions are *(normal? abnormal?)* movements of the chest wall during *(expiration? inspiration?)*.

(c) Infants are likely to do *(mouth? nose?)* breathing during the first month after birth.

(d) Because infants have airways that are *(larger? smaller?)* than those of adults, infant airways offer *(more? less?)* resistance to air flow. Infant airways have *(more? less?)* cartilage than they will later in life; this factor *(increases? decreases?)* risk of collapse.

(e) Adult arterial PO_2 is about _____ mm Hg. This value is _____ mm Hg in a fetus, and about _____ mm Hg in a neonate.

C3. Circle the correct answers or fill in the blanks to contrast respiratory disorders in three children, all 13 months old.

(a) Paulette's respirations are shallow and 38 breaths per minute. She emits audible grunts on expiration. It is likely that she has a(n) *(obstructive? restrictive?)* lung disorder because she cannot adequately inflate her lungs. How does the grunting help her?

_____

(b) Paul has bronchial asthma, which is an *(extra? intra?)*thoracic disorder characterized by *(crowing or stridor? wheezing or whistling?)* as airways collapse during ____piration.

(c) Patrice has croup, which is a(n) *(obstructive? restrictive?)* lung disorder that is *(extra? intra?)*thoracic (larynx). Her respiratory rate is likely to be *(faster? slower?)* than normal because her ____pirations are prolonged. Sounds she makes during inspiration are known as _____.

C4. Zachariah is born by cesarean section at 26 weeks of gestation. He is African American, and his mother has type 1 diabetes mellitus.

(a) Circle the factors above that make Zachariah at high risk for respiratory distress syndrome (RDS).

(b) Surfactant *(increases? decreases?)* lung compliance, *(increasing? decreasing?)* the work of breathing. With surfactant deficiency, Zachariah is at *(higher? lower?)* risk for atelectasis (collapse of lung or part of it).

(c) Explain why RDS is also called hyaline membrane disease.

_____

(d) Neonates with RDS typically *(do? do not?)* exhibit cyanosis and retractions. Grunting and _____pnea are likely to be present as indicators of *(obstructive? restrictive?)* lung disorders. (*Hint:* See Question C3[a].)

(e) Describe possible treatments for Zachariah's RDS.

_____

C5. What factor puts infants at highest risk for bronchopulmonary dysplasia?

_____

Explain why these infants typically develop signs of right-sided heart failure (cor pulmonale).

_____

_____

C6. Respiratory infections are *(common? rare?)* in young children. List two reasons why.

_____

_____

C7. Answer the following questions about croup.

(a) Croup most often occurs in children *(younger? older?)* than 5 years, and it is likely to be *(bacterial? viral?)*.

(b) Circle the interventions most likely to help a child with croup.

(1) Antibiotics

(2) Bronchodilators

(3) Exposure to cold air

(4) Being placed in a bathroom with a warm shower running

(5) Being placed in a supine position

(6) Epinephrine or steroids

C8. Distinguish characteristics of these respiratory conditions in small children. Select from the list to fill in the blanks.

Bronchiolitis   Epiglottitis
Spasmodic croup   Viral croup

(a) The most common form of acute respiratory infection in children; accompanied by a barking cough at night; usually not severe outcome: _____

(b) Immediate hospitalization is required because this condition can be rapidly progressing and life-threatening, possibly fatal within hours of onset; establishing an airway usually is necessary: _____

(c) Caused by the bacterium *Haemophilus influenzae*; less common now because of vaccine against this microbe: _____

(d) Does not respond to antibiotics; but exposure to cold air or steam from a shower can relieve airway spasms: _____

(e) Likely to be triggered by an allergic response rather than a microbe; symptoms are most common late at night; does not involve a fever: _____

(f) Most likely to occur in the trachea in children 3 months to 5 years of age: _____

(g) The child with this disorder has dysphagia and tends to assume a position sitting up with mouth open and chin thrust forward: _____

(h) A lower airway infection; most commonly caused by the RSV virus; severe form most often occurs before the age of 6 months; recovery usually begins after 2 to 3 days, but respiratory failure is possible: _____

(i) Breathlessness, rapid breathing, and retractions of lower ribs and sternum occur in young infants with this disorder: _____

C9. Signs of impending respiratory failure can include:

(a) Very *(rapid? slow?)* respirations *(with? without?)* retractions from use of accessory muscles.

(b) Very *(rapid? slow?)* heart rate.

(c) *(Extreme agitation? Decreased level of consciousness?)*.

CHAPTER 22

Disorders of Ventilation and Gas Exchange

■ Review Questions

A. DISORDERS OF LUNG INFLATION

A1. Review the pleural coverings over lungs, pleural cavity, and intrapleural pressure in Chapter 20, Questions A9 and B2(b).

A2. Mr. Martini has chest pain in the lower left region of the chest. His breathing is shallow, and he splints the left side of his chest while he breathes. He states that it hurts to take a deep breath or to cough. Based on this information, circle the most likely cause of his pain.

(a) Bronchial irritation

(b) Myocardial infarction

(c) Musculoskeletal pain

(d) Pleural pain

A3. The pleura normally secretes a small amount (10 to 20 mL = _____ tsp) of *(mucous? serous?)* fluid into the pleural cavity. Pleural _____ means abnormal fluid in the pleural cavity. One cause is a more negative intrapleural pressure as develops with _____. Identify four other factors that cause edema and can also cause pleural effusions.

_____

_____

_____

A4. Select the term that best fits each description below.

Chylothorax   Empyema   Exudate
Hemothorax   Hydrothorax   Pneumothorax

(a) Conrad has three ribs fractured in a motorcycle accident. Three of his intercostal arteries bleed into the thoracic cavity (or pleural space): _____

(b) Ms. Blanchard has a streptococcal infection of the lungs with rupture into the pleural space: _____

(c) Lymph has accumulated in Mrs. Ivey's chest cavity because her lymph nodes are blocked by metastases: _____

(d) Hospitalized for congestive heart failure, Mr. Schefflein has serous transudate in his pleural cavity: _____

(e) Air in the pleural cavity: _____

A5. Circle the correct answers or fill in the blanks to answer the following questions about pleural effusions.

(a) The most common sign is _____. Other signs include _____ noted on percussion and *(normal? diminished?)* breath sounds.

(b) Define thoracentesis.

_____

_____

A6. Select the type of pneumothorax that best fits each of the following patients' conditions.

Primary spontaneous   Secondary spontaneous
Tension   Traumatic

(a) Conrad's three fractured ribs (see Question A4[a]) have caused _____ pneumothorax; treatment involves insertion of a large-bore needle into the chest for aspiration that allows lung re-expansion.

(b) Mr. DePalma has a life-threatening condition in which air can enter but not leave the right side of his thorax; his trachea has shifted to the left, and his left lung has collapsed: _____

(c) Mick, age 19, is 6' 2" tall and weighs 150 lb. He has a ruptured air-filled bleb on the surface of his left lung: _____

(d) Mrs. McLaughlin has pneumothorax associated with her end-stage emphysema: _____

A7. Circle each of the following that is a sign of tension pneumothorax.

(a) Decreased respiratory rate

(b) Decreased heart rate

(c) Diminished breath sounds

(d) Dyspnea

(e) Hypoxemia followed by vasoconstriction in the affected lung

A8. Identify the type of atelectasis in each case by writing C for compression or O for obstructive.

(a) Caused by mucus plug: ____

(b) Coughing and deep-breathing postsurgery are designed to prevent this type of atelectasis: ____

(c) Pleural effusions, hemothorax, pneumothorax, and tumor all lead to: ____

A9. Signs of atelectasis are typically *(similar to? different from?)* those of pneumothorax (see Question A7).

A10. Treatment for both atelectasis and pneumothorax are aimed at:

_____

B. OBSTRUCTIVE AIRWAY DISORDERS

B1. Circle the two true statements. (Pay particular attention to whether the **bold-faced** word or phrase makes the statement true or false.)

(a) Vagus nerve impulses cause **constriction** of airways.

(b) Sympathetic stimulation tends to cause airways to **constrict.**

(c) Histamine causes airways to **constrict.**

(d) Incidence of bronchial asthma in the United States is **decreasing.**

B2. Circle the correct answers or fill in the blanks to answer the following questions about bronchial asthma.

(a) Asthma is a chronic *(inflammatory? noninflammatory?)* condition. Cough with asthma is typically worse *(in the afternoon and early evening? during the night and early morning?)*.

(b) Write E (extrinsic) or I (intrinsic) to indicate the category of asthma described in each case below.

(b1) Examples of triggers of this type of asthma include animal danders and house dust: ____

(b2) Examples of triggers include exercise, emotions, smoke, aspirin, and respiratory infections: ____

(b3) A type 1 hypersensitivity (atopic) immune response: ____

(b4) Involves early (acute) and late responses: ____

(c) The acute or early response typically occurs within _____ minutes of exposure to an allergen. Airborne antigens bind to *(epithelial? mast?)* cells coated with Ig __ antibodies lining airways. Chemical mediators are then released and cause the three hallmark signs of bronchial asthma:

(c1) Broncho_____

(c2) Mucosal edema related to increased _____ of mucosal blood vessels

(c3) *(Increased? Decreased?)* mucus secretions. All of these effects lead to a(an) *(increase? decrease?)* in the diameter of airways.

(d) The late-phase response recruits more cells such as _____. Resulting chronic inflammation leads to changes that *(are always? may not be?)* reversible.

(e) Of the two subsets of T helper cells, *(T_H1? T_H2?)* cells are more likely to lead to production of IgE associated with allergies and asthma. Children who are exposed to other children early in life (for example, older siblings or being enrolled in day care) are more likely to develop *(T_H1? T_H2?)* cells and *(increase? decrease?)* their risk of developing environmental allergies and asthma.

B3. Answer the following questions about triggers of asthma attacks.

(a) Asthma caused by inhaled allergens typically begins in *(younger? older?)* persons who *(do? do not?)* have a family history. List several common household allergens.

_____

_____

(b) Exercise-induced asthma (EIA) is a *(rare? common?)* form of asthma and is more likely to occur when people exercise in a *(cold? warm?)* environment.

(c) Respiratory infections, especially those caused by *(bacteria? viruses?)*, can lead to asthma attacks.

(d) List several examples of inhaled irritants that can cause asthma attacks.

_____

_____

(e) Emotional upsets and hormonal changes *(appear to? are not known to?)* precipitate asthma attacks.

(f) List medications that can lead to asthma attacks.

_____

B4. Circle each of the following that is a sign of asthma (in addition to those listed in Question B2[c]).

(a) Increased $FEV_{1.0}$

(b) Shortened expiration period

(c) Hyperinflation of lungs as more air is retained in lungs (FRC increases)

(d) Wheezing as air is exhaled through narrowed airways

(e) Increased forced vital capacity (FVC)

(f) Contraction of sternocleidomastoid muscles during ventilation

(g) Cough due to extra mucus production and irritated mucosa

(h) Dyspnea and fatigue

B5. Explain why chronic asthma increases the risk of right-sided congestive heart failure.

_____

_____

_____

B6. Jodi, age 14, has asthmatic symptoms about every other day with episodes at night about once a week. She has had to curtail participation in physical education classes. Her forced expiratory volume in 1 second is about 75% of normal levels.

(a) Jodi's asthma is classified as:

(1) Mild intermittent

(2) Mild persistent

(3) Moderate persistent

(4) Severe persistent

(b) Jodi regularly assesses her asthma by her portable meter that measures her PEF, or

_____ .

B7. Answer the following questions about treatments for asthma.

(a) List several examples of how contributing factors may be controlled.

_____

(b) Circle the correct answers or fill in the blanks to describe categories of medications for asthma. Note that many asthma medications are_____ (preventative).

(b1) Broncho*(constrictors? dilators?)* mimic *(sympathetic or adrenergic? parasympathetic or cholinergic?)* neurotransmitters or block _____ pathways. These drugs *(constrict? relax?)* smooth muscle of airways.

(b2) Anti_____ include cromolyn that help to prevent asthma attacks.

(b3) Another category of drugs known as _____ modifiers inhibit synthesis or action of broncho-constrictor chemicals released from the asthmatic person's own mast cells.

(c) In general, medications that bronchodilate are classified as *(quick relief? long-term?)* medications.

B8. Circle the risk factors for death from asthma listed in the following paragraph:

Marisol has had four visits to the ER over the past year, one 3 weeks ago. She has been hospitalized once in the past year and that stay required intubation. Marisol uses one β_2-stimulator inhaler about every 3 weeks and she knows how to use a peak flow meter.

From an upper-middle-class family with good health insurance, Marisol is a happy, sociable adolescent who does not smoke, drink alcohol, or use other illegal drugs.

B9. Circle the two true statements about asthma. (Pay particular attention to whether the **bold-faced** word or phrase makes the statement true or false.)

(a) Most asthma deaths have occurred **outside** the hospital.

(b) Asthma is a **rare** cause for admission to children's hospitals.

(c) Most children who develop asthma have symptoms **before** they reach school age.

(d) It **is not** recommended that children be involved in developing their own asthma management plans.

B10. What signs might suggest onset of bronchial asthma in an 18-month-old child?

_____

_____

B11. Fill in the blanks or circle the correct answers within each statement about COPD.

(a) COPD is an acronym that refers to

_____.

List the two major forms of COPD: _____ and

_____.

(b) COPD is a *(common? rare?)* cause of death in the United States. The largest single cause of COPD is _____.

(c) Signs or symptoms *(are? are not?)* typically present in early stages of COPD.

(d) Circle the characteristics that are true of both COPD and asthma.

(1) Inflammation

(2) Bronchoconstriction

(3) Excessive secretion of mucus

(4) Loss of elastic fibers in alveolar walls

(5) Difficult expiration

B12. Circle the correct answers or fill in the blanks to answer the following questions about emphysema.

(a) Emphysema involves *(thickening? breakdown?)* of alveolar walls causing a(n) *(increased? decreased?)* surface for gas exchange.

(b) Most people with emphysema develop it as a result of *(smoking? a genetic disorder?)*. Cigarette smoke stimulates movement of _____ cells into lungs, and these cells release the enzyme _____, which digests the *(fat? protein?)* elastin in alveolar walls. Loss of elasticity in alveolar walls causes the characteristic barrel-chested appearance in which lungs are *(hypo? hyper?)*inflated.

B13. Write *CB* (chronic bronchitis) or *Emph* (emphysema) next to descriptions that fit each disorder.

(a) Patients have a productive cough (especially in the morning) of more than 3 months' duration for at least 2 consecutive years, and possibly for many years: ____

(b) The earliest feature of this disorder is excessive mucus production in the trachea and bronchi: _____

(c) Called "blue bloaters": cyanosis results from CO_2 retention, and bloating derives from cor pulmonale (see Question D7): ____

(d) Hypoxemia also results in polycythemia and sluggish blood, with possible clot formation: ____

(e) Called "pink puffers" because they respond to hypoxia by working extra hard to breathe (often using accessory muscles and pursed lips) and they do maintain quite normal blood gas values: ____

(f) More likely to experience major weight loss related to the extra work of breathing: ____

(g) In young adults, the major cause is deficiency of the enzyme α_1-antitrypsin that normally protects alveolar walls from destruction: ____

B14. Mr. Eggers, age 48, complains of shortness of breath (dyspnea) and a productive cough early in the morning. He does not have an infection. Answer the following questions related to his case.

(a) List the components of Mr. Eggers's workup that ultimately lead to his diagnosis of COPD.

_____

_____

(b) Circle the results likely to be found in his diagnostic workup:

  (b1) Prolonged *(ins? ex?)*piration

  (b2) Forced vital capacity (FVC) of *(4 to 5? 7 to 8?)* sec.

  (b3) The volume of air that can be forcibly exhaled in 1 sec ($FEV_{1.0}$) is *(greater? less?)* than normal.

  (b4) The total lung capacity (TLC) is *(greater? less?)* than normal.

B15. Mrs. Rice, age 68, has advanced emphysema. The home health nurse is assessing Mrs. Rice's management of her emphysema. Circle Mrs. Rice's statements that indicate good management of COPD.

  (a) "I got my flu shot this fall."

  (b) "My friend Sadie always seems to have a cold. I ask her if we can talk on the phone then—instead of her visiting me here."

  (c) "My sister still smokes two packs a day, and I just can't ask her to not smoke when she's here."

  (d) "I eat a little something every 2 or 3 hours; I get too tired if I eat big meals."

  (e) "I tried doing those breathing exercises—it's too much for me, so I stopped."

B16. Circle each of the following that is an intervention typically used to treat COPD.

  (a) Adrenergic bronchodilators

  (b) Anticholinergic bronchodilators

  (c) Theophylline

  (d) Oxygen by nasal cannula to maintain PO_2 at 90 mm Hg

B17. Circle the correct answers or fill in the blanks within each statement about bronchiectasis.

  (a) Bronchiectasis involves broncho*(constriction? dilatation?)* associated with _____. Since the introduction of vaccinations and the use of antibiotics, the incidence of bronchiectasis is *(increasing? decreasing?)*.

  (b) Causes of localized bronchiectasis include:
  _____

  (c) Causes of generalized bronchiectasis include: _____

  (d) Generalized bronchiectasis is a *(reversible? permanent?)* condition.

(e) Describe the "vicious cycle" that is likely to occur in bronchiectasis.

_____

(f) Signs and symptoms of bronchiectasis include *(low body temperature? fever?)*, coughing up *(small? large?)* amounts of sputum that contains _____ and *(is? is not?)* foul smelling, weight *(gain? loss?)*, and changes in fingers known as _____ that may occur with cardiac or pulmonary disease.

B18. Circle the correct answers or fill in the blanks to answer the following questions about Brent, age 8, who has cystic fibrosis (CF).

  (a) CF is a *(rare? common?)* fatal hereditary disorder in whites. Both of Brent's parents must have the CF gene because this is a(n) *(autosomal dominant? autosomal recessive? sex-linked?)* disorder. Because they are carriers, it is likely that Brent's parents have *(no? some?)* symptoms of CF.

  (b) Mapped to chromosome ___, the defective gene known as _____ fails to code for a protein needed for *(Ca^{2+}? Cl^-? Mg^{2+}?)* transport. As a result *(endocrine? exocrine?)* secretions are affected. Sweat has *(high? low?)* salt content, which can lead to salt depletion. Mucus becomes extremely *(thin? thick?)* and blocks ducts.

  (c) The most serious effects of CF are on these major organs: _____ and the _____. Initial respiratory signs are _____ of airways, including those caused by *Staphylococcus aureus* and _____. Repeated infections lead to _____ and related destruction.

  (d) Blockage of ducts of the _____ prevents enzymes from this organ from breaking down foods, especially fats. Brent experiences fatty stool, known as _____orrhea, as well as diarrhea and abdominal pain. As a result, Brent's weight, as in most CF patients, tends to be *(higher? lower?)* than normal.

  (e) Brent is at high risk for infertility because bilateral failure of _____ development accompanies CF in most males.

B19. Explain why early diagnosis of cystic fibrosis (CF) is important.

_____

_____

Circle the correct answers or fill in the blanks to describe diagnostic tests for CF.

(a) Newborn screening tests for blood levels of _____, which is produced in the *(lungs? pancreas?)*. Obstruction of ducts prevents passage of the chemical out of the organ, so that blood levels *(drop? elevate?)*.

(b) Confirmatory tests for CF include analysis of _____ collected from skin as well as a genetic test for mutations in the _____ gene.

B20. Currently, the median survival age for persons with cystic fibrosis is *(15? 25? 35?)* years. Treatment of CF focuses on replacement of _____ enzymes and methods of keeping _____ clear. Describe several treatments for airways.

_____

_____

C. INTERSTITIAL LUNG DISEASES

C1. Circle the three true statements about interstitial lung diseases. (Pay particular attention to whether the **bold-faced** word or phrase makes the statement true or false.)

(a) These conditions are classified as **restrictive** rather than **obstructive.**

(b) They have their primary effects on **airways** of lungs.

(c) Interstitial diseases **do** involve injury, inflammation, and formation of scar tissue.

(d) These conditions **are all** rapidly progressive.

(e) Interstitial lung diseases are **rarely** caused by occupational and environmental inhalants.

(f) Such diseases **decrease** lung compliance.

C2. Circle the signs or symptoms typical of interstitial lung diseases.

(a) Rapid, shallow breathing

(b) Bradypnea

(c) Dyspnea with wheezing (as in COPD)

(d) Dyspnea without wheezing

(e) Increase in total lung capacity with hyperinflated lungs (as in COPD)

(f) Hypoxemia and clubbing of fingers

(g) Hypercapnia and cyanosis

C3. Fill in the blanks to list several factors that can lead to interstitial lung diseases.

(a) Inhalation of inorganic dusts such as _____ and _____

(b) Therapeutic procedures to combat cancer: _____ and _____

(c) System connective tissue (collagen) disorders: _____, _____, _____

C4. List several diagnostic techniques for interstitial lung diseases.

_____

_____

_____

C5. Treatments for later stages of interstitial lung disease are *(similar? dissimilar?)* to those for COPD. List several treatments.

_____

_____

D. PULMONARY VASCULAR DISORDERS

D1. Answer the following questions about pulmonary emboli (PEs).

(a) Most PEs are composed of blood clots (or thrombi). List three other substances that can form emboli.

_____

(b) Almost all PEs originate as _____ (DVTs) in *(upper? lower?)* extremities.

(c) Write examples of each of the three major factors that lead to DVTs (and therefore to PEs):

(1) Venous stasis due to:

_____

_____

(2) Injury to the inner lining of veins as occurs in:

_____

_____

(3) Hypercoagulability related to:

_____

_____

(d) PEs affect blood flow through lungs by two mechanisms. Briefly describe these.

_____

_____

(e) List the three most common signs or symptoms of PEs.

_____

(Hypoxemia? Carbon dioxide retention?) is more likely to occur as a result of PEs. *(Small? Medium-sized? Large?)* emboli are most likely to result in collapse, shock, loss of consciousness, and possibly death.

D2. Identify purposes (I–III) of the interventions for PEs listed below.

I. Prevention of clot formation
II. Prevention of movement of clots to lungs
III. Sustaining of life by clot dissolution when PEs are already present

(a) Thrombolytic therapy: ____

(b) Use of an anticoagulant: ____

(c) Use of compression stockings or IPC boots: ____

D3. Fill in the blanks with a typical pulmonary artery (PA) blood pressure: ____/____ mm Hg with a mean PA pressure of ____ mm Hg. Compared with systemic circulation, pulmonary circulation is a *(low? high?)* pressure system with *(thin and compliant? thick and stiff?)* vessels.

D4. Most cases of pulmonary hypertension are *(primary? secondary?)*. Select the category of cause of pulmonary hypertension that fits the related description.

Elevation of pressure in pulmonary veins (EPPV)
Increased pulmonary blood flow (IPBF)
Obstruction of pulmonary vessels (OPV)
Pulmonary hypoxemia leading to reflex pulmonary vasoconstriction (PHPV)

(a) COPDs such as chronic bronchitis or emphysema: ____

(b) Mitral valve stenosis or left-sided heart failure: ____

(c) Living in a town at an elevation of 12,000 feet: ____

(d) Congenital heart defects (VSD, ASD, or PDA) with left-to-right shunting that overloads and stimulates structural damage to the pulmonary artery: ____

(e) Pulmonary embolism: ____

D5. List major signs and symptoms of secondary pulmonary hypertension.

_____

_____

_____

D6. Complete this exercise about Mrs. Budd, who has a diagnosis of primary pulmonary hypertension.

(a) Her mean pulmonary artery blood pressure is most likely to be *(14? 26? 94?)* mm Hg. This value is considerably *(higher? lower?)* than normal.

(b) This is a relatively *(common? rare?)* condition, occurring in about one person in a *(thousand? million?)*. The 5-year survival rate is about ____ %.

(c) What signs or symptoms is Mrs. Budd likely to manifest?

_____

_____

(d) What treatments may help?

_____

_____

D7. Cor pulmonale refers to a heart ("cor") problem resulting from a _____ problem. Arrange in the correct sequence the events in development of cor pulmonale.

(a) Retrograde blood flow from lungs to right ventricle

(b) Pulmonary hypoxemia that causes reflex pulmonary vasoconstriction

(c) Some chronic lung problem such as chronic bronchitis

(d) Right ventricular hypertrophy that soon "outgrows" coronary blood supply

(e) Right ventricular failure with back flow into systemic veins

(f) Increased resistance to flow through pulmonary vessels

(g) Jugular vein distension, ankle edema, hepatomegaly, and ascites

____ → ____ → ____ →
____ → ____ → ____ → ____

D8. Mr. Sokolski has chronic bronchitis and cor pulmonale. Blood work reveals a hematocrit of 56; physical exam indicates presence of "plethora." Explain.

_____

_____

D9. Mr. Ellison suffered severe burns and multiple fractures in the collapse of a burning building. He experienced significant bleeding and has now been diagnosed with ARDS. Answer the following questions about ARDS.

(a) ARDS is an acronym for _____ _____ _____ syndrome. List possible causes of ARDS in Mr. Ellison.

_____

_____

_____

(b) Lung changes resulting from ARDS involve injury to alveoli that cause a(an) *(increase? decrease?)* in permeability of the alveolar-capillary membrane, *(activation? inactivation?)* of surfactant, formation of a _____ membrane inside of alveoli, and *(increase? decrease?)* in gas exchange. Resulting pulmonary edema, alveolar collapse, and fibrosis *(increase? decrease?)* Mr. Ellison's work of breathing.

(c) His treatment involves administration of _____ needed by vital organs and multiple interventions to address the other pathologies associated with his injuries.

E. RESPIRATORY FAILURE

E1. _____ means low level of O_2 in blood, whereas _____ means excess CO_2 in blood.

E2. Recall the three factors necessary for respiration to occur.

(a) _____ of air from the atmosphere into lungs

(b) _____ of blood from heart to lungs and back

(c) _____ between air in alveoli and blood in pulmonary capillaries

E3. Circle the correct answers or fill in the blanks to answer the following questions about normal and abnormal blood gases.

(a) Select the normal value(s) for arterial PO_2:

30   48   72   88   102

(b) In respiratory failure, arterial PO_2 is less than _____ mm Hg. This condition is known as _____.

(c) Select the normal value(s) for arterial PCO_2:

30   38   42   52   64

(d) In respiratory failure, arterial PCO_2 is greater than _____ mm Hg. This condition is known as _____.

E4. Indicate whether each of the following conditions is likely to result in *hypoxemia, hypercapnia,* or *both.*

(a) ARDS: _____

(b) Most cases of advanced COPD: _____

(c) Hypoventilation due to drug overdose: _____

(d) Interstitial lung disease: _____

E5. Circle the three true statements about hypoventilation. (Pay particular attention to whether the **bold-faced** word or phrase makes the statement true or false.)

(a) Hypoventilation refers to a significant reduction of **pure oxygen** moving into or out of the lung.

(b) If alveolar ventilation is **halved,** then $PaCO_2$ is likely to **double** (from 40 to 80 mm Hg).

(c) In patients who are hypoventilating, administration of oxygen can bring PaO_2 **back to normal,** but $PaCO_2$ will remain **high.**

(d) Hypoventilation is **rarely** caused by disorders outside of the lungs, for example, respiratory muscle weakness or abnormal thoracic cage.

(e) Hypoventilation **can** occur in situations in which hypercapnia is not present, but hypercapnia **cannot** occur unless hypoventilation is present.

E6. Match each condition with the related description below. (Use each answer only once.)

Cyanosis   Hypercapnia
Hypoxemia   Impaired diffusion   Shunt

(a) Occurs with atelectasis of a portion of a lung or a congenital heart defect such as tetralogy of Fallot: _____

(b) Pneumonia, pulmonary edema, interstitial disease, and ARDS all increase the thickness of the alveolar-capillary membrane: _____

(c) Bluish discoloration of skin (more readily detected in light skin) and mucosa caused by reduction of at least 5 g/dL of hemoglobin (Hb); can be central (as in tongue and lips) or peripheral (as in extremities); can occur in polycythemia without hypoxia because too many Hb molecules are present to bind with a normal level of O_2 molecules: _____

(d) Indicated by a $PaCO_2$ level greater than 50 mm Hg and a low arterial pH. Occurs with hypoventilation sufficient to cause hypoxia, such as COPD, Guillain-Barré syndrome, or severe scoliosis: _____

(e) If mild, produces few signs or symptoms. Can lead to impairment of vital centers (such as brain) and activation of compensatory mechanisms (such as tachycardia, hyperventilation, cool skin, sweating, erythropoiesis). If not reversed, will lead to bradycardia, hypotension, and death: _____

E7. Describe a noninvasive method for oxygen assessment.

_____

_____

E8. Answer the following questions about Mrs. McLaughlin, who has advanced COPD.

(a) Before developing COPD, Mrs. McLaughlin's respiratory center would have been stimulated by (central? peripheral?) chemoreceptors that sense an increase in (H^+? HCO_3^-?) ions directly related to (low blood levels of O_2? high blood levels of CO_2?).

(b) With chronic hypercapnia (as in COPD), reactivity of those chemoreceptors (increases? decreases?). People with COPD must turn to another mechanism for control

of ventilation—that involving (central? peripheral?) receptors located in the aorta and in _____ arteries.

(c) Mrs. McLaughlin normally inspires 1 to 2 L/min of O_2 by nasal cannula. If she were to breathe higher concentrations of oxygen, her $PaCO_2$ would (increase? decrease?). Explain.

_____

_____

_____

_____

E9. Fill in the blanks to describe mechanisms that can lead to hypercapnia. Respiratory muscles cannot produce normal CO_2 exhalation if they:

(a) Require more energy for breathing than normal, for example: _____

_____

(b) Lack normal energy resources or muscle strength, for example: _____

_____

_____

E10. June has a $PaCO_2$ level of 58 mm Hg and a PaO_2 level of 54 mm Hg. Answer the following questions about her state of hypercapnia.

(a) She is likely to be in respiratory (acidosis? alkalosis?) as indicated by an arterial blood pH of (7.25? 7.45?).

(b) June is likely to manifest signs and symptoms of hypercapnia when $PaCO_2$ is (slightly? markedly?) elevated above the normal level of about _____ mm Hg. One effect is an (increase? decrease?) of central nervous system activity. Manifestations such as skin flushing and headache are related to hypercapnic effects of vaso(constriction? dilatation?).

(c) Treatments for June are likely to focus on:

_____

_____

_____

CHAPTER 23

Control of Kidney Function

■ Review Questions

A. KIDNEY STRUCTURE AND FUNCTION

A1. Circle the correct answers or fill in the blanks to answer the following questions about kidney structure.

(a) Kidneys are normally situated *(at waist level? in the pelvis?)*. They are located *(in the anterior of the abdomen? retroperitoneally?)*. State the significance of this location.

_____

(b) Arrange these renal structures in correct sequence from outermost to innermost:

Medulla   Capsule   Cortex

_____ → _____ →

_____

(c) Urine formed in the cortex and medulla flows into the renal _____ from which urine enters the *(ureters? urethra?)* and passes to the urinary bladder.

(d) Refer to Figures 23-3 and 23-4 in *Essentials of Pathophysiology* and arrange these blood vessels in correct sequence from first to and through the kidneys:

Afferent arteriole   Efferent arteriole
Glomerular capillary   Intralobular artery
Intralobular vein   Peritubular capillary
Renal artery   Renal vein

_____ → _____ →
_____ → _____ →
_____ → _____ →
_____ → _____

A2. Answer the following questions about the structure of a nephron.

(a) Fill in the blanks show that a nephron consists of:

(1) A cluster of capillaries known as a _____ in which blood is filtered and collected into _____'s capsule. Taken together, the glomerulus and capsule are known as a renal

_____.

(2) A _____, which transports the filtrate (or "forming urine") and allows reabsorption of much of the filtrate into _____ capillaries.

(b) Glomeruli consist of three layers. The middle layer, which is the *(basement membrane? endothelium? epithelium?)*, determines the permeability of the glomerulus. Normally, this membrane *(allows? prevents?)* passage of red blood cells and plasma protein from blood into filtrate. It is responsible for leakage in many glomerular diseases.

(c) _____ cells cover areas of glomeruli lacking a basement membrane. State two functions of these cells.

_____

(d) Refer to Figure 23-4 in *Essentials of Pathophysiology* and arrange the following portions of the renal tubule in correct sequence from first to last:

Ascending limb of the loop of Henle (ALLH)
Collecting duct (CD)
Distal convoluted tubule (DCT)
Descending limb of the loop of Henle (DLLH) Proximal convoluted tubule (PCT)

_____ → _____ →
_____ → _____ →
_____

(e) About 85% of nephrons have *(long? short?)* loops of Henle located only in the renal cortex. The remaining 15% are known as *(cortical? juxtaglomerular?)* nephrons as their long loops of Henle extend into the renal medulla. These nephrons help to produce *(concentrated? dilute?)* urine.

A3. Refer to Study Guide Figure 23-1 and identify the three steps in urine formation. Note the direction of movement of substances in each step. (Note that glomerular filtrate and tubular fluid are different stages of "forming urine.")

(a) Step I: _____ is the movement of substances out of blood into filtrate ("forming urine").

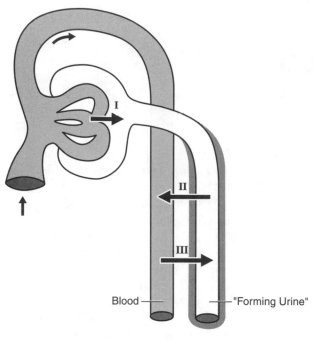

Blood ———   ——— "Forming Urine"

FIGURE 23-1

(b) Step II: _____ is the return of substances from filtrate ("forming urine") now present in tubular fluid back into blood (in peritubular capillaries).

(c) Step III: _____ is the movement of substances out of peritubular blood via kidney tubule cells into tubular fluid ("forming urine").

A4. Answer these questions about urine formation in Julian, age 46, whose kidneys and blood pressure are normal.

(a) Julian's kidneys are likely to move about ____mL/min of substances from blood to filtrate (forming urine). This is known as his _____ _____ rate (GFR). The filtrate formed is similar to his blood plasma except that filtrate lacks _____ and _____.

(b) His kidneys are likely to reabsorb about ____ mL/min back into his blood. In other words, Julian's urinary output will be about ____ mL/min (or ____ mL/hour or ____ mL/day).

(c) Normal glomerular capillary blood pressure (BP) is about ____ mm Hg; this is considerably (*higher? lower?*) than BP in all other capillaries of the body. When Julian is highly stressed, his sympathetic nerves will cause (*vasoconstriction? vasodilation?*) of his afferent and efferent

arterioles. This leads to (*increased? decreased?*) GFR and (*increased? decreased?*) urine production, as well as (*increased? decreased?*) blood volume and BP.

A5. Answer the following questions about Steps II and III (from Question A3) of urine formation.

(a) Refer to Figure 23-7 in *Essentials of Pathophysiology* and trace the path of Na^+ from right to left in the figure. This process depends on the "sucking" of Na^+ from renal tubule cells into the (*lumen of the tubule? interstitial fluid and blood?*), a process driven by the _____ pump (shown on the left side of the figure). In fact, most ATP used by kidneys is devoted to the (*filtration? reabsorption? secretion?*) of Na^+ from tubular fluid via tubule cells to blood. Simultaneously, glucose and amino acids are (*co? counter?*)transported in the same direction. The latter is also known as (*primary? secondary?*) active transport.

(b) H^+ ions move the (*same? opposite?*) direction as Na^+ and therefore undergo ATP-dependent (*co? counter?*)transport. This results in (*reabsorption? secretion?*) of H^+ into urine, a mechanism that reduces acidity of blood. Name three buffers that assist in secretion of H^+ ions: _____, _____, and _____.

(c) Movement of H_2O in the same direction as Na^+ occurs during the (*active? passive?*) process of osmosis. Most such resorption of H_2O and Na^+, as well as that of glucose and amino acids, normally occurs in the (*PCT? DCT?*). This process helps prevent dehydration and loss of nutrients in urine.

(d) In uncontrolled diabetes, blood levels of glucose are (*higher? lower?*) than normal, so (*more? less?*) glucose than normal is filtered in glomeruli. If the amount of glucose in tubular fluid surpasses the _____ (reabsorption) maximum for glucose as shown in Figure 23-8 in *Essentials of Pathophysiology*, then glucose (*does? does not?*) appear in urine.

A6. Philippe runs 10 miles on a sweltering day. As a cooling mechanism, his sweat glands become (*more? less?*) active. Answer the following questions about how his kidneys respond to help prevent dehydration.

(a) His kidneys produce a (*larger? smaller?*) amount of (*concentrated? dilute?*) urine.

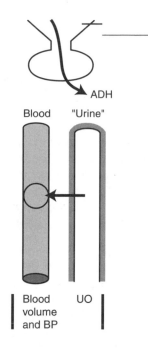

FIGURE 23-2

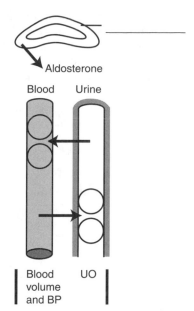

FIGURE 23-3

(b) The mechanism involved is known as the _____ mechanism, which is based on the flow of fluids in *(the same? opposite?)* direction(s) within the two limbs of the loop of Henle and also in the parallel capillaries known as _____. This arrangement causes the renal medulla to become *(hyper? hypo?)*tonic (comparable to a desert) so it draws water out of urine.

A7. Refer to Study Guide Figures 23-2 through 23-4 and describe the effects of hormones on kidneys. Fill in lines to show where hormones are produced, complete arrows to show their impact on urinary output (UO) as well as blood volume and blood pressure (BP), and fill in names of electrolytes (Na^+, K^+, H^+, or Ca^{2+}) or H_2O in circles.

(a) ADH (Figure 23-2) causes insertion of water channels into membranes of renal tubules. The result is a(an) *(increase? decrease?)* in permeability of the medullary collecting ducts and reabsorption of water.

(b) Principal cells in the late *(PCT? DCT?)* and cortical collecting tubules are sensitive to aldosterone (Figure 23-3), which causes resorption of *(Na⁺? K⁺?)* and water, and secretion of ____ into urine. Intercalated cells here secrete ____ into urine.

(c) Although aldosterone and ADH work by different mechanisms, they both *(increase? decrease?)* urinary output and *(lower?*

raise?) BP. The hormone ANP, produced by the _____, *(mimics? opposes?)* release and action of ADH and aldosterone.

(d) Parathyroid hormone (Figure 23-4) acts on the *(PCT? DCT?)* to increase reabsorption of ____ ions. Vitamin D *(mimics? opposes?)* effects of PTH as both chemicals "pull" from several sources to *(increase? decrease?)* blood levels of Ca^{2+}.

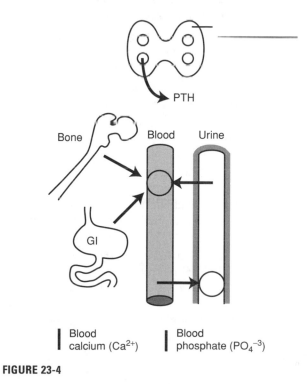

FIGURE 23-4

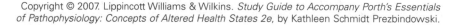

(e) Thiazide diuretics inhibit NaCl reabsorption in the *(PCT? DCT?)*, whereas loop diuretics inhibit reabsorption of Na^+ and H_2O in the *(thin? thick?)* portion of the loop of Henle.

A8. Normally about *(2.5%? 25%?)* of cardiac output flows into kidneys each minute. Answer the following questions about variations in blood flow through the kidneys (with direct effects on GFR and urinary output).

(a) Match each of the following neural or chemical factors with their effects on the kidneys.

Antidiuretic hormone (ADH or vasopressin)
Angiotensin II   Atrial natriuretic peptide
Nitric oxide   (ANP)
Dopamine   Endothelin I
Sympathetic nerve   Prostaglandin
   activity $(PG)E_2$ and I_1

(a1) Cause renal vasoconstriction, decreased GFR, and decreased urinary output: _____, _____, _____

(a2) Cause renal vasodilation, increased GFR, and increased urinary output: _____, _____

(b) When renal blood pressure increases, for example when blood pressure is high, the process of _____ causes renal vessels to dilate, increasing GFR and urinary output, and *(increasing? decreasing?)* blood pressure.

(c) The juxtaglomerular (JG) complex (Figure 23-10 in *Essentials of Pathophysiology*) consists of two types of cells:

(c1) _____ cells in the distal tubule that monitor NaCl levels.

(c2) JG cells in the walls of _____ arterioles that respond to stretching of these vessels. JG cells then release renin, which leads to the production of _____, a vasoconstrictor that regulates glomerular flow. Angiotensin II also stimulates release of the hormone _____. (See also Question A7[b].)

(d) ANP *(increases? decreases?)* the volume of urine. In addition to its action as a vasodilator (so less blood flows into kidneys), it also *(stimulates? inhibits?)* production of aldosterone (which then

causes more sodium and water to exit in urine) and *(stimulates? inhibits?)* release of ADH.

A9. "Renal clearance" means the volume of plasma that is "cleared" (or cleaned) of a given chemical each minute. Renal clearance is greatest for substances that are *(well? poorly?)* filtered from blood and *(well? poorly?)* reabsorbed back into blood. An example is *(inulin? insulin? glucose?)*; its clearance is directly related to the person's GFR because this chemical is *(highly? slightly? not at all?)* reabsorbed.

A10. Mr. Charles has gouty arthritis. This is related to increased blood levels of _____ acid. Name two types of medications that Mr. Charles should avoid because they lead to hyperuricemia and exacerbate gout.

_____

A11. Answer the following questions about Ms. Jensen, age 55, who has a history of rheumatoid arthritis and diabetes mellitus. Her BUN level is 67 mg/dL and her GFR is 24 mL/min. Ms. Jensen's blood calcium level is low.

(a) BUN refers to blood _____ nitrogen. Normal values range from _____ to _____ mg/dL; Ms. Jensen's BUN is *(low? normal? high?)*.

(b) High levels of BUN can result from increased breakdown of *(fats? proteins?)*, which contain about 16% nitrogen (N), *(increased? decreased?)* ability of kidneys to clear nitrogen-containing wastes, or *(de? over?)*hydration.

(c) Breakdown of protein leads to production of ammonia in the *(intestine? kidney? liver?)*, which is converted to urea in the _____, which is then eliminated by _____.

(d) List several reasons why Ms. Jensen's BUN levels may be high.

_____

_____

_____

_____

(e) If the cause of Ms. Jensen's high BUN is related to renal failure, blood levels of some of her medications may *(increase? decrease?)*. Explain the clinical significance.

(f) Ms. Jensen's hematocrit level is 18. Her physician prescribes "epoetin-a." Explain why.

_____

_____

(g) What might explain Ms. Jensen's hypocalcemia?

_____

_____

_____

B. TESTS OF RENAL FUNCTION

B1. Conrad has a urinalysis performed. Circle those findings that are abnormal.

Casts   Specific gravity of 1.015
Glucose   90 mg protein in a 24-
Pink color   hour urine sample
400 mL total volume
     in a 24-hour urine
     sample

B2. Answer the following questions about renal function tests involving urine.

(a) On a day when a person produces a large amount of sweat, specific gravity is likely to be *(1.010? 1.025?)*. Urine with a specific gravity of 1.003 is likely to appear *(yellow-amber? colorless?)*. Urine with such low specific gravity can occur when ADH level is *(higher? lower?)* than normal as in *(SIADH? diabetes insipidus?)*.

(b) Explain why a specific gravity 1.060 may be found in a person with diminished renal function.

_____

(c) Casts are more likely to be found in urine that has a *(high? low?)* concentration of

proteins, as in nephrotic syndrome, and is *(acidic? alkaline?)*.

B3. Creatinine is a(n) *(abnormal? normal?)* product of muscle metabolism. Answer the following questions about its role in renal function testing.

(a) Because it is filtered out of blood and *(is? is not?)* reabsorbed, creatinine clearance directly reflects GFR levels. Normal creatinine clearance is about *(120? 90? 60?)* mL/minute. In other words, a high level of creatinine clearance indicates *(good? poor?)* kidney function.

(b) As kidneys fail, *(more? less?)* creatinine will end up in ("be cleared into") urine, so blood levels of creatinine *(increase? decrease?)*. Therefore, a high serum creatinine level indicates *(good? poor?)* kidney function.

(c) Circle the normal serum creatinine level (see Table 23-1 in *Essentials of Pathophysiology*): *(1.0? 5.0?)* mg/dL of blood. If the serum creatinine level is three times normal (such as 3.0 mg/dL), then GFR is *(three times? one third of?)* normal. Serum creatinine level tends to be *(higher? lower?)* among elderly persons.

(d) The normal BUN:creatinine ratio is about *(10:1? 1:1? 1:10?)*, such as 12 mg/dL of BUN to ___ mg/dL of creatinine. A high BUN:creatinine ratio, such as 17:1, is more likely to accompany:

(1) Congestive heart failure or GI bleeding

(2) Liver disease or chronic renal dialysis

B4. High blood levels of *(BUN? creatinine? K^+? H^+?)* is the most specific indicator of renal failure. Explain.

_____

_____

_____

_____

_____

CHAPTER 24

Disorders of Renal Function

■ Review Questions

A. CONGENITAL DISORDERS OF THE KIDNEYS

A1. Choose the three true statements. (Pay particular attention to whether the **bold-faced** word or phrase makes the statement true or false.)

(a) Fetal kidneys can be detected by ultrasound by about **12 weeks'** gestation.

(b) **Unilateral** renal agenesis is incompatible with life.

(c) Renal hypoplasia is considered **more** serious than renal agenesis.

(d) Potter syndrome refers to **facial features** that accompany renal agenesis.

(e) If fetal kidney function is less than normal, the volume of amniotic fluid is likely to be **greater** than normal.

(f) Horseshoe kidneys are **fused** kidneys.

A2. Jenny Rose was born with her kidneys located within her bony pelvis. Explain the clinical significance.

_____

_____

A3. Circle the correct answers or fill in the blanks to answer the following questions about renal cysts and polycystic kidney disease (PKD).

(a) Renal cysts are *(solid? fluid-filled?)* cysts located between nephrons. Cysts may range in size from 1 or 2 mm to 5 cm (about ___ inch[es]). Signs and symptoms range from none to fatality. What are typical effects of larger cysts?

_____

(b) Polycystic kidney disease is one of the most *(common? rare?)* hereditary diseases in the United States and such disease is *(commonly? rarely?)* fatal. Match the type of cystic kidney disease with the correct description below. Choose from these answers:

ADPKD: Autosomal dominant polycystic kidney disease
ARPKD: Autosomal recessive polycystic kidney disease

(b1) Also known as adult PKD, the disorder is transmitted by different PKD genes; systemic effects are common and often serious, such as colon, liver or mitral valve disease, portal hypertension, or cerebral aneurysm: _____

(b2) Infantile or childhood form of PKD and relatively rare; usually bilateral and fatal because enlarged kidneys limit lung expansion: _____

(c) About five out of six cases of adult PKD involve the gene *(PDK1? PDK2?)* located on chromosome ____. This gene codes for *(carbohydrate? protein?)* known as _____. Such mutated genes contribute to formation of faulty *(glomeruli? renal tubules?)*.

A4. Explain why each of the following signs or symptoms may accompany polycystic disease.

(a) Hypertension

_____

(b) Hematuria

_____

(c) Flank pain

_____

(d) Infected kidneys

_____

B. OBSTRUCTIVE DISORDERS

B1. Identify possible causes of obstructions to urine flow.

_____

_____

_____

B2. Fill in the blanks to list the two major problems that arise from urinary tract obstructions.

(a) _____ of urine leading to _____ (discussed in section C below) and formation of kidney _____

(b) Back pressure that predisposes to _____

B3. Circle the correct answers or fill in the blanks within each statement about manifestations of urinary tract obstructions.

(a) Pain is more likely to occur with *(acute? chronic?)* obstructions. Severity of pain is more related to the *(degree? rate?)* of distension of urinary tract structures. Obstruction of the upper ureter is likely to cause pain in the *(flank area? testes of male or labia of female?)*.

(b) Hypertension is more likely to occur with *(bilateral? unilateral?)* obstruction in which renin secretion is *(increased? decreased?)*.

(c) The most common cause of upper urinary tract obstruction is _____. Stone formation requires a nucleus or _____ around which the stone forms. Identify the theory of stone formation in each of the following cases. Choose from these theories:

Inhibitor   Matrix   Saturation

(c1) The _____ theory proposes that the risk of stone formation increases when urine contains high levels of salts that form stones.

(c2) The _____ theory holds that mucopolysaccharides form the nidus of stones.

(c3) The _____ theory states that a lack of chemicals such as cephrocalcin or uropontin leads to crystal formation.

B4. Select the type of kidney stone that fits each description.

Calcium oxalate or calcium phosphate
Cystine   Struvite   Uric acid

(a) Occur in patients with gout when urine is abnormally acidic; these stones are not visible on x-rays: _____

(b) Known as "staghorn stones" because they conform to the shape of the renal pelvis (much like a stag's horns); almost always occur in the presence of UTIs and alkaline urine: _____

(c) About three quarters of all kidney stones are of this type: _____

B5. Mr. Laredo, age 68, has recently recovered from a fractured tibia that required immobilization for 2 months. He has benign prostatic hyperplasia (BPH) and a history of kidney stones. He is transported to the emergency room with excruciating pain in his left flank. Describe his condition by circling the correct answers or filling in the blanks.

(a) Mr. Laredo says his pain "comes and goes" and it intensifies. This is *(colicky? noncolicky?)* pain that suggests *(left? bilateral?)* kidney stones. Kidney stones are typically *(bi? uni?)*lateral.

(b) Mr. Laredo reports: "I tried drinking about a quart of water an hour ago—thought it might help this stone pass. But the pain just got worse." Explain.

_____

(c) Radiographs with intravenous dye *(are? are not?)* likely to help diagnose kidney stones. Mr. Laredo's stone is 1.2 cm and lodged in the left ureter. Because of its size, his stone *(is? is not?)* likely to "pass" on its own. The treatment of choice is:

(1) Extracorporeal shock wave lithotripsy
(2) Open stone surgery

(d) How may Mr. Laredo's stone be related to his BPH?

_____

(e) How may his stone be related to his fracture?

_____

(f) If Mr. Laredo were not treated promptly, he would be at increased risk for *(bilateral? unilateral?)* hydronephrosis. Prolongation of this condition causes *(reversible? irreversible?)* kidney damage.

C. URINARY TRACT INFECTIONS

C1. Choose the three true statements. (Pay particular attention to whether the **bold-faced** word or phrase makes the statement true or false.)

(a) Urinary tract infections (UTIs) are the **most common** type of bacterial infection seen in health care settings.

(b) Infections of the bladder (cystitis) are considered **less** serious than renal pelvis (pyelonephritis) infections.

(c) **Most** uncomplicated UTIs are caused by the gram-negative bacteria, *E. coli*.

(d) Most UTIs occur from spread of infections from **the bloodstream**.

(e) The urine present in the kidneys and in the bladder is usually **sterile**.

C2. Circle the person who is at greater risk of UTIs in each case and then give a brief rationale.

(a)
  (1) A 12-year-old girl
  (2) An 82-year-old woman

  _____

(b)
  (1) A sexually active 21-year-old woman
  (2) A sexually active 21-year-old man

  _____

(c)
  (1) A 60-year-old man with benign prostatic hyperplasia (BPH)
  (2) A 60-year-old woman

  _____

(d)
  (1) A healthy 40-year-old woman
  (2) A 40-year-old woman with multiple sclerosis who is regularly catheterized

  _____

C3. Circle the correct answer in each case to indicate whether the following factors cause *(C)* or help to prevent *(P)* UTIs. Then explain your answer.

(a) Bacterial fimbriae or pili: C P
  _____

(b) Vesicoureteral reflux (backflow from bladder to ureter): C P_____

(c) Mucin: C P _____

(d) IgAs: C P _____

C4. Rochelle, age 20, reports that she "has been urinating two or three times an hour, and it burns and itches and smells something awful. And my belly feels yucky." When the nurse asks more about pain, Rochelle states: "It's not sharp pain, my belly just feels really bad." She denies any pain "at the back of her waist." Her temperature is 99.8°F. A clean-voided urine sample is positive for leukocytes (pyuria) and the bacterium *E. coli*. Answer the following questions related to Rochelle's case.

(a) Rochelle's UTI is most likely to be a(n):
  (1) Lower UTI: cystitis (bladder infection) and possibly lower ureters
  (2) Upper UTI (pyelonephritis)

(b) UTIs are more common in women between ages *(15 and 24? 35 and 44?)*.

(c) Because Rochelle's diagnosis is an acute fungal UTI involving the urethra and bladder, treatment is likely to include an antifungal drug and *(increased? decreased?)* fluid intake. How does the latter help?

  _____

C5. Repeated urinary tract infections (UTIs) *(can? cannot?)* lead to scarring of urine pathways. Explain how this change leads to further UTIs.

  _____
  _____

C6. Explain why it is recommended that a pregnant woman have a urine culture performed at her first prenatal obstetric visit.

  _____
  _____

C7. Explain why early diagnosis of UTIs is especially important in each of these populations.

(a) Three-year-old children with febrile upper UTIs

  _____
  _____

(b) Elderly residents of nursing homes

  _____
  _____
  _____

D. DISORDERS OF GLOMERULAR FUNCTION

D1. Refer to Chapter 23, Questions A2(b) and (c), to review glomerular structure. Name the three layers: _____,
_____, _____.
In addition, mesangial cells cover areas of the glomerulus that *(have? lack?)* a basement membrane.

D2. Circle the correct answers in this overview of glomerular disorders and use the list of terms to complete the statements about major signs and symptoms. (One term will be used twice.)

Azotemia	Coagulation disorders
Edema	Infections
Oliguria	Hematuria
Hypertension	Hypoalbuminemia
Proteinuria	Pyuria

(a) Glomerulonephritis is a *(nephritic? nephrotic?)* condition that is a *(rare? common?)* cause of chronic renal failure (CRF) in the United States. The suffix "-itis" indicates that this *(is? is not?)* an inflammatory disorder that reduces GFR. But, paradoxically, the inflamed membrane does allow blood cells into urine.

   (a1) Because of decreased GFR, BUN and serum creatinine levels increase: _____

   (a2) Decreased GFR tends to decrease urinary output (_____) with fluid retention that leads to _____ and _____.

   (a3) Imagine gaping holes in inflamed glomerular membranes; these allow red blood cells to pass into urine, leading to the classic sign of cola-colored urine (_____). Presence of white blood cells in urine (_____) can also occur.

(b) *(Nephritic? Nephrotic?)* syndromes (or nephroses) involve damage to the glomerular membrane that allows protein and possibly lipids to escape into urine.

   (b1) The passage of proteins from blood to urine results in _____ and _____.

   (b2) Because depleted plasma proteins are not sufficient to create the osmotic "pull" of water into vessels, _____ occurs.

   (b3) Loss of immunoglobulin proteins into urine increases risk for _____, and loss of fibrinogen can cause _____.

D3. Ms. Gowland has a form of glomerulonephritis. Her urinary output is higher than normal with a specific gravity of 1.005. Explain.

_____

_____

_____

D4. Circle the correct answers or fill in the blanks to answer the following questions about causes and categories of glomerulonephritis.

(a) Most of these conditions *(are? are not?)* immune-related. Glomerular damage results from anti_____ that react with anti_____ on glomerular membranes (or from antigen-antibody complexes). These cause inflammatory changes in the membranes. List two or more sources of such antigens.

_____

(b) Glomerular disease that is widespread throughout kidneys is called *(diffuse? focal?)*. If it affects only certain segments of the glomerulus, it is called _____.

(c) Identify the type of damage to the glomerular wall that occurs in each of these categories of glomerulonephritis.

   Membranous   Proliferative   Sclerotic

   (c1) Increased collagen between cells: _____

   (c2) Increased number of cells in the glomerular wall: _____

   (c3) Increased thickness by deposits of antigen-antibody complexes: _____

D5. Match the selected types of glomerular disease with their descriptions. One answer will not be used.

Acute proliferative glomerulonephritis (APGN)
Chronic glomerulonephrosis
Focal segmental glomerulosclerosis (FSGS)
IgA nephropathy
Membranous glomerulonephritis (MGN)
Minimal change disease
Nephrotic syndrome
Rapidly progressive glomerulonephritis

(a) Dramatically increased permeability of glomeruli to proteins leads to the hallmark sign of this disorder: proteinuria more than 3.5 g/day causing systemic and pulmonary edema; altered lipid metabolism also occurs; usually primary in children; may occur as MGN or FSGS, or secondary to diabetes or lupus: _____

(b) Involves increased collagen laid down in some but not all glomeruli; occurs in sickle cell disease, some congenital heart defects, with drug use or HIV; usually does lead to renal failure: _____

(c) Most commonly occurs 1 or 2 weeks post–strep infection as antigen-antibody complexes build up; occurs mainly in children and has a 95% survival rate; cola-colored urine is a typical first sign:

_____

(d) Involves severe glomerular injury that progresses within months; no known cause, but can be associated with SLE or with Goodpasture syndrome; involves formation of crescent-shaped structures that fill Bowman's space: _____

(e) May occur as a primary disorder affecting only kidneys, from lack of resolution of acute glomerular disease (such as APGN), or secondary to systemic disorders like diabetes or hypertension; gradual progression to end-stage renal disease:

_____

(f) Involves fusion of foot processes from the epithelial layer of the glomerular membrane; peak incidence is between 2 and 6 years of age: _____

(g) Involves deposition of antigen-antibody complexes in the glomeruli; most common cause of glomerular nephritis in Asians: _____

D6. André, age 17, was diagnosed with diabetes mellitus at age 12. Answer the following questions related to his case.

(a) About 1 in *(3? 6? 10?)* people with type 1 diabetes develops diabetic nephropathy. Diabetes more commonly damages the *(glomerulus? renal tubule?).*

(b) It is likely that André's glomerular membrane is becoming *(thinner? thicker?)* or sclerosing (see Question D4[c1]). At least part of this change results from incorporation of excessive blood _____ into the glomerular wall.

(c) At this early stage of glomerulosclerosis, André's GFR is likely to be abnormally *(high? low?),* enlarging glomerular pores. Protein in his urine then becomes *(dramatically? slightly?)* elevated, a predictor of future nephropathy. Such changes *(are? are not?)* likely to be minimized by control of blood sugar and blood pressure.

(d) André has taken up smoking. Smoking cessation *(is? is not?)* likely to reduce his degree of diabetic nephropathy.

D7. Is glomerular disease a cause or effect of chronic hypertension?

_____

E. TUBULOINTERSTITIAL DISORDERS

E1. Answer the following questions about tubulointerstitial disorders.

(a) Circle the areas in nephrons that are most affected by tubulointerstitial disorders.

DCT   Glomerulus   PCT
Interstitium   Loop of Henle

(b) Tubulointerstitial disorders can have rapid onset (acute disorders) or gradual onset (chronic disorders). Circle the examples of acute disorders:

Acute hypersensitivity reaction to drugs
Acute pyelonephritis
Chronic pyelonephritis
Interstitial fibrosis
Mononuclear infiltrates

(c) Select the type of tubulointerstitial disorder (listed in part [b]) that fits each description.

(c1) Bacterial infection superimposed on obstructive urinary tract abnormalities; can result in renal scarring and atrophy; responsible for up to 20% or all cases of end-stage renal disease (ESRD): _____

(c2) Abrupt onset with chills, fever, headache, back pain and general malaise; possibly dysuria and urgency; treatment includes antimicrobial drugs with possible hospitalization:

_____

(c3) First noted 2 to 40 days after administration of sulfonamide drugs (in medications such as thiazide diuretics) to allergic persons; accompanied by fever, high eosinophil count, blood in urine, elevated protein levels in urine, and possibly rash; recovery usually follows withdrawal of the drug: _____

E2. List several other drugs that can be nephrotoxic.

_____

_____

E3. Define the following terms that are manifestations of early stage tubulointerstitial disorders and explain causes.

(a) Polyuria and nocturia

_____

_____

(b) Edema of renal interstitium

_____

E4. Explain why kidneys are at high risk for damage by toxic drugs.

_____

_____

E5. Mrs. Stein, age 75, has rheumatoid arthritis and hypertension. Explain why she may be at increased risk for drug-related nephropathy.

_____

_____

F. NEOPLASMS

F1. Wilms tumor is a kidney tumor of *(young children? adults?)*. Incidence is *(higher? no greater?)* in children with congenital genitourinary anomalies. Almost all cases are *(bi? uni?)*lateral. Most common presenting symptoms are abdominal mass and *(hyper? hypo?)*tension. With aggressive treatment, survival is about ___%.

F2. Adult renal carcinoma (kidney cancer) is most likely to affect persons who are *(20? 40? 60?)* years old. The most common presenting sign is *(an abdominal mass? hematuria?)*. It is most commonly detected in *(early? late?)* stages. The treatment of choice is _____ectomy. Persons in stage *(I? IV?)* of the disease are likely to have a 5-year survival rate of 65% to 85%.

CHAPTER 25

Renal Failure

■ Review Questions

A. ACUTE RENAL FAILURE

A1. Choose the two true statements. (Pay particular attention to whether the **bold-faced** word or phrase makes the statement true or false.)

(a) Acute renal failure (ARF) is potentially **reversible,** whereas chronic renal failure (CRF) **is not.**

(b) The mortality rate of patients with ARF in intensive care units is about **4% to 8%.**

(c) The most common sign of ARF is increase in blood levels of **BUN and creatinine.**

(d) ARF is most likely to be caused by **postrenal** causes.

(e) Mortality rate from ARF **has** decreased markedly over the past 40 years.

A2. Refer to Chart 25-1 in *Essentials of Pathophysiology* and identify the category or cause of acute renal failure in each case. Select from these answers:

Intrinsic (intrarenal)   Postrenal   Prerenal

(a) Decreased renal perfusion as by hemorrhage, shock, or renal vasoconstriction: _____

(b) Prostatic hyperplasia or bladder cancer: _____

(c) Long-term use of NSAIDs for control of arthritis pain or acute pyelonephritis: _____

(d) Most commonly caused by acute tubular necrosis (ATN): _____

(e) Heart failure: _____

A3. Circle the correct answers or fill in the blank within each statement about acute renal failure (ARF).

(a) In ARF, both glomerular filtration rate (GFR) and urinary output *(increase? decrease?).* The ratio of BUN to creatinine is more likely to be *(10:1? 25:1?)* because

the small amount of creatinine that is filtered is *(largely? not?)* reabsorbed.

(b) Signs and symptoms of renal failure do not typically occur until renal perfusion falls to about _____% of normal. Ischemia is more likely to destroy cells of *(glomeruli? tubules?)* because of their greater oxygen demands. Toxins are also more damaging to *(glomeruli? tubules?).* An early sign of tubular damage is inability of kidneys to _____ urine, a condition that may mask a decrease in GFR.

A4. Identify the most likely cause of acute tubular necrosis (ATN) in each case.

Ischemia   Intratubular obstruction
Nephrotoxic

(a) Mr. Barkley is undergoing cisplatin chemotherapy for his cancer: _____

(b) Elena's urinary output decreases while she is taking the aminoglycoside kanamycin to treat her infection: _____

(c) Nate completes his first marathon but is hospitalized shortly after this extreme exertion with severely reduced urinary output and tea-colored urine: _____

(d) Allesandra has been in the children's burn unit for 2 weeks following severe burns and multiple fractures: _____

(e) Mrs. Daugherty's recovery from open-heart surgery for valve replacement is complicated by prolonged renal hypoperfusion that requires her to be on renal dialysis: _____

A5. Mr. Yoho's 24-hour urine output is 640 mL; his BUN is 32 g/dL, and his creatinine level is 1.7 g/dL. His potassium level is 6.2 mEq/L. Mr. Yoho is likely to be in the _____ of acute tubular necrosis (ATN).

(a) Initial phase

(b) Maintenance phase

(c) Recovery or repair phase

A6. Explain why early diagnosis of acute renal failure is critical, especially for elderly persons.

_____

_____

_____

B. CHRONIC RENAL FAILURE

B1. Circle the correct answers or fill in the blanks to answer the following questions about kidneys.

(a) Kidneys have *(a high level of? very limited?)* compensatory abilities.

(b) In chronic renal failure (CRF), which functions decrease?

(1) Glomerular filtration

(2) Reabsorption

(3) Renal endocrine function

(c) The outlook for chronic renal failure (CRF) patients has *(improved? gotten much worse?)* over the past three decades.

(d) Which is a more accurate indicator of GFR?

(1) BUN

(2) Serum creatinine level

Explain.

_____

(e) Write a normal value for serum BUN: _____ mg/dL. In renal failure, this value can rise as high as _____ mg/dL.

(f) Write a normal value for serum creatinine: _____ mg/dL. When renal function is 10% of normal, this value can rise as high as _____ mg/dL.

(g) Write a normal value for glomerular filtration rate (GFR) for a healthy 25-year-old: _____ mL/min.

B2. Arrange the four phases of renal failure listed here from least serious to most serious.

Diminished renal reserve (DRR)
End-stage renal disease (ESRD)
Renal failure (RF)   Renal insufficiency (RI)

_____ → _____ → _____ → _____

Identify the phase of chronic renal failure demonstrated in each case below.

(a) Mr. Ash, age 49, has type 2 diabetes. His blood pressure is 148/92 even when taking antihypertensive medication; his GFR is 32% of normal and he has signs of azotemia: _____

(b) Mrs. LaRocca, age 61, has only one kidney following nephrectomy for renal carcinoma 5 years earlier. Her blood pressure is 136/82, GFR is 60%, BUN is 21 mg/dL, and her creatinine level is 1.1 mg/dL: _____

(c) Mrs. Rodriguez-Rivera's GFR is 14% of normal. Her feet and ankles are so swollen that she can wear only large slippers on her feet. Her hematocrit is 27, her arterial pH is about 7.25, and she is lethargic: _____

B3. Contrast *azotemia* with *uremia*.

_____

_____

_____

B4. Explain why patients with CRF may become overhydrated and edematous or may become dehydrated.

_____

_____

_____

B5. Insert arrows to indicate how blood levels, chemicals, or other factors change with chronic renal failure ($\uparrow$ = increase; $\downarrow$ = decrease).

(a) Na^+: ____

(b) K^+: ____ when in severe CRF (GFR = 5 mL/min)

(c) H^+: ____ (so pH ____) with buffering by bone leading to ____ in bone density

(d) PO_4^{-3} ____, which may be treated by *(increasing? decreasing?)* intake (especially in dairy products)

(e) Active vitamin D levels ____, which causes ____ in blood levels of Ca^{2+}

(f) Ca^{2+}: ____, which causes ____ secretion of PTH, which causes ____ in bone density

(g) Red blood cell count and hematocrit: ____

B6. Circle the correct answers or fill in the blanks within each statement about CRF.

  (a) Blood levels of PO_4^{-3} and Ca^{2+} are *(directly? inversely?)* related. Because kidneys fail to excrete ____, they excrete excessive amounts of ____.

  (b) Most people with end-stage renal disease (ESRD) tend to develop *(hyper? hypo?)*parathyroidism.

  (c) Osteodystrophy derives from the electrolyte changes shown in Question B5(d–f) and involves *(increased? decreased?)* bone mineralization. One form of this bone disorder, osteitis fibrosa, involves *(over? under?)*active bone cells; cysts may form in porous spaces.

  (d) Osteomalacia is another form of renal osteodystrophy, in which bones are *(softer? more brittle?)* than normal, which is related to a *(high? low?)* turnover of bone, as osteoblast activity *(increases? decreases?)*. Two factors that cause this condition are _____ deficiency and high blood _____ that occur with CRF. Until recently, osteomalacia was common among CRF patients on _____ who developed high blood levels of _____ from the procedure.

B7. Identify which system involves the signs and symptoms below. Choose from these answers:

Cardiovascular   Gastrointestinal
Hematologic   Immune
Integumentary   Neurologic
Reproductive

  (a) Uremic encephalopathy caused by toxic substances in blood: _____

  (b) Restless legs syndrome and asterixis: _____

  (c) Pruritus resulting from presence of phosphate or urea crystals; Terry's nails, in which nails are thin and brittle with dark and white bands: _____

  (d) Impotence (in half of men on dialysis) and amenorrhea: _____

  (e) Failure to develop a fever in the presence of infection: _____

  (f) Metallic taste in the mouth that may lead to anorexia: _____

  (g) The system most responsible for death in end-stage renal disease: _____

  (h) Decreased erythropoietin production by kidneys: _____ and _____

B8. Give rationales for the following interventions for chronic renal failure.

  (a) rhEPO and iron supplements

  _____

  _____

  (b) Salt and water restriction

  _____

  (c) Adjustment (often lowering) of medication dosages and caution taking over-the-counter (OTC) drugs

  _____

  (d) Restriction of dairy products

  _____

  (e) Caution about types of antacids used

  _____

B9. Explain why the outlook for chronic renal failure (CRF) patients has improved in recent years.

  _____

  _____

B10. Contrast forms of dialysis for end-stage renal failure patients by writing *H* for hemodialysis or *P* for peritoneal dialysis.

  (a) A cellophane membrane is involved in the dialysis: ___

  (b) A sterile dialyzing glucose solution (usually 2 L) is instilled into the abdominal cavity for a period of time as the glucose osmotically draws metabolic wastes from blood vessels in the peritoneal membrane: ____

  (c) Usually requires an arteriovenous fistula and heparin: ____

  (d) Dialysis usually is performed three times a week to remove impurities and restore electrolytes: ____

B11. Answer the following questions about Hye-Sun, age 35, who has ESRD that was caused by glomerulonephropathy. She is receiving hemodialysis.

  (a) Hye-Sun's diet is likely to be relatively *(high? low?)* in protein and phosphates. Are eggs and meats likely to be contraindicated in her diet? *(Yes? No?)* Explain.

  _____

(b) Why should Hye-Sun avoid taking penicillin for infections and consuming foods such as orange juice and chocolate?

_____

(c) She experiences nausea and vomiting as well as muscle cramps during the dialysis. Are these normal side effects of the procedure? _____

(d) Hye-Sun is constantly thirsty. Explain.

_____

(e) The fact that she has gained 13 lb since her last dialysis treatment 3 days ago suggests edema involving retention (possibly from drinking) of ___ liters of fluid.

C. RENAL FAILURE IN CHILDREN AND ELDERLY PERSONS

C1. Billy, age 17 months, has chronic renal failure from a congenital kidney disorder. He is currently on dialysis therapy as he awaits a transplant. Answer the following questions related to his case.

(a) Renal osteodystrophy is *(more? less?)* likely to exert damaging effects in a child than in an adult. Explain.

_____

(b) *(Nutrition? Gonadotropic hormone?)* is the key factor in bone maturation during infancy.

(c) Billy is having CAPD treatment; CAPD refers to _____ _____ _____ dialysis that *(does? does not?)* allow him to walk around (ambulate) during his treatments.

(d) After Billy does receive a transplant, he is likely to be at increased risk for infections. Explain why.

_____

C2. Circle the correct answers or fill in the blank within each statement.

(a) GFR *(does? does not?)* tend to decrease with normal aging; as a result, nephrotoxic drugs are likely to exert *(greater? fewer?)* effects on older adults.

(b) In an 80-year-old, a decreased GFR *(is? is not?)* as likely to increase blood creatinine to high levels as in a 30-year-old. Explain.

_____

(c) Oliguria and cola-colored urine are more likely the first signs of renal failure in *(elderly? younger?)* persons.

(d) State one factor that may increase survival rate from kidney transplant in elderly persons.

_____

CHAPTER 26

Disorders of Urine Elimination

■ Review Questions

A. CONTROL OF URINE ELIMINATION

A1. The elimination of urine from the bladder is a process known as _____. Circle the correct answers or fill in the blanks to answer the following questions about the structures involved in this process.

  (a) The floor of the bladder is composed of the triangular muscle known as the *(detrusor? trigone?)* with its three corners marked by openings. Two corners have openings from *(ureters? urethra?)*, structures about 30 cm (___ inches) long, that carry urine from kidneys to bladder. These openings *(do? do not?)* have valves. Explain.

  _____

  _____

  (b) The other opening empties into the *(ureter? urethra?)* and is surrounded by the internal sphincter; it is longer in *(females? males?)*.

  (c) The empty bladder *(is smooth? has folds known as rugae?)*.

  (d) Arrange the layers of the bladder wall in correct sequence from outside to inside.

Mucosa (transitional epithelium)
Submucosa   Muscle
Serous membrane (continuous with peritoneum)

  _____, _____,

  _____, _____

  (e) Most of the bladder wall consists of the _____ muscle, which has *(great? little?)* distensibility. When it does contract, micturition is *(stimulated? inhibited?)*. The detrusor muscle can be thought of as the *("stop"? "go"?)* muscle. Simultaneously, the *(internal? external?)* sphincter is pulled open, causing urine to *(flow out of? stay within?)* the bladder.

  (f) Contraction of the *(internal? external?)* sphincter at the base of the bladder causes urine to *(flow out of? stay within?)* the bladder. It helps to maintain *(continence? incontinence?)*, which is the ability to

  _____.

A2. Refer to Table 26-1 as well as Figure 26-2 in *Essentials of Pathophysiology.* Answer the following questions about regulation of micturition.

Table 26-1 Innervation of Urinary Structures Regulating Micturition

Type of Nerves (Motor)	Source of Nerves	Voluntary or Involuntary	Structure Innervated	Effect on Micturition (Stop/Go)
Parasympathetic (pelvic nerves) (cholinergic)	S2-S4	Involuntary	Detrusor	Stimulates ("go")
Sympathetic (sympathetic nerves) (adrenergic)	T11-L2	Involuntary	Trigone and internal sphincter	Inhibits ("stop")
Lower motorneurons (pelvic nerves)	S2-S4	Voluntary (somatic)	Detrusor	Stimulates ("go")
Lower motorneurons (pudendal nerves)	S2-S4	Voluntary (somatic)	External sphincter	Inhibits ("stop")

(a) The (*parasympathetic? sympathetic?*) division of the autonomic nervous system inhibits ("stops") micturition. These nerves stimulate contraction of the trigone and the ___ternal sphincter, and relax the _____. In other words, during stress, when the sympathetic nerves predominate, the focus (*is? is not?*) on urinating, and urine is allowed to distend the bladder. _____ drugs mimic sympathetic nerves.

(b) Parasympathetic nerves arise from levels (*T11 to L2? S2 to S4?*) of the cord and pass to the detrusor through (*pelvic? pudendal?*) nerves. These cause the flow of urine to (*"stop"? "go"?*). These nerves are (*adrenergic? cholinergic?*). Medications that relax detrusor muscles (to slow down "hyperactive bladder") and therefore "stop" micturition (in persons with "overactive bladder") are (*cholinergic? anticholinergic?*).

(c) External sphincter control is (*involuntary? voluntary?*) or somatic and carried by (*pelvic? pudendal?*) nerves. External sphincter action is (*increased? decreased?*) by skeletal muscle relaxants.

(d) All the nerves discussed in A2(a–c) are (*motor? sensory?*). Afferent (sensory) nerves accompany (*sympathetic? parasympathetic? voluntary?*) nerves. They alert the CNS (including the micturition center in the _____) of bladder distention. In infants, reflex contraction of the (*detrusor? external sphincter?*) and relaxation of the _____ results. After further growth of sphincters and bladder training, overriding nerve impulses initiated from the _____ can inhibit micturition until the appropriate time and setting are reached.

A3. Circle the correct answers to explain why a man is not likely to expel semen and urine at the same time. During ejaculation, (*sympathetic? parasympathetic?*) nerves contract the (*detrusor? trigone and internal sphincter?*) so that urination (*does? does not?*) accompany ejaculation.

A4. Normal capacity of the bladder is about _____ mL. The sensation of fullness is normally perceived at about _____ mL. When the bladder is emptied adequately, less than _____ mL should remain (postvoided residual volume, or PVR).

A5. Match each method for evaluating bladder function with the correct description.

Cystoscopy   Excretory urography
Postvoided residual volume (PVR)
Ultrasound bladder scan

(a) Uses radiopaque dye plus CT, MRI, or US: _____

(b) Measures the volume of urine left in the bladder after urination: _____

(c) Noninvasive method for evaluating bladder volume: _____

(d) Direct visualization of the inside of the bladder: _____

A6. Fill in the blanks about bladder control.

(a) Joshua is a healthy 5-year-old; his bladder capacity is likely to be _____ oz (____ mL).

(b) By 5 years of age, _____ % of children are continent during the day, and _____ % are likely to be continent at night.

(c) List several factors that regulate conscious control of bladder function.

_____

_____

_____

B. ALTERATIONS IN BLADDER FUNCTION

B1. List the two major categories of alterations in bladder function. Then write the two mechanisms that can lead to either B1(a) or B1(b).

(a) _____

(b) _____

_____

B2. Explain how each of the following factors can obstruct urine outflow through the urethra.

(a) Myelomeningocele

_____

(b) Gonorrhea

_____

(c) Fecal impaction

_____

(d) Prostatic hyperplasia

_____

B3. In response to urinary obstruction, two major compensatory mechanisms relieve distention of the bladder. Answer the following questions about these mechanisms.

(a) Bladder wall *(a? hyper?)*trophy occurs. Ultimately, the thickened wall becomes ischemic and _____ sets in before the bladder is emptied. *(Frequent? Infrequent?)* attempts at urination result. The bladder wall may form pockets known as diverticulas that increase risk for _____. Hypertrophy can also cause back pressure against ureters, leading to _____.

(b) *(Hypo? Hyper?)*sensitivity of the bladder to filling and stretching occurs. This leads to _____ and _____.

B4. List five signs of acute retention of urine.

_____

_____

_____

B5. Circle the correct answers or fill in the blanks to answer the following questions about spastic or flaccid bladder disorders resulting from neural dysfunction.

(a) Name two or more cerebral disorders that can cause neurogenic bladder.

_____

(b) Neurogenic bladder can produce two opposite effects. One is failure to *(store? empty?)* urine; this is a *(spastic? flaccid?)* bladder dysfunction that is likely to accompany spinal cord injury (SCI) *(above? at?)* S2–S4 levels of the cord. This condition, called bladder *(a? hyper?)*reflexia, also occurs during the first few months immediately after SCI, regardless of level of injury.

(c) Another form of neurogenic bladder, failure to store urine, is more likely to occur with *(higher? lower?)* SCI, such as at level *(T6 to T7? S2 to S4?)* of the cord. In such cases, the bladder is being controlled by *(spinal cord? brainstem?)* reflexes and is *(a? hyper?)*reflexic.

(d) Decreased perception of bladder filling can lead to bladder overfilling. Name two disorders that cause such afferent nerve neuropathies and also affect motor neurons leading to flaccid bladder. _____,

_____

(e) In detrusor-sphincter dyssynergia, when the bladder wall contracts, the external sphincter *(constricts? dilates?)*, causing intravesicular pressure to *(increase? decrease?)*.

(f) Sabrina gave birth to a baby a week ago and she has a vaginal infection. Otherwise, she is in good health. Which disorder of urinary elimination is she most likely to have?

(1) Flaccid bladder dysfunction

(2) Bladder dysfunction caused by peripheral neuropathy

(3) Nonrelaxing external sphincter

(g) List several interventions for flaccid bladder.

_____

_____

B6. Complete Table 26-2.

Table 26-2. Medications to Treat Neurogenic Bladder Incontinence

Type of Medication	Mimics (P?S?)	Effect on Detrusor	Useful to Treat
(a) Cholinergic	__	Stimulates	_____
(b) Anticholinergic	__	_____	Spastic bladder
(c) Adrenergic	__	Relaxes	_____

B7. Select the category of urinary incontinence that fits each case.

Overflow Urge (overactive bladder)
Stress Other cause

(a) Mr. Laredo, age 68, has benign prostatic hyperplasia (BPH): _____

(b) Ms. Patterson, age 56, has given birth to six children; she states that urine "leaks a little" when she coughs or laughs: _____

(c) Mrs. Winston, age 93 and a resident of a skilled nursing facility, has recurrent fecal impaction: _____

(d) Mr. Aguilar has been diagnosed with Alzheimer disease. He was transferred to an Alzheimer unit yesterday: _____

(e) Ms. Marshall-Petersen, age 61, has osteoarthritis and early stages of Parkinson disease. She is aware of the urge to urinate, but she cannot get to the toilet in time; her physician has just prescribed an anticholinergic medication (oxybutynin): _____

(f) Mrs. Aufman takes a diuretic for her heart failure; she also takes a "sleeping pill": _____

B8. Describe the following interventions for incontinence.

(a) Kegel's exercises that strengthen pelvic floor muscles

_____

_____

_____

(b) Habit training (voiding on a regular schedule)

_____

_____

_____

(c) Surgically implanted inflatable cuff

_____

_____

_____

B9. Urinary incontinence occurs more often in *(elderly? younger?)* persons. Explain.

_____

_____

_____

_____

C. CANCER OF THE BLADDER

C1. Choose the three true statements. (Pay particular attention to whether the **bold-faced** word or phrase makes the statement true or false.)

(a) Bladder cancer is a **rare** form of urinary tract cancer.

(b) Almost all bladder cancers derive from the **epithelial** lining of the bladder.

(c) The 5-year survival rate for noninvasive bladder cancer is **24%.**

(d) Cigarette smoking **is** associated with bladder cancer.

(e) Chronic bladder infections **increase** risk of bladder cancer.

C2. Answer the following questions about bladder cancer.

(a) State the most common sign of bladder cancer.

_____

List other signs.

_____

_____

(b) State possible complications of bladder cancer other than metastases.

_____

(c) Treatment with diathermy involves *(electrocautery? external beam radiation?).* Intravesicular chemotherapy refers to administration of cytotoxic drugs into the *(urinary bladder? pelvic cavity?).* If the bladder is removed (a procedure known as _____), urinary diversion is typically effected by creating an alternative urine reservoir from the part of the small intestine known as the _____.

CHAPTER 27

Structure and Function of the Gastrointestinal System

■ Review Questions

A. STRUCTURE AND ORGANIZATION OF THE GASTROINTESTINAL TRACT

A1. Complete this overview of the digestive system.

(a) Write a brief description of functions of the digestive system.

_____

_____

_____

(b) Contrast the gastrointestinal (GI) tract with its accessory organs.

_____

_____

_____

(c) What is the lumen of the GI tract?

_____

_____

A2. Refer to text Figure 27-1 in *Essentials of Pathophysiology* and answer these questions about parts of the GI tract.

(a) Name the organs of the upper GI tract.

_____

The *(pharynx? esophagus?)* is the throat.

(b) The esophagus is about *(10? 25?)* inches long. Its *(upper? lower?)* sphincter normally prevents gastric reflux. The esophagus empties into the *(cardiac? fundic? pyloric?)* portion of the stomach.

(c) The wall of the stomach normally offers *(minimal? great?)* distensibility. The _____ portion of the stomach is attached to the small intestine.

(d) Arrange the parts of the small intestine from first to last in the pathway of food.

Duodenum   Ileum   Jejunum

_____ → _____ → _____

(e) Arrange these parts of the large intestine from first to last in the route of wastes.

Ascending colon   Anus
Cecum   Descending colon
Rectum   Sigmoid colon
Transverse colon

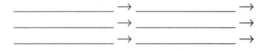

_____ → _____ →
_____ → _____ →
_____ → _____ →
_____

(f) The appendix normally arises from the _____. (Select an answer from the list in Question A2[e].)

A3. Answer these questions about the GI wall.

(a) Arrange the layers of the wall from the deepest to the most superficial.

Mucosa   Muscularis
Peritoneum   Submucosa

_____ → _____ →
_____ → _____

(b) Match the layers of the GI wall (from Question A3[a]) with the following descriptions:

(b1) The largest serous membrane in the body: _____

(b2) Epithelial cells in this layer are replaced every 4 to 5 days: _____

(b3) Composed largely of blood vessels, nerves, and glands: _____

(b4) Consists of circular and longitudinal layers; the myenteric (Auerbach) nerve plexus is located between these layers: _____

A4. Circle the correct answer or fill in the blanks within each statement about the peritoneum and its extensions.

(a) The *(parietal? visceral?)* layer of peritoneum adheres to the outside of organs of the abdomen and pelvis, whereas the _____ layer lines the abdominopelvic cavity. The accumulation of abnormally large volumes of fluid between these membranes is a condition known as

_____.

(b) The *(greater omentum? lesser omentum? mesentery?)* supports loops of small intestine and provides routes for blood and lymph vessels and nerves. The *(greater? lesser?)* omentum anchors the stomach to the liver.

B. INNERVATION AND MOTILITY

B1. Circle the correct answers or fill in the blanks within each statement about control of movement of the GI tract wall.

(a) Most of the wall of the GI tract contains *(skeletal? smooth?)* muscle. Peristalsis is an example of *(rhythmic? tonic?)* movement of this muscle.

(b) Of the two plexuses that control the GI tract, the *(myenteric? submucosal?)* regulates both motility and secretion.

(c) The *(parasympathetic? sympathetic?)* division of the autonomic nervous system (ANS) stimulates motility and secretion of most of the GI tract. The _____ nerves transmit such impulses to the stomach, small intestine, cecum, and the first half of the colon. The _____ nerves carry parasympathetic fibers to the last portions of the colon. Excessive vagal or other parasympathetic nerve impulses *(overexcite? inhibit?)* GI activity.

(d) Sympathetic nerves *(decrease? increase?)* blood flow to the GI tract, *(stimulate? inhibit?)* contractions of the GI wall, and *(stimulate? inhibit?)* contractions of the GI sphincters. The overall effect of the sympathetic nerves is to *(decrease? increase?)* GI activity.

(e) Enteric nerves exert local control because they *(are located within? extend outside of?)* the GI wall. Afferent nerves carry *(sensory? motor?)* impulses.

B2. Choose the two true statements about swallowing. (Pay particular attention to whether the **bold-faced** word or phrase makes the statement true or false.)

(a) The three phrases of the swallowing process are **oral, pharyngeal,** and **esophageal.**

(b) During swallowing, the **soft palate** normally prevents the bolus of food from entering the nasopharynx.

(c) The control center for swallowing is located in the **cerebral cortex.**

(d) Cranial nerve X (the vagus) regulates the **oral** and **pharyngeal** phases of swallowing.

B3. Describe the major factor that normally prevents esophageal reflux.

_____

_____

B4. Fill in the blanks or circle the correct answers to complete this exercise about gastric and intestinal motility.

(a) Typically, gastric peristaltic contractions are initiated by a "pacemaker" in the stomach wall at a rate of _____ contractions per minute; each contraction lasts up to _____ seconds.

(b) List several factors that normally prevent premature emptying of chyme from the stomach.

_____

_____

(c) Diabetic neuropathy is more likely to lead to gastric *(atony and retention? dumping?)*.

(d) *(Propulsive movements? Segmentation waves?)* move chyme alternately forward and backward. Explain how these movements help digestion.

_____

(e) Propulsive movements ultimately convey chyme through the *(pyloric? ileocecal?)* sphincter into the large intestine.

(f) Explain how motility of the small and large bowel can be easily assessed.

_____

(g) Where do haustration movements occur?

_____

(h) Mass movements of the colon involve propulsion of *(small? large?)* amounts of wastes. How often do these typically occur?

_____

B5. Circle the correct answers or fill in the blank within each statement about defecation.

(a) Defecation is initiated by movement of feces into the *(rectum? anus?)*. Afferent impulses travel into the _____ segments of the spinal cord. Reflex *(sympathetic?*

parasympathetic?) impulses then travel to relax the *(external? internal?)* sphincter to allow feces to be expelled.

(b) Simultaneously sacral impulses pass to the cerebral cortex, which can send impulses to the *(external? internal?)* sphincter to override the process and stop defecation if the timing is not appropriate.

C. HORMONAL AND SECRETORY FUNCTION

C1. A total of approximately ___ liters (quarts) of fluid is secreted into the GI tract each day. List the three major mechanisms that regulate GI secretion.

_____

_____

_____

As described earlier, the *(sympathetic? parasympathetic?)* division of the ANS plays the major role in stimulating motility and secretion.

C2. Select the hormone that fits each description.

Cholecystokinin (CCK)   Gastrin
Ghrelin   Glucose-dependent
Secretin   insulinotropic
                                           polypeptide (GIP)

(a) Stimulates production of alkaline pancreatic secretions that neutralize acids from the stomach:

_____

(b) Stimulates production of pancreatic secretions rich in digestive enzymes; also stimulates contraction of the gallbladder:

_____

(c) Stimulates gastric secretion and motility; enhances blood flow to the stomach:

_____

(d) Inhibits food intake, so helps to control meal size: _____

(e) An incretin hormone, it increases insulin release: _____

(f) Stimulates appetite and digestion as well as release of growth hormone: _____

(g) Hormones in this list that are not made by the intestine: _____

C3. Choose the two true statements. (Pay particular attention to whether the **bold-faced** word or phrase makes the statement true or false.)

(a) Sympathetic activity, for example, during stressful times, **decreases** salivary flow and duodenal mucus production.

(b) The salivary glands produce a **protein-digesting** enzyme.

(c) Mumps is an inflammation of the **sublingual** glands.

(d) Most of the GI secretions produced each day are made by combined efforts of the **stomach** and the **small intestine.**

(e) Brunner glands are **gastric** cells that produce **mucus.**

C4. Select the gastric secretion that fits each description.

Gastrin   Ghrelin
Hydrochloric acid   Intrinsic factor
Mucus   Pepsinogen

(a) The only chemical listed that is a hormone; secreted by cells lining the pylorus:

_____

(b) Produced by chief cells within gastric pits, this is the inactive form of the protease pepsin: _____

(c) Deficiency causes a type of anemia resulting from lack of vitamin B_{12}:

_____

(d) Cells that produce this chemical are harmed by chronic use of "barrier breakers," such as aspirin or nonsteroidal anti-inflammatory drugs (NSAIDs): _____

(e) Two secretions produced by parietal cells in gastric pits: _____ and

_____

(f) A newly discovered hormone involved with gut-brain regulation:

_____

C5. Match the organ with the chemicals it produces.

Large intestine   Small intestine
Salivary glands   Stomach

(a) Enzymes that complete digestion by breakdown of dipeptides and disaccharides:

_____

(b) Mucus and a starch-digesting enzyme:

_____

(c) Enzymes that produce pepsinogen and HCl, which initiate protein digestion:

_____

(d) Mucus but no digestive enzymes:

_____

D. DIGESTION AND ABSORPTION

D1. Answer the following questions about digestion.

(a) Explain why foods must be digested.

_____

_____

(b) Almost all digestion occurs in the *(stomach? small intestine? colon?)*. List three structural features of the small intestine that enhance its ability to carry out digestion.

_____

_____

_____

(c) Distinguish the functions of these cells on villi:

(c1) Goblet cells

_____

(c2) Enterocytes and brush border enzymes

_____

(d) Describe the roles of lacteals.

_____

D2. Refer to Table 27-1. Fill in the blanks or circle the correct answer within each of the following statements.

(a) Digestion of starch begins in the _____. Name two organs that produce amylase to digest starch into disaccharides: _____ , _____

(b) The disaccharide lactase normally breaks down lactose into _____ and _____. Describe the effects of lactase deficiency.

_____

_____

(c) _____ and _____ are the products of the disaccharide sucrose. Which of these simple sugars does not require adenosine triphosphate (ATP) for absorption? _____ Which requires ATP and a sodium-dependent carrier for absorption? _____

(d) Which organ secretes virtually all of the enzymes that digest fats? _____ In which part of the small intestine does most fat absorption take place? _____ Which chemical is needed for absorption of fat-soluble vitamins and products of fat digestion? _____ Circle the fat-soluble vitamins: A B C D E K

(e) Steatorrhea refers to _____ in the stool. What does this condition indicate?

_____

(f) Most proteases are produced in *(active? inactive?)* form. Explain.

_____

_____

Table 27-1 Roles of Digestive Organs in Secreting Enzymes and Other Chemicals*

Organ	Carbohydrates	Proteins	Lipids	Other Functions
Salivary glands	Amylase	—	—	Mucus
Stomach	—	Pepsinogen	—	HCl, intrinsic factor
Pancreas	Amylase	Trypsinogen, chymo-trypsinogen, carboxypeptidase	Lipase	Bicarbonate
Liver	—	—	—	Bile
Small intestine	Brush border enzymes: disaccharidases (lactase, maltase, sucrase)	Brush border enzymes: dipeptidases	—	Mucus
Large intestine	—	—	—	Mucus

*Note: Hormones are not included.

(g) Name two inactive precursors of proteases and their active counterparts.

_____

_____

(h) Circle the two types of products of digestion that are absorbed into blood capillaries within villi.
   (1) Amino acids from protein digestion
   (2) Monosaccharides from carbohydrate digestion
   (3) Fatty acids from fat digestion

E. ANOREXIA, NAUSEA, AND VOMITING

E1. Define anorexia.

_____

List three or more factors than can trigger anorexia.

_____

_____

_____

E2. Explain links among nausea, vomiting, and anorexia.

_____

_____

Circle the correct answers or fill in the blanks to answer the following questions about nausea, vomiting, and anorexia.

(a) Control centers for appetite are located in the *(hypothalamus? medulla? thalamus?),*

whereas centers for nausea and vomiting are in the _____.

(b) Mary Lizbeth is feeling nauseous. What signs is she likely to manifest?

_____

_____

(c) Emesis means _____.
As Mary Lizbeth vomits, how are her heart rate and blood pressure likely to change?
_____

(d) Describe the "good news and bad news" of vomiting.

_____

_____

_____

_____

(e) Use the following key words to describe triggers for vomiting.
   (e1) Vestibular apparatus

_____

_____

   (e2) Hypoxia

_____

_____

   (e3) Inflammation or distention

_____

_____

   (e4) The neurotransmitter dopamine

_____

_____

CHAPTER 28

Disorders of Gastrointestinal Function

■ Review Questions

A. DISORDERS OF THE ESOPHAGUS

A1. Fill in the blank within each statement about gastrointestinal disorders.

(a) Disorders of the digestive system rank third in _____ in the United States.

(b) It has been estimated that _____ million Americans have gastrointestinal disorders.

A2. Match the esophageal disorder with the correct description.

Achalasia   Aspiration   Diverticulum
Dysphagia   Odynophagia

(a) Outpouching of the esophagus (or other organ) caused by muscle weakness of the wall: _____

(b) Failure of the lower esophageal sphincter to relax; an entire meal or two may lodge in the esophagus: _____

(c) Movement of esophageal contents into the lung, potentially leading to infection there: _____

(d) Painful swallowing: _____

(e) Difficulty in swallowing, possibly caused by stroke, esophageal cancer, or scarring: _____

A3. Choose the three true statements about gastroesophageal reflux disease (GERD). (Pay particular attention to whether the **bold-faced** word or phrase makes the statement true or false.)

(a) **Most** people **do** occasionally experience gastroesophageal reflux.

(b) Even small hiatal hernias **are** considered causes of GERD.

(c) The most frequently occurring symptom of gastroesophageal reflux is **heartburn** within an **hour** after eating.

(d) Sitting up and antacids typically **do not** relieve symptoms of gastroesophageal reflux.

(e) A large percentage of people with GERD also have **asthma.**

(f) The severity of heartburn is an indicator of the extent of esophageal mucosal injury.

A4. Describe these two complications of gastroesophageal reflux.

(a) Esophageal strictures

_____

(b) Barrett esophagus

_____

_____

A5. Describe treatments for gastroesophageal reflux.

(a) Prevention methods

_____

_____

_____

(b) Medications

_____

_____

A6. Gastroesophageal reflux is *(common? rare?)* in infants. Explain why.

_____

_____

A7. Explain why iron-deficiency anemia and failure-to-thrive (FTT) can be manifestations of gastroesophageal reflux in infants.

_____

_____

_____

A8. Circle each of the following that is a risk factor for esophageal cancer:

(a) Alcohol

(b) Barrett esophagus

(c) Age younger than 30 years

(d) Female gender

(e) Smoking

A9. _____ is the most common sign of esophageal cancer. This type of cancer typically is diagnosed *(early? late?)* in the course of the disease and is associated with a *(good? poor?)* prognosis.

B. DISORDERS OF THE STOMACH

B1. List the major factors that contribute to the "gastric mucosal barrier."

_____

_____

_____

B2. Mrs. Snyder, age 54, has "been plagued with arthritis for years." Describe mechanisms by which the following practices have contributed to her current diagnosis of "stomach ulcers."

(a) "I've taken aspirin and ibuprofen for as long as they've made them."

_____

_____

_____

_____

(b) "I know my drinking and smoking don't help, but they get me through the day with all my pain."

_____

_____

_____

B3. Stephen ate *Staphylococcus*-contaminated food at a picnic about 4 PM today. He is likely to experience an abrupt onset of vomiting at about *(6 PM? 9 PM? 1 AM?)*. His gastritis is *(acute? chronic?)*.

B4. What is *Helicobacter pylori* and to what has it been linked?

_____

Explain how each of the following factors contributes to the "success" of *H. pylori*.

(a) Flagella

_____

(b) Enzymes

_____

(c) Urease

_____

(d) Cytokines

_____

B5. Fill in the blanks and circle correct answers in this exercise about chronic gastritis.

(a) List three methods for identifying *H. pylori* infection.

_____

_____

_____

(b) Which medication increases gastric pH, creating an environment that reduces bacterial growth?

(A) Proton pump inhibitors

(B) Bismuth

B6. Explain why the following two conditions may be linked in patients with chronic gastritis: achlorhydria and pernicious anemia.

_____

_____

_____

B7. Choose the two true statements about peptic ulcers. (Pay particular attention to whether the **bold-faced** word or phrase makes the statement true or false.)

(a) Peptic ulcers can affect **either** the stomach or the duodenum.

(b) Duodenal ulcers are **much more common** than gastric ulcers.

(c) The incidence of peptic ulcer is about four times higher in **women than in men.**

(d) Since the 1980s, stress **has** been considered the causative factor of peptic ulcer.

B8. Fill in the blanks or circle the correct answers in this exercise about peptic ulcers.

(a) _____ and _____ are the two most common causes of peptic ulcer.

About ____% of people with gastric ulcer have *H. pylori* infection and ____ % of people using nonsteroidal anti-inflammatory drugs (NSAIDs), such as Mrs. Snyder in Question B2, have these ulcers develop.

(b) Circle the times when burning or gnawing pain is likely to be experienced by patients with peptic ulcer.

(1) 8 AM

(2) 3 PM

(3) 6 PM

(4) 1 AM

Peptic ulcer pain tends to recur at *(hourly? daily? weekly or monthly?)* intervals.

(c) Mrs. Snyder (Question B2) passed loose, tarry stools in the past 24 hours and has felt dizzy, weak, thirsty, and cold. What do these symptoms suggest?

_____

(d) What symptoms signal the possibility of a perforated ulcer?

_____

(e) List several treatments for peptic ulcers.

_____

B9. Identify the gastric condition most likely in each patient described.

Curling ulcer   Cushing ulcer
Zollinger-Ellison syndrome   Rotavirus

(a) Ms. Innes has second- and third-degree burns over 50% of her body. _____

(b) Mr. Edwards has a gastrin-secreting tumor of his stomach (gastrinoma). _____

(c) Timothy is admitted with severe head trauma and elevated intracranial pressure after being hit by a car. _____

B10. Circle the correct answers within each statement about stomach cancer.

(a) The incidence of stomach cancer is *(decreasing? increasing?)* in the United States. Worldwide, stomach cancer is *(common? rare?)*.

(b) Like esophageal cancer, stomach cancer often is diagnosed *(early? late?)* in the course of the disease.

(c) The treatment of choice for stomach cancer is *(chemotherapy? subtotal gastrectomy?)*.

C. DISORDERS OF THE SMALL AND LARGE INTESTINES

C1. Circle the three true statements about irritable bowel syndrome (IBS). (Pay particular attention to whether the **bold-faced** word or phrase makes the statement true or false.)

(a) In Western countries, approximately **1 person in 1,000** has the disorder.

(b) This disorder **is** explained by structural abnormalities (such as inflammation) of the wall of the intestine.

(c) IBS involves abdominal pain that **is not** relieved by defecation.

(d) Manifestations of irritable bowel syndrome include abdominal pain, bloating, diarrhea and/or constipation, **and anorexia.**

(e) Patients with IBS **do** experience a change in consistency (hard, loose, or watery) or frequency of stools.

(f) IBS is associated with **stress.**

C2. Identify which of the two major forms of inflammatory bowel disease fits each description below. Mark *CD* for Crohn disease and *UC* for ulcerative colitis. (In some cases both CD and UC will apply, or neither may apply.)

(a) A familial predisposition is present: Susan is at increased risk because both her mother and aunt have this disorder. _____

(b) Leonard states that he has been in "a vicious cycle for weeks" of diarrhea and fecal urgency that subsides, then recurs; he also has a "stiff, sore back," with fatigue (showing anemia) and recurrent eye inflammation (uveitis). _____

(c) Rhoda has two fistulas connecting portions of her jejunum and ileum and strictures in several areas of the small bowel. _____

(d) Polly received a diagnosis of this inflammatory bowel disease when she was 14 years old; the surface of her ascending colon resembles cobblestones and exhibits "skip lesions" with thickened areas that resemble lead pipes. _____

(e) Charles averages 30 to 40 bowel movements a day; his stools are bloody (derived from mucosal inflammation). _____

(f) A stool culture demonstrates that Mr. Okerson has a parasitic infection. _____

(g) Faith, age 8, is small for her age, and she eliminates fatty stools (steatorrhea) (both indicators of malabsorption); she requires a high-calorie, high-protein diet. _____

(h) J. T.'s diagnosis is proctosigmoiditis with confluent, necrotic lesions and pseudopolyps; his disorder is classified as acute, fulminating with increased risk for toxic megacolon. _____

C3. Choose the two true statements. (Pay particular attention to whether the **bold-faced** word or phrase makes the statement true or false.)

(a) Ulcerative colitis **does significantly** increase risk for colon cancer.

(b) Crohn disease occurring in childhood **is not** likely to retard growth.

(c) Fiber supplements are likely to **decrease** the diarrhea of ulcerative colitis.

(d) Toxic megacolon refers to abnormal **strictures** that **narrow** the colon.

C4. List several types of medications used to treat ulcerative colitis.

_____

C5. Identify the large bowel condition most likely to occur in each patient's case.

C. difficile colitis   Diverticulosis
E. coli O157:H7 infection   Rotavirus

(a) Melinda has eaten a hamburger that was not fully cooked. _____

(b) Monique has just completed a course of broad-spectrum antibiotics. _____

(c) Bryan eats a low-fiber diet and often "fails to respond to nature's call" to defecate. _____

(d) Nicholas, age 9 months, was infected in day care and continues rehydration several days later. _____

C6. Answer the following questions about C. difficile colitis.

(a) What characteristics of C. difficile warrant its name ("difficult")?

_____
_____

(b) The pseudomembranous form of this colitis is typically (more? less?) severe. Explain.

_____
_____

(c) Patients with C. difficile colitis should (continue? discontinue?) the broad-spectrum antibiotic that leads to this infection. (See Question C5[b].)

_____

C7. Answer the following questions about E. coli O157:H7 infection.

(a) Identify two settings in which person-to-person transmission of this infection is likely. _____

(b) List two serious complications of E. coli O157:H7 infection and explain why they are potentially life-threatening.

_____
_____

(c) Describe treatment that is most effective against E. coli O157:H7 infection.

_____
_____

C8. Circle the correct answers and explain where indicated.

(a) Diverticular disease is (more? less?) common in the United States than in developing countries. Explain.

_____

(b) (Diverticulitis? Diverticulosis?) is an inflammatory disease. A common complaint of this condition is pain in the:

(1) Lower left quadrant (LLQ)

(2) Lower right quadrant (LRQ)

(3) Upper left quadrant (ULQ)

(4) Upper right quadrant (URQ)

(c) What condition is indicated by air in the urine (pneumaturia)?

_____
_____

(d) Treatment includes (increasing? decreasing?) bulk in the diet and bowel retraining so that the person has at least one bowel movement per (day? week?).

C9. Circle the correct answers or fill in the blanks in the following questions about appendicitis.

(a) Appendicitis is *(common? rare?)* in the United States, with greater incidence among *(young? elderly?)* persons.

(b) Pain within 12 hours of onset is likely to be *(colicky? steady?)* and eventually locates in the *(LLQ? LRQ? ULQ? URQ?)*. Temperature and white blood cell count both typically *(decrease? increase?)*.

(c) Describe the rebound tenderness that is likely to accompany appendicitis.

_____

(d) State the usual treatment of appendicitis.

_____

C10. Circle the correct answer or fill in the blank within each statement about changes in intestinal motility.

(a) Intestinal motility increases as a result of myenteric nerve action (meaning nerves located within the _____), as well as from *(sympathetic? parasympathetic?)* stimulation.

(b) Typically, the colon eliminates about _____ g (or mL) of stool each day. Increased frequency of stool passage is known as *(constipation? diarrhea?)*. Increased volume of feces is known as _____ diarrhea.

(c) Diarrhea is *(sometimes? always?)* pathological. Diarrhea of 10 days' duration is considered *(acute? chronic?)*. Most cases of food poisoning lead to *(acute? chronic?)* diarrhea.

(d) Classify each of the following cases of diarrhea according to categories of cause.

Large volume
Small volume: infectious
Small volume: inflammatory

(1) Rebecca has been diagnosed with *Salmonella* food poisoning after eating infected chicken.

_____

(2) Polly (Question C2[d]) has Crohn disease with colicky diarrhea, urgency, and straining upon defecation (tenesmus).

_____

(3) Luther has lactose intolerance, in which indigestible lactose attracts water to the intestinal lumen.

_____

(e) Most acute diarrhea *(is? is not?)* serious. Explain when diarrhea may become serious and even lethal.

_____

(f) Feeding *(should? should not?)* be continued during diarrhea. Write the meaning of the treatment known as ORT: _____ Circle food or drink that should be avoided in the treatment of diarrhea:

(1) Apple juice

(2) Fatty foods

(3) Cola

(4) Starchy foods

(g) Explain how medications such as Lomotil and Imodium are effective against diarrhea.

_____

C11. Answer the following questions about constipation.

(a) What is considered "normal" for frequency of bowel movements?

_____

(b) List several examples of causes of constipation in each category.

(b1) Drugs

_____

(b2) Disease

_____

(b3) Aging

_____

(c) List several health behaviors that can help prevent constipation.

_____

_____

_____

C12. Match the terms related to intestinal obstruction with the descriptions that follow.

Borborygmus   Intussusception
Paralytic ileus   Strangulation
Volvulus

(a) Complete twisting of the bowel:
_____

(b) Seen most often after surgery; indicated by absence of bowel sounds in all four quadrants: _____

(c) Mechanical obstruction complicated by ischemia, necrosis, and possibly gangrenous bowel:
_____

(d) Telescoping of the bowel into an adjacent segment; most common in infants:
_____

(e) Rumbling sounds related to intestinal gas propulsion: _____

C13. Interruption of blood flow (strangulation) due to intestinal obstruction can lead to growth of *(aerobic? anaerobic?)* bacteria that release potentially lethal endotoxins. *(Mechanical? Paralytic?)* intestinal obstruction is more likely to involve severe, colicky pain. List two treatments for intestinal obstruction.

_____

_____

C14. Describe the location of the peritoneum.

_____

_____

What makes infection of this membrane (peritonitis) potentially serious?

_____

_____

C15. List four or more causes of peritonitis.

_____

_____

_____

_____

C16. Circle the typical early manifestations of peritonitis.

(a) Pain that is:

(1) Diffuse

(2) Localized over the inflamed area

(b) The person is likely to appear:

(1) Highly restless and active

(2) Subdued

(c) The abdominal wall becomes:

(1) Rigid

(2) Soft

(d) Blood work indicates:

(1) Leukocytosis

(2) Leukocytopenia

C17. Give a rationale for each of the following treatments of peritonitis.

(a) Intravenous fluids and electrolytes

_____

_____

(b) "Holding fluids" (n.p.o. = nothing by mouth) and nasogastric suctioning

_____

_____

C18. Identify the cause of intestinal malabsorption in each case. Select from this list of causes:

Lymphatic obstruction   Maldigestion
Transepithelial transport disorder

(a) Deficiency of pancreatic enzymes, as in cystic fibrosis: _____

(b) Metastasis that blocks the thoracic duct or periaortic nodes; interferes with fat absorption: _____

(c) Celiac disease or sprue:

_____

C19. Answer the following questions about two patients with intestinal malabsorption.

(a) Mary Ellen, age 9, has received a diagnosis of celiac disease (sprue). Circle the dietary restrictions likely for Mary Ellen.

Barley   Corn   Rye   Rice   Wheat

(b) Adam, age 4, has steatorrhea.

(b1) Explain why Adam's stools float in the toilet.

(b2) Explain the possible connection between his steatorrhea and his tendency to bleed and bruise excessively.

_____

(b3) Adam is small and weak for his age. Explain.

_____

C20. Circle the correct answers or fill in the blank within each statement about intestinal neoplasms.

(a) Adenomatous polyps of the intestine are *(common? rare?)*. These are *(benign? cancerous?)* and may be pedunculated, meaning _____.

(b) These polyps consist of excessive growth of *(mucosa? submucosa?)*. There also may be *(excessive? deficient?)* apoptosis (normal cell death). Removal of suspect polyps *(does? does not?)* reduce the incidence of colorectal cancer.

C21. Mildred is undergoing tests to rule out colorectal cancer.

(a) This form of cancer is *(common? rare?)* in the United States.

(b) Circle the factors in Mildred's personal and family history that increase her risk for colorectal cancer.

(1) She is 58 years old.

(2) Her mother died of breast cancer.

(3) Her younger brother has had a total colectomy for familial adenomatous polyps of the colon.

(4) Her husband has kidney cancer.

(5) Mildred has ulcerative colitis.

(6) She regularly takes aspirin or ibuprofen for her "stiffness."

(7) Her favorite snack foods (which she says she "eats too much") are ice cream, chocolate, and chips.

(c) List signs related to Mildred's bowel movements that would suggest colorectal cancer.

_____

_____

(d) Signs such as those just listed typically appear *(early? later?)* in the course of the cancer.

CHAPTER 29

Disorders of Hepatobiliary and Exocrine Pancreas Function

■ Review Questions

A. THE LIVER AND HEPATOBILIARY SYSTEM

A1. Choose the two true statements about the liver. (Pay particular attention to whether the **bold-faced** word or phrase makes the statement true or false.)

    (a) In healthy persons, the liver **can** be palpated inferior to the rib cage.

    (b) The bulk of the liver lies in the **upper right quadrant.**

    (c) The liver receives blood from the **portal artery** and the **portal vein.**

    (d) Bile is formed in the **liver** and is emptied into the **small intestine.**

A2. The portal vein transports blood from _____ into the liver. This vein and the hepatic veins *(have? lack?)* valves. Explain the significance.

_____

_____

_____

A3. Identify the term that fits the related description.

    Bile canaliculi   Hepatocytes
    Kupffer cells   Lobules
    Sinusoids

    (a) Phagocytic cells that remove bacteria, old blood cells, and other debris from blood that enters the liver: _____

    (b) Functional units of the liver; up to 100,000 per liver: _____

    (c) Liver cells that perform the many roles of the liver: _____

    (d) Wide channels between hepatocytes that contain blood supplied by hepatic artery and portal vein; lined with Kupffer cells: _____

A4. Arrange in correct sequence (from first to last) the structures that carry bile.

    Ampulla of Vater   Bile canaliculi
    Common hepatic   Sphincter of Oddi
    duct
    Right and left hepatic ducts

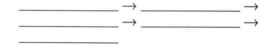

A5. Identify the chemical involved in liver metabolism that fits the related description.

    Amino acid   Albumin   Bile   Glycerol
    Glycogen   Ketone   Lactic acid   Urea

    (a) Acetoacetic acid produced when **fat** breakdown is excessive: _____

    (b) The type of chemical used for protein synthesis: _____

    (c) Most is formed in the liver and later excreted by kidneys or converted to ammonia within the intestine: _____

    (d) Yellow-green secretion produced by the liver and required for digestion and absorption of fats and fat-soluble vitamins: _____

    (e) The most abundant protein synthesized by the liver. Contributes greatly to colloidal osmotic pressure; if inadequate, leads to edema: _____

    (f) Carbohydrate formed when blood glucose levels rise: _____

    (g) Deamination and transamination are processes involved in conversion of these chemicals to glucose or use of them as sources of energy: _____

    (h) Chemicals that can be converted to glucose when blood glucose level is low (three answers): _____, _____, _____

A6. Answer the following questions about drug-induced liver disease.

(a) Explain how chemicals that enter the body, including drugs and alcohol, can injure the liver.

_____

_____

_____

(b) Drugs should be altered or detoxified by bio_____; this occurs in two phases:

   (b1) Phase 1: The drugs are chemically modified or _____.

   (b2) Phase 2: Additional reactions convert _____-soluble drugs to _____-soluble ones that can be eliminated by _____.

(c) Many hormones produced by the body also are normally metabolized by the liver. Name several.

_____

_____

Liver damage is likely to (decrease? increase?) circulating levels of hormones. Describe the effects of this.

_____

_____

_____

(d) Explain how polypharmacy in an 84-year-old woman can affect her liver.

_____

_____

_____

A7. Answer the following questions about bile pathways and blockage.

(a) Describe the route bile takes once it has reached the duodenum (see Question A4).

_____

_____

This is known as _____ circulation.

(b) Define cholestasis and list two of its causes.

_____

_____

(c) List the common manifestations of cholestasis.

_____

_____

_____

A8. Arrange in correct sequence the chemicals formed in the "life cycle" of bilirubin.

Biliverdin   Conjugated bilirubin
Free bilirubin   Hemoglobin
Urobilinogen

Red blood cells → _____ →
_____ → _____ →
_____ → _____

Put an asterisk (*) next to the chemical that is present in bile.

Put a double asterisk (**) next to the chemical that is reabsorbed into portal circulation or is excreted in feces.

A9. Circle the correct answers or fill in the blanks in the following questions about jaundice. Jaundice refers to an abnormally high serum level of _____ .

(a) Circle serum levels of bilirubin that are higher than normal: ____ mg/dL

   (1) 0.2
   (2) 1.0
   (3) 1.8
   (4) 2.5

(b) At which blood levels of bilirubin will sclerae (and also white skin) appear yellow? _____

(c) Match the types of jaundice with the related descriptions:

Intrahepatic   Posthepatic   Prehepatic

   (c1) Gallstones or tumors block bile ducts; cholestatic jaundice with pruritus; stools are clay colored because of lack of bilirubin in bile; also called cholestatic jaundice: _____

   (c2) Cirrhosis, hepatitis, liver cancer, or drugs such as halothane, anabolic steroids, or estrogen impair liver function, preventing removal of bilirubin from blood as quickly as it is formed: _____

   (c3) Excessive destruction of red blood cells in sickle cell anemia or in an Rh disorder (hemolytic disease of the newborn): _____

(c4) Serum bilirubin is elevated; stools appear normal in color:

_____

(c5) Urine may appear dark, indicating high levels of bilirubin:
_____ or _____

A10. Explain why serum levels of liver enzymes increase with liver damage.

_____

Which enzyme level is specific for hepatic injury? _____

B. DISORDERS OF THE LIVER

B1. List six or more causes of liver disease.

_____

_____

B2. Circle the correct answers or fill in the blanks in the following questions about hepatitis. Hepatitis refers to _____ of the liver.

(a) Circle possible causes of hepatitis.

   Autoimmune disease   Drugs
   Toxins   Viruses

(b) Explain the basis of naming the following types of this disorder: hepatitis A, hepatitis B, and hepatitis C.

_____

B3. Refer to Table 29-1. Circle the correct answers or fill in the blanks within each statement about the five major types of viral hepatitis.

(a) Hepatitis *(A? B?)* typically is a more serious health problem with longer duration.

(b) Relatively rare in the United States, hepatitis ___ has the highest mortality in infected pregnant women.

(c) Hepatitis ___ occurs only when it accompanies hepatitis ___.

(d) Hepatitis ___ typically has mild signs or symptoms; however, it is the most common cause of chronic hepatitis, cirrhosis, and primary liver cancer worldwide.

(e) Most likely to be transmitted by improper hand-washing techniques: ___ ___

(f) Health care workers are at greatest risk for these two types of hepatitis via accidental needle sticks: ___, ___

(g) Janelle is born of an HBV-infected mother. Janelle's risk of being a chronic carrier is approximately *(10%? 50%? 90%?)*. Her risk of dying of chronic liver disease as an adult is ___ %. The presence of *(anti-HBs? HBV DNA?)* in serum is the most certain indicator of HBV infection.

(h) It *(is? is not?)* recommended that Janelle receive hepatitis B vaccine. List other categories of candidates for HBV vaccine.

_____

B4. Complete this exercise about the clinical course of viral hepatitis.

(a) One major mechanism of liver injury in hepatitis is direct cellular injury. What is the other?

_____

Circle the correct answers within each statement about two types of immune responses.

(a1) A prompt and intense immune response during acute injury *(does? does not?)* cause cellular injury (and possible liver necrosis), and it *(does? does not?)* eliminate the virus. This type of response is *(more? less?)* likely to lead to fulminant hepatitis than the response described in B4(a2).

(a2) A more moderate immune response produces *(more? fewer?)* immediate symptoms and *(eliminates the virus? leads to a chronic or carrier state?)*. Carriers *(always? sometimes?)* have symptoms.

   Circle the types of hepatitis that can produce carriers.

   Hepatitis A   Hepatitis B
   Hepatitis C   Hepatitis D

(b) The three phases of acute symptomatic hepatitis are characterized partially by whether icterus (or _____) is present. Answer the following questions about manifestations of the phases.

(b1) The prodromal phase or *(icterus? preicterus?)* phase occurs first. Circle typical manifestations.

   Sense of well-being   Hearty appetite
   Jaundice   High blood
   Malaise   bilirubin
   Myalgia   Severe anorexia
   Nausea, vomiting, diarrhea

Table 29-1 Types of Hepatitis

Type: Virus	Distinguishing Characteristic; Incidence	Mode of Transmission; Risk Factors	Manifestations	Serological Markers; Vaccine
A: HAV (RNA virus)	Brief incubation period (15 to 45 days)	Fecal–oral route via contaminated water or shellfish (usually not by blood). At risk: pre-schoolers; those practicing rectoanal sex; persons in regions with poor sanitation	A benign, self-limited (acute, not chronic) disease with duration <2 months. Virus replicates in the liver, is excreted into bile and then into stool. 90% of adults develop jaundice	IgM anti-HAV indicates acute hepatitis; IgG anti-HAV documents past exposure and provides long-term protection against HAV. Vaccine: HAV is available for prevention
B: HBV (DNA virus); virion is Dane particle	A more serious health problem than hepatitis A. In the U.S. >1 million persons are carriers, with 300 million globally	Through blood or other body secretions. At risk: infants of HBV-infected mothers, persons who have rectoanal sex and/or multiple sex partners, IV drug users and health care workers with accidental needle sticks	Can be acute, fulminant with massive liver necrosis; can be chronic, carrier state, and develop into cirrhosis. Jaundice is present in <30% of cases	HBV vaccine is effective long term; immune globulin helps if given within a week of HBV exposure
C: HCV (RNA virus with many subtypes)	Greatest concern is high risk for chronic hepatitis, cirrhosis, or cancer of the liver	Injected drug use is most common source; may be transmitted by tattoos, body piercing, or acupuncture	Most infected persons do not know they are ill: symptoms are absent or mild, such as malaise or weight loss. Becomes chronic in 3 out of 4 cases	Tests for serum HCV and anti-HCV are available. No vaccine related to diverse subtypes
D: HDV (RNA virus)	Coinfection with hepatitis B	Routes of transmission similar to those of HBV. Mostly seen in drug users and hemophiliacs and in persons infected with (or carriers of) HBV	HDV can exacerbate HBV infection and cause it to become chronic or progress to cirrhosis	Detected by anti-HDV or HDV RNA in serum
E: HEV (RNA virus)	High mortality rate (20%) if occurs in pregnant women. Seen mostly in developing countries	Fecal–oral route	Fulminating manifestations similar to those of HBA. Does not lead to chronic or carrier state	

High serum levels of liver enzymes (AST and ALT)   Severe pruritus

(b2) Identify signs or symptoms of the icterus phase; choose from the list in (b1).

_____

(b3) Identify signs of the convalescent phase; choose from the list in (b1).

_____

(c) Complete clinical recovery is likely for hepatitis A within ___ months and for hepatitis B within ___ months.

B5. Circle correct answers or fill in the blanks within each statement about the chronic viral hepatitis.

(a) Chronic viral hepatitis is likely to have a duration longer than ___ months.

(b) Three forms of hepatitis that are known to become chronic: ___, ___, ___. Most cases of chronic hepatitis are of type ___.

(c) Persons with chronic viral hepatitis *(are? are not?)* likely to be carriers who *(can? cannot?)* transmit the disease. With which forms of viral hepatitis can infected persons become carriers? *(A? B? C? D? E?)*

(d) There *(are? are not?)* simple, effective treatments for chronic viral hepatitis. List possible treatments in each category below:

    (d1) Medications:_____

    (d2) Surgical: _____

B6. Fulminant hepatitis tends to progress *(rapidly? slowly?)*. *(HAV? HBV? HCV?)* accounts for most cases of viral hepatitis that lead to fulminant hepatitis and liver failure.

B7. List two factors that contribute to autoimmune hepatitis.

_____

B8. Write *PBC* (for primary biliary cirrhosis), *PSC* (for primary sclerosing cholangitis), or *SSC* (secondary sclerosing cholangitis) next to each description.

(a) Inflammation and obstruction of large bile ducts either inside or outside of the liver; retention of bile leads to hepatic necrosis with potential liver failure; occurs more in males:____

(b) Incidence is greater in persons with autoimmune disease; scarring of the liver leads to accumulated bile with green hue to the liver: _____

(c) The most common cause is gallstones (cholelithiasis): _____

(d) Liver transplantation is the only treatment of advanced disease: _____

B9. The United States has an estimated _____ alcoholics. About ___ % of alcoholics develop cirrhosis.

B10. List the three major disorders of the liver associated with chronic alcoholism in the sequence in which they are likely to appear:

_____ → _____ → _____.

Answer the following questions about these disorders.

(a) A fatty liver appears _____ in color. Presence of fat in hepatocytes is known as _____. Hepatic changes during the fatty liver stage *(are? are not?)* likely to be reversible.

(b) List four or more causes of fatty liver disease other than chronic alcoholism.

_____

_____

(c) List triggers for alcoholic hepatitis.

_____

Circle each of the following that is a sign typical of alcoholic hepatitis:

(1) Anorexia and nausea

(2) Fever

(3) Compression of hepatic veins by hepatic nodules

(4) Upper right quadrant (URQ) tenderness

(5) Accumulation of fluid within the peritoneal cavity (ascites)

During the acute phase of alcoholic hepatitis, mortality rate is ____ %.

(d) Early stages of alcoholic cirrhosis involve *(small? large?)* nodules. How do these nodules injure the liver?

_____

_____

Is cirrhosis considered a serious disorder?

_____

B11. Mr. Nardella has been diagnosed with hepatic failure. About *(10% to 15%? 45% to 50%? 80% to 90%?)* of liver function must be lost before liver failure occurs. Answer the following questions about his case.

(a) Mr. Nardella states: "I've never taken a drink in my life." List several factors other than alcohol that can lead to liver failure.

_____

_____

(b) Mr. Nardella's liver is palpable and tender. He is weak and has no appetite; he speaks about having a "belly for the first time in my life," yet he has not gained weight; his ankles are swollen. Explain these signs and symptoms.

_____

_____

_____

(c) Mr. Nardella has enlargement of breast tissue.

_____

B12. Mr. Roderick has advanced-stage hepatic failure related to chronic alcoholism. Explain the manifestations of his illness.

(a) Mr. Roderick has had an esophageal balloon tamponade inserted to compress his bleeding esophageal veins.

_____

_____

(b) He cannot breathe well when he lies down; he is taking diuretics and has had a number of paracentesis treatments.

_____

_____

(c) Mr. Roderick's prothrombin time has doubled, indicating decreased ability to clot blood, and his hemoglobin level is 7 g/100 mL.

_____

_____

_____

(d) Mr. Roderick's skin is yellow and he has clubbing of fingers.

_____

_____

(e) Mr. Roderick also has hemorrhoids.

_____

B13. Describe possible treatments for Mr. Roderick (Question B12).

_____

_____

B14. Select the category of portal hypertension that applies to each of the following patients.

   Intrahepatic   Prehepatic   Posthepatic

(a) Mrs. Daugherty has right-sided heart failure: _____

(b) Mr. Roderick (Question B12) has liver failure due to cirrhosis:

_____

B15. Match the condition associated with portal hypertension and liver failure with the correct description.

   Asterixis   Azotemia
   Caput medusae   Esophageal varices
   Fetor hepaticus

(a) Large, red veins in the skin around the umbilicus related to backup of portal vein blood into collateral vessels: _____

(b) Sweet, musty breath resulting from bacterial degradation of toxins within the intestine: _____

(c) Flapping of wrists related to the effects of hepatic encephalopathy; exacerbated by high-protein meals that increase production of ammonia: _____

(d) Highly elevated blood urea nitrogen (BUN) and serum creatinine levels, indicating renal failure: _____

(e) Occur in about two thirds of persons with advanced cirrhosis; in 50% of cases, lead to rupture, hypovolemic shock and death; may be treated by the TIPS (transjugular intrahepatic portosystemic shunt) surgery:

_____

B16. Circle the correct answer or fill in the blank within each statement about liver cancer.

(a) Primary liver cancer accounts for approximately ___ % of all cancers. It is more common in (*the United States? developing countries?*)

(b) Which type of primary liver cancer is more common: cancer of (*bile ducts? hepatocytes?*). Almost all hepatocellular carcinoma in the United States is associated with _____. Which forms of chronic hepatitis are associated with this type of cancer? _____

(c) What is a cholangiocarcinoma? _____ This type of liver cancer (*is? is not?*) associated with chronic alcoholism.

(d) Primary liver cancers typically are diagnosed in (*early? late?*) stages. The 5-year survival rate is approximately ___ %.

(e) Most liver cancers are *(primary? metastatic?)*. In which organs are metastatic cancers likely to originate?

_____

C. DISORDERS OF THE GALLBLADDER AND EXOCRINE PANCREAS

C1. Circle the correct answer within each statement about the gallbladder.

(a) The major function of the gallbladder is to *(produce? concentrate?)* bile.

(b) The hormone *(cholecystokinin? secretin?)* stimulates contractions of the gallbladder.

(c) Bile exits from the gallbladder directly into the *(cystic? common bile?)* duct.

(d) The sphincter of the bile duct regulates entrance of bile into the *(large? small?)* intestine.

C2. Answer the following questions about gallstones.

(a) The primary chemical component of almost all gallstones is _____; the secondary chemical component is _____.

(b) List the three major factors that contribute to formation of gallstones.

_____

(c) Circle each factor that increases risk for formation of gallstones.

(1) Male

(2) Lean body

(3) Multiparous women

(4) Women taking oral contraceptives

(5) Native American heritage

(6) Medications that lower blood cholesterol levels

(7) Young age (teens or twenties)

(8) Formation of gallbladder sludge

(9) Sickle cell anemia

(d) At what point is pain likely to accompany gallstones?

_____

Name two areas to which gallstone pain is likely to refer: _____, _____

(e) Jaundice is more likely to accompany *(large? small?)* stones in bile ducts.

C3. Match the term with the related description.

Cholangitis   Cholecystitis
Cholelithiasis   Choledocholithiasis

(a) Gallstones: _____

(b) Stones in the common bile duct:

_____

(c) Inflammation of the common bile duct:

_____

(d) Inflammation of the gallbladder:

_____

C4. Mrs. Jorgenson, age 52, has a history of cholelithiasis and now has cholecystitis. Circle the correct answer or fill in the blank within each statement related to her case.

(a) A history of gallstones *(is? is not?)* associated with both acute and chronic cholecystitis.

(b) What types of foods should Mrs. Jorgenson avoid in attempts to reduce acute attacks of cholecystitis?

_____

(c) Pain that accompanies inflammation of the gallbladder is likely to begin as *(steady? colicky?)* pain.

(d) The most widely used tool for diagnosing cholecystitis and cholelithiasis is:

(1) CT (computed tomography) scan

(2) MRI (magnetic resonance imaging)

(3) US (ultrasonography)

(e) One of Mrs. Jorgenson's gallstones blocks her common bile duct; the purulent infection she now has is acute

_____.

Explain why this condition may lead to emergency surgery.

_____

C5. Cholecystectomy performed by the laparoscopic method involves:

(a) An incision through the wall of the upper right quadrant of the abdomen

(b) Entrance into the abdominal cavity via the umbilicus

C6. Cancer of the gallbladder is *(common? rare?)*, typically with *(acute? insidious?)* onset. The 5-year survival rate is approximately ___ %.

C7. Circle the correct answers or fill in the blanks within each statement about the pancreas and its disorders.

(a) The "head" of this fish-shaped organ rests against the *(duodenum? liver? spleen?)*, whereas the "tail" rests against the _____. Symptoms of pancreatic disorders are notable *(when changes are small? only when changes are great?)*. Explain.

_____

_____

(b) Exocrine ducts of the pancreas empty into

_____

(c) The pancreas produces *(many? few? no?)* digestive enzymes. Pancreatic amylases digest _____, whereas lipases digest _____.

(d) Explain why the protease trypsin produced by the pancreas normally does not cause the pancreas to digest itself.

_____

(e) The pancreas also secretes *(acid? alkaline?)* fluids that neutralize the *(acid? alkaline?)* gastric materials that enter the small intestine.

C8. Mr. Lowheide, age 61, has a history of alcoholism. He is being examined for a possible diagnosis of acute pancreatitis. Answer the following questions related to his case.

(a) The two major causes of acute pancreatitis are _____ and _____.

(b) Mr. Lowheide states that he "knocked off just a few beers last night with my buddies." Explain how alcohol triggers pancreatitis.

_____

_____

(c) Mr. Lowheide refuses to lie on his back; he wants to sit up and lean forward in bed. Explain.

_____

(d) Acute pancreatitis is likely to be *(mild? life-threatening?)*. Explain.

_____

_____

(e) Explain why Mr. Lowheide has a rapid heart rate, low blood pressure, and cool and clammy skin.

_____

(f) Mr. Lowheide's wife is informed that her husband's "blood levels of pancreatic enzymes" are high. Which two enzymes are likely to be high?

_____

How do these test results point to pancreatic damage?

_____

(g) Explain why each of these treatments is ordered for Mr. Lowheide:

(g1) Intravenous fluid and electrolytes

_____

(g2) Nothing by mouth and nasogastric suction

_____

(g3) Antibiotics

_____

C9. Brad, age 13, was diagnosed with cystic fibrosis (CF) as an infant. Answer the following questions related to his case.

(a) Explain how CF can lead to chronic pancreatitis in the head of the pancreas.

_____

_____

(b) Describe signs and symptoms that Brad is likely to manifest.

_____

_____

(c) Explain why Brad is put on a low-fat diet.

_____

_____

(d) Why does Brad receive pancreatic enzymes orally?

_____

C10. Answer the following questions about pancreatic cancer.

(a) The 5-year survival rate associated with pancreatic cancer is approximately *(1%? 10%? 50%? 90%?)*. Incidence is especially high in *(young adult? elderly?)* persons. Pancreatic cancer typically is identified *(before? after?)* metastases have occurred.

(b) List dietary factors that appear to increase the risk for pancreatic cancer.

_____

(c) What other factors are associated with the increased risk of pancreatic cancer?

_____

(d) Onset typically is *(acute? insidious?)*. List typical manifestations.

_____

_____

(e) What health practices might help prevent pancreatic cancer?

_____

CHAPTER 30

Organization and Control of the Endocrine System

■ Review Questions

A. THE ENDOCRINE SYSTEM

A1. Describe the chemical links among these three systems: endocrine, nervous, and immune.

_____

_____

_____

A2. Give one example for each of the following statements.

(a) A single hormone can affect several different organs.

_____

_____

(b) A single function can be regulated by several different hormones.

_____

_____

A3. *(Auto? Juxta? Para?)*crine chemicals exert effects on the same cell that made the chemical, whereas _____crine chemicals act on cells adjacent to those that produce the chemical. Many hormones exert effects on distant organs; these hormones travel through *(blood plasma? ducts?)*.

A4. Classify the following hormones according to chemical category. Select from this list:

Amines or amino acids
Fatty acid derivatives
Peptides, polypeptides, glycoproteins, and proteins
Steroids

(a) Eicosanoids including prostaglandins (involved with inflammation) and thromboxanes (active in hemostasis):

_____

(b) The smallest of all these molecules; include the catecholamines such as epinephrine, norepinephrine, and dopamine:

_____

(c) Derived from cholesterol; include sex hormones, cortisone, and aldosterone:

_____

(d) Comprise the largest category of hormones; include follicle-stimulating hormone (FSH), luteinizing hormone (LH), adrenocorticotropic hormone (ACTH), thyroid-stimulating hormone (TSH), antidiuretic hormone (ADH), oxytocin, releasing hormones, and insulin:

_____

(e) Thyroid hormone:

_____

A5. Circle the correct answers or fill in the blank within each statement about synthesis and transport of hormones.

(a) Steroids are synthesized in *(rough? smooth?)* endoplasmic reticulum (ER), whereas _____ hormones are formed on ribosomes located on *(rough? smooth?)* ER.

(b) Insulin is an example of a *(steroid? protein?)* hormone that is formed as a prohormone in rough ER. Then this chemical is converted to active insulin in *(Golgi? mitochondria?)*.

(c) Carrier-bound hormones are *(active? inactive?)* in that state. Circle the hormones that are normally carried in blood bound to carriers.

Aldosterone   Cortisone
Estrogen   Growth hormone
Insulin   Parathyroid hormone
Thyroid hormone
   (thyroxine)

(d) About ____% of thyroxine in blood is bound to protein carriers. What effect does aspirin exert on the effectiveness of thyroxine?

_____

_____

_____

(e) Thyroxine has a half-life of 6 *(minutes? hours? days?)*. This means that 50% of the thyroid hormone molecules in the body on Monday will be out of the body by the following Sunday.

A6. Answer the following questions about metabolism of hormones.

(a) How does metabolism of hormones affect hormone activity?

_____

(b) Where does metabolism of hormones normally occur?

_____

(c) Name an enzyme that degrades and destroys catecholamines such as epinephrine or norepinephrine.

_____

(d) How are steroid hormones inactivated?

_____

A7. Explain how a specific hormone "knows" which cells to affect.

_____

_____

Circle the correct answers or fill in the blanks within each statement about receptors.

(a) How many receptor molecules are present on (or in) one cell? _____

(b) Joyce has a decreased blood level of a particular hormone. As a result, her cells are likely to *(decrease? increase?)* the number of receptors for that hormone by *(induction? repression?)* of transcription of receptor genes. This mechanism is known as *(down-regulation? up-regulation?)*.

(c) Refer to Table 30-2 in *Essentials of Pathophysiology*. The hormones in the left two columns of the table are likely to be more *(water? lipid?)* soluble. As a result, these *(can? cannot?)* penetrate the highly lipid cell membrane. As these hormones attach to *(surface? intracellular?)* receptors, they serve as *(first? second?)* messengers that trigger production of _____ (or a similar chemical) known as the *(first? second?)* messenger. The _____ messenger then triggers events within the cell that cause the effects of the specific hormone.

(d) Steroid hormones *(can? cannot?)* penetrate the cell membrane. These hormones attach to *(surface? intracellular?)* receptors that initiate the effects of the steroid hormone.

A8. Match the bodily location with the hormone(s) released there. Refer to Table 30-1 in *Essentials of Pathophysiology*.

Adrenal cortex   Adrenal medulla
Anterior pituitary   Gastrointestinal tract
Hypothalamus   Kidney
Ovaries   Posterior pituitary
Testes

(a) Releasing hormones such as corticotropin-releasing hormone (CRH), gonadotropin-releasing hormone (GnRH), or thyrotropin-releasing hormone (TRH): _____

(b) Tropic hormones such as ACTH, FSH, LH, or TSH: _____

(c) Growth hormone (GH): _____

(d) Cortisol and aldosterone: _____

(e) ADH and oxytocin: _____

(f) Erythropoietin: _____

(g) Androgens such as testosterone: _____ and _____

A9. Select the hormone(s) listed in Table 30-1 in *Essentials of Pathophysiology* that fit(s) each description.

(a) Lowers blood calcium: _____

(b) Lowers blood glucose: _____

(c) Stimulate release of hormones from the anterior pituitary: _____

(d) Mimic effects of the sympathetic nervous system: _____

(e) Promotes protein synthesis in bones and muscles: _____

(f) Stimulates secretion of HCl by the stomach: _____

B. CONTROL OF HORMONE LEVELS; DIAGNOSTIC TESTS

B1. Circle the correct answers or fill in the blanks within each statement about regulation of hormone levels.

(a) The hypophyseal portal system is a system of _____ that transport hormones from the _____ to the _____. (Select from the list in Question A8.) These hormones are known as *(releasing? tropic?)* hormones such as TRH.

(b) Tropic hormones are produced by the *(anterior? posterior?)* pituitary. For example, the tropic hormone TSH stimulates its target gland (_____) to release the target hormone _____. Increasing levels of thyroxine have a *(positive? negative or opposite?)* feedback effect, causing a(n) *(decrease? increase?)* in TRH and TSH.

(c) ACTH is the tropic hormone that stimulates adrenal *(cortex? medulla?)* production of the hormone *(cortisol? epinephrine?)*. Cortisol is known as a glucocorticoid because one of its functions is to regulate levels of _____ in blood. Cortisone injections are *(endo? exo?)*genous forms of cortisol, which will cause a(n) *(decrease? increase?)* in production of CRH and

ACTH and *(stimulation? suppression?)* of adrenocortical function.

(d) The *(anterior pituitary? posterior pituitary? hypothalamus?)* is called the master gland because it regulates so many target organs and cells.

(e) Name two or more hormones that are regulated by blood levels of the chemicals that these hormones control.

_____

_____

B2. Answer the following questions about tests of hormone levels.

(a) Circle the tests that require use of radiolabeled forms of the hormone being tested:

Enzyme-linked immunosorbent assay (ELISA)
Immunoradiometric assay (IRMA)
Magnetic resonance imaging (MRI)
Radioimmunoassay (RIA)

(b) Describe advantages and disadvantages of assessing endocrine function by urine testing.

_____

_____

(c) Explain how imaging tests such as CT scans, MRIs, or ultrasound (US) are used to assess the endocrine system.

_____

_____

CHAPTER 31

Disorders of Endocrine Function

■ Review Questions

A. GENERAL ASPECTS OF ALTERED ENDOCRINE FUNCTION

A1. *(Hyper? Hypo?)*function refers to a decrease in function of an endocrine gland. List six or more possible causes of such an alteration.

_____

_____

_____

_____

A2. Identify the category of endocrine hypofunction in the following cases.

   1° = Primary   2° = Secondary   3° = Tertiary

   (a) Mr. Bagley's radiation treatments for brain cancer have led to his adrenal cortex hypofunction: _____

   (b) Marguerite has a bilateral oophorectomy related to her ovarian cancer: _____

   (c) Seth's low thyroid hormone level is linked to a defect in TSH production: _____

B. PITUITARY AND GROWTH HORMONE DISORDERS

B1. Refer to Figure 30-3 and Table 30-1 in *Essentials of Pathophysiology*. Fill in the blanks to identify these acronyms for hormones produced by the anterior pituitary:

   (a) ACTH:

   _____

   (b) FSH:

   _____

   (c) LH:

   _____

   (d) _____: thyroid-stimulating hormone

   (e) GH: _____

   (f) PRL: _____

   Circle (in a–f, above) all anterior pituitary hormones that control the release of other hormones in the body.

B2. Choose the three true statements about the pituitary gland. (Pay particular attention to whether the **bold-faced** word or phrase makes the statement true or false.)

   (a) The pituitary gland is located within the **sella turcica,** just **inferior** to the hypothalamus portion of the brain.

   (b) The **posterior pituitary** produces releasing and inhibiting hormones that regulate release of anterior pituitary hormones.

   (c) Manifestations of hypopituitarism are apparent by the time **25%** of the pituitary is destroyed.

   (d) Hypopituitarism is **always** acquired (not congenital).

   (e) **Adrenal cortex** hypofunction is the most serious endocrine deficiency secondary to hypopituitarism.

   (f) Cortisol and thyroid hormone replacement therapy **can** help clients with hypopituitarism.

B3. List the anterior pituitary hormones in the sequence in which they are lost as a result of hypopituitarism.

   ACTH   FSH   GH   LH   TSH

   _____ → _____ → _____ → _____ → _____

B4. Answer the following questions about factors that regulate growth and maturation.

   (a) List four hormones required for normal growth and maturation.

   _____

   (b) Circle each of the following that is a function of growth hormone (GH).

      (1) Increases protein in body cells

(2) Increases blood glucose levels

(3) Acts directly on bones and muscles to increase growth of these tissues

(4) Decreases use of fats and increases use of carbohydrates as major fuel sources

B5. Circle the three true statements related to growth factors. (Pay particular attention to whether the **bold-faced** word or phrase makes the statement true or false.)

(a) Growth hormone (GH) normally is produced **only during childhood.**

(b) Insulin-like growth factors (IGFs) are also known as **somatomedins.**

(c) IGFs normally are produced by the **liver.**

(d) Anterior pituitary release of growth hormone (GH) is **stimulated** by somatostatin.

(e) Release of GH is greatest during **deep** sleep.

(f) Hypoglycemia, starvation, stress, and the amino acid arginine all **decrease** production of GH.

B6. Answer the following questions about stature (height).

(a) List the three factors that can most accurately diagnose short stature.

_____

(b) Troy, age 5, is in the fourth percentile for his age and sex; he (is? is not?) classified as having growth retardation.

(c) Explain why lateral skull x-rays as well as CTs and MRIs of Troy's head may help to diagnose causes of his short stature.

_____

_____

(d) Children with congenital GH deficiency typically have (short? tall?) stature with (normal? abnormal?) intelligence. Growth hormone deficiency typically is treated with GH replacement therapy derived from (cadaver pituitary? recombinant DNA?).

(e) Determine the "midparental height" for children of Cindy (5'7") and Alex (6'2"). Male children: _____

Female children: _____

B7. Match the short stature condition with the related description.

Congenital GH deficiency
Constitutional short stature
Genetically short stature

Laron-type dwarfism
Psychosocial dwarfism   Panhypopituitarism

(a) Caused by hereditary deficiency in insulin-like growth factor (IGF) production with normal GH production: _____

(b) Most likely to occur in severely neglected or abused children: _____

(c) Well-proportioned child who has short parents: _____

(d) Condition in which all pituitary hormones are deficient, including GH:

_____

(e) Richard's condition with short stature, thin build, delayed skeletal and sexual maturation, and absence of other causes of decreased growth: _____

(f) Eric was 20 inches long at birth, but at 2 years, looked short and fat; he also had a low GnRH level and developed a smaller than normal penis: _____

B8. Match the condition to the related description.

Acromegaly   Gigantism   Somatopause

(a) Mr. Gordon, age 67, is the same height he was at age 20. He has gained weight, and he comments, "I have a belly that I never had before." He is fatigued and his blood GH levels are subnormal for a person his age: _____

(b) During the past 3 years, Mr. George's shoe size has increased, and his ring finger has outgrown his wedding ring. His lower jaw protrudes, and his voice has deepened. Mr. George is 46 years old and 6'1". Lateral skull x-rays and CTs reveal an enlarged pituitary gland: _____

(c) Billy, age 8, is in the 99th percentile for his age and parental height; his serum GH levels are extremely high: _____

B9. Complete this exercise about Mr. George (Question B8[b]).

(a) Mr. George's height (is? is not?) likely to increase. Explain.

_____

(b) His condition is a quite (common? rare?) disorder with an (acute? insidious?) onset. Almost all cases of acromegaly are caused by (benign? malignant?) tumors of the pituitary that increase GH production.

(c) Mr. George has increased risk of heart failure. Explain.

_____
_____
_____

(d) Headaches and visual defects also have plagued Mr. George recently. Explain how these are related to his acromegaly.

_____
_____

(e) Mr. George will have his pituitary tumor removed. The nurse tells Mr. George that his sense of smell may be diminished after the surgery. Explain why this may happen.

_____

B10. Roberta, age 8, is diagnosed with a tumor of her hypothalamus. Match each condition to the description that relates to this tumor.

Isosexual precocious puberty
Menarche   Thelarche

(a) She began to develop breasts at age 6: _____

(b) Her first menstrual period took place at age 7: _____

(c) Her sexual development has occurred much earlier than normal: _____

C. THYROID DISORDERS

C1. Select from the list of terms to fill in the blanks within each statement about the thyroid gland and its hormone. (Not all terms will be used.)

De-	Four
Free	Follicles
Iodide	In-
Lobules	Larynx
TBG	Protein
Thyroglobulin	Three
Triiodothyronine (T_3)	Thyroxine (T_4)
	Tyrosine

(a) The thyroid is a shield-shaped structure located just inferior to the _____ . This endocrine gland is composed of tiny saclike _____ filled with _____ .

(b) Thyroglobulin consists of long chains of the amino acid _____, to which the ion _____ is attached. The most active form of thyroid hormone appears to be _____, in which _____ iodides are attached to tyrosine.

(c) Almost all thyroid hormone exists bound to _____, primarily the binding protein named _____. Only the _____ form of thyroid hormone can enter cells and affect their metabolism.

(d) Corticosteroids, protein malnutrition, kidney disorders such as nephrosis (in which protein is lost in the urine), and aspirin all _____crease T_3T_4 binding to TBG, causing a(n) _____crease in active thyroid hormone.

C2. Review negative feedback mechanisms that regulate thyroid hormone in Chapter 30, Question B1(b). High thyroid hormone levels are likely to (stimulate? inhibit?) production of TRH and TSH. Cold temperature (triggers? inhibits?) thyroid production by stimulating TRH release from the (anterior pituitary? hypothalamus? thyroid gland?).

C3. Thyroid hormone exerts effects on (all major? only a few specific?) organs of the body. In general, it (decreases? increases?) metabolism. Write IN (for increase) or DE (for decrease) to indicate the specific effects of thyroid hormone.

(a) _____creases blood levels of cholesterol as fats are used for fuel.

(b) Gastrointestinal absorption of glucose from food is _____creased, providing more fuel for metabolism.

(c) Muscle mass is _____creased as muscle proteins are used for fuel. However, if thyroid hormone is excessive, muscle action _____creases, leading to tremor.

(d) Gastrointestinal tract motility and secretion _____crease, providing more nutrients for metabolism. Risk for diarrhea _____creases related to intestinal motility.

(e) Weight _____creases and body temperature _____creases as calories are "burned" for metabolism. Blood vessels of the skin dilate in attempts to _____crease body temperature associated with increased metabolism.

(f) Heart rate, cardiac output, and ventilation _____crease, providing oxygen for metabolism.

(g) Nerve activity _____creases, leading to anxiety and restlessness if thyroid hormone is excessive. Infants with thyroid deficiency are likely to experience _____creased brain development.

C4. Consider the normal functions of thyroid hormone (Question C3) and also refer to Table 31-2 in *Essentials of Pathophysiology*. Now determine whether each of the following descriptions better applies to hypothyroidism *(hypo)* or hyperthyroidism *(hyper)*.

(a) Neonatal retardation and developmental delay in infants: _____

(b) Sluggishness, sleeping more than normal: _____

(c) Bradycardia and low cardiac output: _____

(d) High blood cholesterol: _____

(e) Weight gain related to accumulation of a mucopolysaccharide that presents as edema; may lead to life-threatening coma: _____

C5. Identify the thyroid condition that affects each of the following patients. (One condition will be used twice.)

Cretinism   Goiter
Graves disease   Hashimoto disease
Myxedema   Thyroid storm

(a) Mrs. Ruiz has an enlargement in her neck in the area of her "Adam's apple." The growth is pressing against her trachea, esophagus, and veins of her neck, causing difficulty breathing and eating as well as facial edema. Mrs. Ruiz lives in a region where iodized salt is not readily available: _____

(b) Screening of Jesus Gomez, born this week, indicates subnormal levels of T_4 and TSH. Additional tests indicate that he has congenital absence of a thyroid gland. Jesus is treated with T_4 to prevent mental retardation and short stature: _____

(c) Mrs. Jones has a history of thyroid cancer with radiation therapy 15 years ago. She has a "puffy" appearance with nonpitting edema. Mrs. Jones states that she "feels cold all of the time": _____

(d) Nan has begun taking lithium carbonate for her bipolar disorder, diagnosed 2 months ago; she is weak and fatigued and her response to her weight gain is exacerbation of her depression: _____

(e) Ms. Mason initially presents with a goiter; with time her T_4 levels decrease as a result of her antithyroid antibody production. Her skin is dry and rough; her hair is coarse and brittle. Ms. Mason is treated with T_4: _____

(f) Mrs. Yokum, with type 1 diabetes mellitus, has undiagnosed hyperthyroidism that is exacerbated as she experiences diabetic ketoacidosis. Her high fever, congestive heart failure, and delirium require rapid treatment to prevent death: _____

(g) Dr. Oxford, age 37, has lost 30 lb during the past month. Her eyes bulge so much that her eyelids barely close over her eyes. Her partner has noted that Dr. Oxford seems "anxious and restless." Dr. Oxford has experienced episodes of palpitations, dyspnea, and irritability that she attributes to her insomnia: _____

C6. Choose the two true statements about the thyroid gland. (Pay particular attention to whether the **bold-faced** word or phrase makes the statement true or false.)

(a) Radiation of the neck is more likely to cause **primary** (rather than secondary) hypothyroidism.

(b) Graves disease is **a rare** form of hyperthyroidism.

(c) Thyroid storm is **a mild** form of hyperthyroidism.

(d) The stress of emotional trauma or infection **increases** risk for occurrence of thyroid storm.

D. DISORDERS OF ADRENAL CORTICAL FUNCTION

D1. Answer the following questions about the adrenal glands.

(a) Where are these glands located? _____

(b) Indicate whether each of the following characteristics describes the adrenal cortex *(C)* or the medulla *(M)*.

(b1) Produces the hormones epinephrine and norepinephrine that both mimic sympathetic nerves: _____

(b2) Most of the hormone production here is stimulated by the anterior pituitary hormone, ACTH: _____

(b3) Critical for stress responses needed for survival: _____

(b4) Its hormones are steroids (derived from cholesterol): _____

D2. Select the adrenocorticoid hormone that fits each description.

Dehydroepiandrosterone (DHEA)
Aldosterone   Cortisol

(a) The chief mineralocorticoid; causes kidneys to retain Na^+ and H_2O and to eliminate K^+ into urine (see Study Guide Figure 6-1, *C*):

_____

(b) Regulated by the renin-angiotensin mechanism and blood levels of K^+:

_____

(c) The most important adrenal sex hormone; especially significant in women for whom an analogue of this hormone can be used to treat adrenal insufficiency (Addison disease):

_____

(d) The major glucocorticoid; controlled by corticotropin-releasing hormone (CRH) and adrenocorticotropic hormone (ACTH) (see Chapter 30, Question B1[c]):

_____

D3. Describe the diurnal variations in cortisol production.

_____

_____

D4. Circle the correct answer within each statement about the effects of cortisol.

(a) *(Decreases? Increases?)* blood glucose levels (see Study Guide Figure 32-1, *B*)

(b) Causes *(synthesis? breakdown?)* of muscle proteins, which can lead to striae (lines) in the skin

(c) Enhances conversion of amino acids into glucose, a process known as *(glycogenesis? gluconeogenesis?)* (see Study Guide Figure 32-1, *B*)

(d) *(Decreases? Increases?)* capillary permeability and action of B and T cells

(e) *(Decreases? Increases?)* fever

(f) *(Decreases? Increases?)* formation of scar tissue

(g) The effects described above (in D4[d], [e], and [f]) are all examples of cortisol's function as an *(anti-inflammatory? inflammation-enhancing?)* hormone.

D5. Vanessa has been taking steroid medications for a year. Explain the following effects.

(a) She has become emotionally labile (has dramatic mood swings).

_____

(b) Her own production of adrenal hormones is diminished.

_____

(c) Vanessa suddenly decides to stop taking her steroid medications.

_____

_____

D6. Describe the following tests related to the adrenal cortex.

(a) Screening test for Cushing syndrome

_____

(b) Dexamethasone suppression test:

_____

D7. Sophie is born with congenital adrenal hyperplasia. Answer the following questions related to her case.

(a) Congenital adrenal hyperplasia *(is? is not?)* a genetic disorder. Sophie lacks the enzymes necessary to synthesize *(ACTH? aldosterone? cortisol? sex hormones?)*.

(b) Decreased cortisol activates the negative feedback mechanism that *(decreases? increases?)* blood levels of ACTH. As a result, Sophie's adrenal cortex *(decreases? increases?)* in size (hyperplasia). In addition, her adrenal cortex *(decreases? increases?)* production of androgen. Describe the effects.

_____

D8. Select the name of the disorder of the adrenal cortex that best applies in the case of each of the following patients. (Some disorders may be used more than once.)

Addison disease   Adrenogenital syndrome
Cushing disease   Cushing syndrome
Secondary adrenal cortical insufficiency

(a) Mrs. Tappin's deficiency of adrenocortical hormones is precipitated by removal of her pituitary gland: _____

(b) Vanessa's adrenal insufficiency (Question D5) caused by cessation of exogenous cortisol is an example of this type of disorder: _____

(c) Aileen is born with this syndrome, which causes enlargement of the clitoris and partial fusion of the labia; most serious is her deficiency in aldosterone which causes her to lose sodium and water and (unless treated) go into hypovolemic shock:

_____

(d) Mr. Fitzgerald is a 41-year-old white man whose adrenal cortex was destroyed by autoimmune mechanisms. His blood levels of cortisol are deficient, causing increased ACTH levels: _____

(e) Lieutenant Jackson has a pituitary tumor with excessive ACTH production that stimulates adrenal production of cortisol:

_____

(f) Mrs. Reed has a small cell lung carcinoma that is producing ectopic ACTH; adrenocorticoid replacement is required:

_____

D9. Answer the following questions related to Mr. Fitzgerald's condition (Question D8[d]).

(a) His disorder is a (*primary? secondary?*) adrenal insufficiency. He is likely to manifest signs of adrenal insufficiency once

these hormones drop to approximately (*10%? 90%?*) of normal.

(b) Circle each of the following that is a typical manifestation of Addison disease.

(1) Increased urinary output with low cardiac output and low blood pressure

(2) Decreased urinary output with high cardiac output and high blood pressure

(3) Excessive loss of salt in urine with abnormal craving for salt

(4) Hyperglycemia with high energy level

(5) Pale skin

(c) Mr. Fitzgerald (*will? will not?*) require lifetime replacement of adrenocortical hormones. Mr. Fitzgerald (*should? has no need to?*) wear a medical alert bracelet or medal.

D10. Signs and symptoms of Cushing syndrome are related to (*deficient? excessive?*) cortisol production. Circle each of the following that is a common manifestation of Cushing syndrome.

(a) Lean trunk with obesity in extremities

(b) Excessive distribution of fat in the face and back

(c) Stretch marks in skin

(d) Osteosclerosis

(e) Hypotension

CHAPTER 32

Diabetes Mellitus and the Metabolic Syndrome

■ Review Questions

A. HORMONAL CONTROL OF GLUCOSE, FAT, AND PROTEIN METABOLISM

A1. Explain why diabetes mellitus (DM) is a major health problem in the United States.

_____

_____

_____

A2. Select the chemical category that best fits each description below.

Carbohydrates   Fats   Proteins

(a) Because the brain can neither synthesize nor store more than a few minutes' supply of this source of energy, normal cerebral function requires a continuous supply from the circulation: _____

(b) The body's most efficient form of fuel storage: _____

(c) Triglycerides are a major type of molecule in this chemical category: _____

(d) In situations that favor breakdown of this category of chemicals, such as diabetes mellitus and prolonged fasting, large amounts of ketones are released into the bloodstream: _____

(e) Makes up most of body tissues, such as muscles; forms most of the structure of enzymes; makes up many enzymes, including insulin; composed of amino acids: _____

(f) Together, these chemicals provide about 80% of the calories in the typical American diet (two answers): _____ _____

A3. Pancreatic hormones are produced by _(acinar cells? islets of Langerhans?)_. Fill in the blanks or circle the correct answer within each statement about the hormones synthesized by the islet cells.

(a) Alpha cells produce _____, which _(decreases? increases?)_ blood glucose.

(b) Beta cells produce _____, which _(decreases? increases?)_ blood glucose, and also _____, which complements action of insulin.

(c) Delta cells produce _____, which inhibits release of both _____ and _____ and _(decreases? increases?)_ gastrointestinal activity.

A4. Describe the _incretin effect_: _____ _____. Name two hormones with this effect: _____ and _____. Circle the organ that produces these hormones: _(Pancreas? Stomach? Small intestine?)_. Type 2 diabetics may take an injectable GLP-1 analogue that _(mimics? opposes?)_ the action of insulin.

A5. Answer the following questions about blood glucose regulation in Simon, who is a healthy 30-year-old man (without DM).

(a) It is 7 AM and Simon has not eaten for 12 hours. Which blood glucose level(s) would be considered normal at this time? _____ mg/dL

36   76   136   780

Which value would indicate hypoglycemia?

_____

(b) Circle the processes that increase Simon's blood glucose level between meals and help maintain his blood glucose level to prevent hypoglycemia:

(1) Glycogenolysis

(2) Glycogenesis

(3) Gluconeogenesis

(c) Which one of these processes (in A5[b]) involves conversion of amino acids or parts of fats into glucose? _____ Where does this process occur? _____

(d) Which process (in A5[b]) releases glucose by breakdown of glycogen? _____

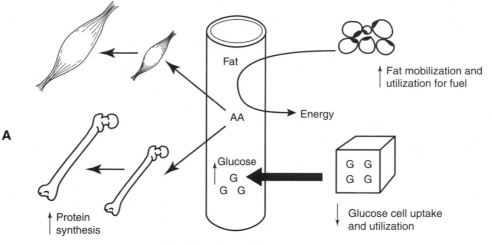

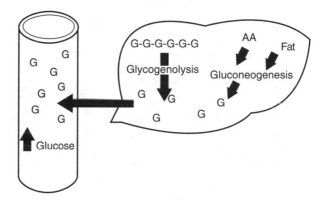

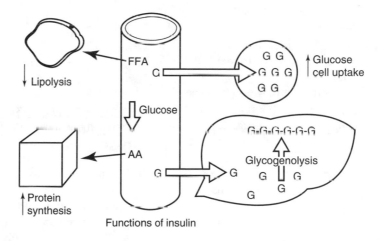

FIGURE 32-1

(e) Circle hormones that promote glycogenesis or gluconeogenesis to help maintain Simon's blood glucose throughout the night (see Study Guide Figure 32-1, *B*).

Cortisol	Epinephrine
Glucagon	Insulin

(f) Which of Simon's tissues relies on glucose as its fuel source and depends on a constant blood supply of glucose because this tissue can neither synthesize nor store much glucose?

    (1) Adipose tissue

    (2) Brain

    (3) Skeletal muscle

    (4) Liver

(g) Skeletal muscle *(lacks? has much of?)* the enzyme glucose-6-phosphatase. State the significance of this fact.

_____

_____

_____

(h) When Simon eats a hearty breakfast, his blood glucose level *(decreases? increases?)*. High blood glucose stimulates the pancreas to release *(glucagon? insulin?)*. This hormone promotes movement of glucose from *(blood into cells? cells into blood?)* and also *(stimulates? inhibits?)* liver storage of glucose as _____. In other words, insulin *(raises? lowers?)* blood glucose. (See Figure 32-1, *C*.)

(i) Refer to Figure 32-1. Which hormones shown there have the effect of increasing blood glucose level? _____
Which one hormone lowers blood glucose level? _____ (Commit this sentence to memory: *Insulin decreases blood glucose level*.) Diabetes mellitus is a condition in which insulin is absent, deficient, or ineffective, so blood glucose *(increases? decreases?)* to an abnormal level.

A6. Answer the following questions about insulin and its functions.

(a) Insulin is a *(carbohydrate? lipid? protein?)* composed of two peptide chains. *(A? B? C?)* chain is removed when active insulin is formed in the pancreas.

(b) Pancreatic release of insulin is signaled by entrance of _____ into beta cells. Glucose enters cells by means of the glucose transporter named _____. Within

minutes, *(preformed? newly synthesized?)* insulin is released.

(c) Insulin released from the pancreas passes into the *(inferior vena cava? portal vein?)* and travels to the liver. Once in general circulation, insulin has a half-life ($T_{1/2}$) of approximately _____ minutes.

(d) GLUT-4 is the glucose transporter for glucose entrance into (circle two answers) *(adipose? brain? liver? skeletal muscle?)* cells; this transporter requires the presence of _____. GLUT-_____ is the transporter for glucose available in all body cells, including neurons; this glucose transporter *(does? does not?)* require insulin.

(e) Insulin also promotes transport of _____ into cells, which facilitates _____ synthesis needed for normal growth and healing. Insulin also stimulates movement of _____ into cells and inhibits fat breakdown known as lipo-_____. (See Figure 32-1, *C*.)

(f) Catecholamines such as epinephrine *(stimulate? inhibit?)* insulin release, and growth hormone (GH) *(antagonizes? mimics?)* the effects of insulin. As a result (and because of other actions shown in Figure 32-1, *A* and *B*), these hormones *(decrease? increase?)* blood glucose.

(g) Explain why acromegaly and chronic stress can lead to hyperglycemia and DM.

_____

_____

_____

B. DIABETES MELLITUS: CLASSIFICATION, ETIOLOGY, MANIFESTATIONS, DIAGNOSIS, AND MANAGEMENT

B1. Choose the two true statements about diabetes mellitus (DM). (Pay particular attention to whether the **bold-faced** word or phrase makes the statement true or false.)

(a) Diabetes mellitus primarily is a problem of **unavailability of insulin**.

(b) The term "mellitus" in DM refers to **urine**.

(c) A value of 108 mg/dL on a fasting blood glucose test is considered **normal**.

(d) Type 1 diabetes accounts for **more** cases of DM than type 2 does.

B2. Answer the following questions about diabetes mellitus (DM).

(a) Consult Table 32-3 in *Essentials of Pathophysiology* and then select from the following answers to identify the best diagnostic classification in each case below.

A. Normal

B. Impaired fasting glucose (IFG)

C. Impaired glucose tolerance (IGT)

D. Provisional diabetes mellitus

(a1) Leanne's blood glucose level is 170 mg/dL on a 2-hour postload glucose tolerance test (OGTT): _____

(a2) Maddie's FPG is 94 mg/dL: _____

(a3) Mr. Belmont's FPG is 130 mg/dL and his OGTT results are 190 mg/dL:

_____

(b) Most type 1 DM is type *(1A? 1B?)*, which is *(idiopathic? immune-mediated?)*. This form of DM formerly was known as *(insulin? noninsulin?)* dependent because patients with type 1 diabetes *(do? do not?)* require exogenous insulin replacement. It was also called *(adult? juvenile?)* diabetes based on its most common age at onset.

(c) Insulin normally *(stimulates? inhibits?)* lipolysis (see Study Guide Figure 32-1, C). With absolute absence of insulin, as in type *(1? 2?)* DM, formation of _____ is more likely to occur as a result of excessive fat breakdown.

(d) There *(is? is not?)* evidence of a genetic predisposition for type 1 diabetes. About *(5? 95%?)* of people with type 1 diabetes possess human leukocyte antigens (HLA) DR3 or DR4.

(e) In type 1 diabetes mellitus, *(beta cells are destroyed? body cells are resistant to insulin?)*. The presence of destructive insulin autoantibodies (IAAs) can be used to detect more than *(25%? 50%? 85%?)* of present and future cases of type 1 diabetes.

(f) After diagnosis of type 1 diabetes, there is often a short time known as the _____ period when beta cells regenerate and produce insulin so that insulin injections are not needed.

(g) *(Most? Few?)* people with type 1 diabetes have type 1B. State the cause of type 1B:

_____

B3. Fill in the blanks or circle the correct answers within each statement about type 2 diabetes.

(a) Describe the three major metabolic abnormalities that lead to type 2 diabetes:

(a1) Peripheral insulin _____: muscle, fat, and other cells are insensitive to insulin, leading to decreased glucose uptake or glycogen storage.

(a2) Pancreatic secretion of insulin may be *(absent? abnormal?)*.

(a3) *(Increase? Decreased?)* production of glucose by the liver, for example by glycogenolysis or gluconeogenesis. (See Study Guide Figure 32-1.)

(b) Four of five persons with type 2 diabetes are *(obese? underweight?)* and tend to have a *(high? low?)* waist-to-hip ratio. The condition of having this kind of obesity and also type 2 diabetes is known as _____ and is related to the _____ syndrome. (See Question B5.) Weight loss and exercise in obese persons *(can? cannot?)* help to protect from and manage type 2 DM.

B4. Write a short essay relating obesity to insulin resistance in diabetics. Include these terms in your essay: *free fatty acids (FFAs), adipokines* such as *adiponectin*, and *peroxisome proliferated-activated receptor-gamma*.

_____

_____

_____

B5. Circle the correct answers within each phrase that describe characteristics of the *metabolic syndrome* (also known as *insulin resistance syndrome*).

(a) *(Lean weight? Obesity?)*

(b) *(High? Low?)* serum triglycerides and *(high? low?)* serum HDLs

(c) *(Increased? Decreased?)* likelihood of inflammation as indicated by high CRP level and *(increased? decreased?)* tendency to break down fibrin clots

(d) *(Hypertension? Hypotension?)* and *(increased? decreased?)* tendency of developing arterial disease

B6. The many types of DM are classified by *(cause? treatment?)*. Refer to Table 32-2 in *Essentials of Pathophysiology* and identify the class of DM present in each of the following patients.

Maturity onset diabetes of the young (MODY)

Drug disorder   Endocrine disorder

Gestational diabetes
mellitus

(a) Clarissa, age 34, is pregnant. At 25 weeks of pregnancy, her glucose tolerance test reveals a blood glucose of 202 mg/dL:

_____

(b) Annette has pheochromocytoma, and Allison has Cushing syndrome, both of which cause hyperglycemia: _____

(c) Harry is taking steroids for a severe case of pneumonia and also is taking Lasix (a loop diuretic) to reduce fluid in his lungs:

_____

B7. Circle each of the following that is a risk factor for gestational DM.

(a) African American

(b) Native American

(c) 23 years old

(d) Previously delivered a healthy 10-pound baby

(e) Third pregnancy

(f) Family history of DM

(g) Weight of 105 lb

(h) Absence of glucose in urine

(i) History of two miscarriages

B8. Explain why early diagnosis and management of gestational DM are essential.

_____

_____

Women with GDM *(are? are not?)* at increased risk for future diagnosis of diabetes.

B9. Answer the following questions about signs and symptoms of DM.

(a) Type *(1? 2?)* DM typically has a more insidious onset.

(b) One sign of diabetes is *(decreased? increased?)* urinary output. Explain the mechanism.

_____

_____

How does polyuria contribute to the fatigue of DM?

_____

_____

(c) Which of the three "polys" of DM refers to excessive thirst and drinking?

Polydipsia   Polyphagia   Polyuria

(d) Polyphagia is more likely to accompany type *(1? 2?)* DM. Explain.

_____

_____

(e) Weight loss is more likely to be a sign of type *(1? 2?)* DM. List three factors that may account for weight loss.

_____

_____

_____

(f) Infections are *(more? less?)* common in people with diabetes. Explain.

_____

_____

_____

(g) How is hyperglycemia related to blurred vision?

_____

_____

_____

B10. Match the blood tests designed for diagnosing or monitoring diabetes with the descriptions that follow.

Fasting blood glucose test
Glycated hemoglobin (A1C test)
Oral glucose tolerance test
Casual blood glucose test
Self-monitoring test

(a) After a "load" (such as 75 g of glucose) is given, blood samples are drawn; individuals without diabetes exhibit normal blood glucose levels within 2 to 3 hours:

_____

(b) The preferred diagnostic test; easily administered and low cost:

_____

(c) Administered at any time regardless of last meal; glucose 200 mg/dL is considered an unequivocal elevation when accompanied by classic signs or symptoms of diabetes:

_____

(d) Measures percentage of hemoglobin that has combined permanently with glucose during the past 3 months since the time when those red blood cells were formed; a measure of diabetes control (and patient compliance) with a value less than 7.0%:

_____

(e) Involves placing a drop of blood on a strip then read by a glucometer; allows rapid, low-cost testing several times a day:

_____

B11. Answer the following questions about nonpharmacologic management of diabetes.

(a) Which type of testing for glucose is considered more accurate? *(Blood? Urine?)* Explain why the diabetic should check urine also.

_____

(b) List three or more mechanisms for control of type 2 diabetes other than by insulin.

_____

_____

_____

(c) The American Diabetic Association (ADA) *(does? does not?)* recommend a specific diet for individuals with diabetes. However, eating foods at *(consistent? varied?)* times is recommended.

(d) Describe the benefits and risks of regular exercise for individuals with diabetes, including the potential problem of delayed hypoglycemia for those with type 1 diabetes.

_____

B12. Oral hypoglycemic drugs can be effective for individuals with type *(1? 2?)* diabetes. Select from this list to identify the mechanisms by which the following drugs act:

IHC: Inhibits hepatic glucose production (by glycogenolysis or gluconeogenesis)

ISC: Increases sensitivity of cells of liver, skeletal muscle, and fat to insulin; thus, enhances uptake of glucose

SBC: Stimulates beta cells to release insulin (which works only for patients with some functional beta cells); can lead to hypoglycemia

(a) Thiazolidinediones (TZDs): _____ and _____

(b) Biguanides: _____ and _____

(c) Sulfonylureas: _____ and _____

B13. Answer the following questions about Melissa, age 19, who has type 1 diabetes.

(a) The medication she takes is more likely to be *(insulin? an oral hypoglycemic?)*. She takes her medication by injection, not by mouth. Explain.

_____

_____

(b) Identify the types of insulin that may possibly be prescribed for Melissa. Choose from these types:

Short-acting   Intermediate-acting
Long-acting

(1) Its effects begin within 30 minutes and typically have a duration of 5 to 8 hours: _____

(2) Ultralente and the human insulin analogue Glargine:

_____

(3) Lente and NPH: _____

(c) If Melissa is to take an intermediate- or long-acting insulin, she *(is? is not?)* likely to take a short-acting insulin also.

C. DIABETES MELLITUS: COMPLICATIONS (ACUTE OR CHRONIC)

C1. Identify the major acute complications of DM that fit descriptions that follow.

Diabetic ketoacidosis (DKA)
Hyperglycemic hyperosmolar state (HHS)
Hypoglycemia

(a) An insulin reaction caused by an insulin level in excess of the body's current needs:

_____

(b) Most associated with excessive fat breakdown (lipolysis) when insulin is lacking: _____

(c) Associated with high blood glucose levels:

_____

(d) Condition with the most rapid onset:

_____

(e) Precipitated by stress: _____

(f) Involves movement of water out of brain cells as extremely high blood glucose exerts an osmotic effect; may involve severe neurological alterations:

_____

(g) Involves dehydration of mucosa (leading to extreme thirst) and dry skin:

_____

(h) Seen most often in association with type 2

DM: _____

C2. Melissa (Question B13) is more likely to have diabetic ketoacidosis (DKA) develop when her blood glucose level is *(35? 100? 260?)* mg/dL. Answer the following questions about her episode of DKA.

(a) Circle the factors that increase Melissa's risk for DKA. She:

(1) Has type 1 diabetes

(2) Is 7 months pregnant

(3) Is a college student and approaching midterm examinations

(4) Has had a respiratory infection this week

(5) Self-monitors her blood glucose three or four times a day

(b) In DKA, excessive fat breakdown leads to formation of _____ in the liver. These chemicals are *(acids? bases?)*, so they *(decrease? increase?)* blood pH. Blood levels of bicarbonate *(decrease? increase?)* as bicarbonate buffers acids.

(c) How can Melissa's ketonemia be readily detected?

_____

(d) Melissa's blood pressure is likely to *(decrease? increase?)* in DKA; *(brady? tachy?)*cardia also may occur. Explain.

_____

(e) Her breathing is likely to be *(slow and shallow? rapid and deep?)*. Explain.

_____

_____

(f) Melissa is admitted to the hospital. List three major goals of her treatment.

_____

_____

C3. Nick, age 17, has type 1 DM and is a football player. He self-monitors to carefully balance his insulin doses with his meals and football practice. Today he had an insulin reaction. Answer the following questions related to his case.

(a) Circle each of the following that is a factor most likely to trigger such a reaction:

(1) Skipping an insulin injection

(2) Taking too large a dose of insulin

(3) Working harder than usual at practice

(4) Skipping a meal

(b) Circle each of the following that is a sign of hypoglycemic effects on his cerebrum:

(1) Making a mistake on a play at practice

(2) Headache

(3) Hunger

(4) Rapid heart rate and cool, clammy skin

(5) Starting a fight with another player

(c) Nick is unconscious and lying on the field. Which treatments for his insulin reaction are most helpful right now?

(1) Insulin injection

(2) Glucagon injection

(3) Hard candy

(4) Orange juice

C4. Colleen, a 50-year-old woman with type 2 DM, recently has increased carbohydrates and calories in her diet. Answer the following questions about her experience.

(a) Her recent changes in diet are likely to *(decrease? increase?)* her blood glucose level.

(b) Colleen notices this change as she self-monitors. She decides to increase her insulin dosage to "cover" the extra blood glucose. The extra insulin puts her into a mild *(hyper? hypo?)*glycemia.

(c) As a result, four counterregulatory hormones are released; all of these will *(decrease? increase?)* her blood glucose. Name these four hormones. (See Study Guide Figure 32-1, *A* and *B*.)

_____

_____

(d) Colleen then may increase her insulin dosage further, creating a vicious cycle. This cycle is known as the *(dawn? Somogyi?)* phenomenon, in which "_____glycemia begets _____glycemia."

(e) If Colleen also exhibits the dawn phenomenon, her blood glucose level will increase in early *(morning? evening?)*; this can *(exacerbate? reduce the effects of?)* her Somogyi phenomenon.

C5. Choose the two true statements about chronic complications of DM. (Pay particular attention to whether the **bold-faced** word or phrase makes the statement true or false.)

(a) Research indicates that intensive treatment for type 1 DM **can** reduce chronic complications.

(b) Nephropathies refer to alterations in **nerves**.

(c) Kidney damage is a **rare** complication of DM.

(d) Most diabetic kidney damage involves **renal tubules**.

(e) **Elevated protein in urine** is an early sign of diabetic nephropathy.

C6. Answer the following questions about chronic complications of DM in Colleen, Daniel, and Melissa.

(a) Colleen (Question C4) is showing signs of peripheral neuropathies. These are most likely to start in her *(hips and shoulders? feet and hands?)* and progress *(proximally? distally?)*. This is known as the _____ pattern and is likely to be *(bilateral? unilateral?)*.

(b) Explain why Colleen's peripheral neuropathies can lead to further complications.

_____

_____

(c) Daniel, age 65, received a diagnosis of type 2 DM 9 years ago. Circle each of the following that is a manifestation associated with autonomic nerve damage:

(1) Pain in his hands

(2) Burning pain in his legs

(3) Urinary tract infections

(4) Constipation

(5) Erectile dysfunction

(6) Feeling dizzy when he stands up quickly

(d) Circle factors that increase Daniel's risk for diabetic nephropathy and end-stage renal disease (ESRD).

(1) Daniel is Native American

(2) His father had diabetic nephropathy

(3) Daniel smokes a pack of cigarettes a day

(4) His blood pressure typically is 150/92 mm Hg

(5) His HbA$_{1c}$ usually is 6%

(6) His total cholesterol is 246 mg/dL

(e) List three regions of Daniel's body particularly at risk for macrovascular disease.

_____

_____

(f) Daniel is tested with a Semmes-Weinstein monofilament. What is being tested?

_____

In addition to decreased circulation, what factors might contribute to foot ulcers in Daniel?

_____

_____

(g) Blindness in individuals with diabetes most commonly results from:

Cataracts   Glaucoma   Retinopathy

Which factors listed in Question C2(a) increase Melissa's risk for diabetic retinopathy?

_____

_____

C7. Summarize measures that can best prevent chronic complications of DM.

_____

_____

_____

CHAPTER 33

Organization and Control of Neural Function

■ Review Questions

A. NERVOUS TISSUE CELLS

A1. Review Chapter 1, questions D10 and D11 on divisions of the nervous system and neuron cell structure.

A2. Schwann cells are found in the *(central? peripheral?)* nervous system. Complete this exercise about Schwann cells.

(a) Schwann cells wrap around axons ("jelly roll" fashion) to form _____ sheaths. Composed of lipid, myelin gives nerves their *(gray? red? white?)* color.

(b) Myelin functions as an _____ for axons. Myelin *(decreases? increases?)* the velocity of nerve conduction as impulses are forced to "jump" between nodes of Ranvier, where myelin is *(extra thick? lacking?)*. This type of conduction is known as _____.

(c) Myelin *(is? is not?)* required for survival of axons. Explain how this fact is related to multiple sclerosis (MS) and Guillain-Barré syndrome.

_____

_____

_____

(d) The endoneurial sheath (see Figure 33-3 in *Essentials of Pathophysiology*) around Schwann cells is required for the process of _____ of axons. This sheath is absent in the *(central? peripheral?)* nervous system. Explain the significance.

_____

_____

A3. Match the supporting cells of the nervous system with the description of their functions.

Astroglia	Ependymal cells
Microglia	Oligodendroglia
Satellite cells	Schwann cells

(a) Together with endothelial cells, they form the blood-brain barrier: _____

(b) Link neurons to blood vessels, therefore critical for nourishing neurons; form scar tissue (gliosis) when CNS tissue is destroyed: _____

(c) Form cerebrospinal fluid (CSF): _____

(d) Phagocytic "clean-up" cells: _____

(e) Form myelin around axons of the brain and spinal cord: _____

(f) Surround and protect cell bodies in ganglia of the peripheral nervous system (PNS): _____

(g) Supporting cells of the PNS: _____, _____

A4. Mr. Jenkins, who has type 1 diabetes, has experienced a "small stroke," in which the blood supply to his brain was interrupted for approximately 90 seconds. Answer the following questions related to his case.

(a) The brain makes up approximately _____ % of body weight, yet uses approximately _____ % of the body's oxygen. Brain cells are *(hyper? hypo?)*metabolic.

(b) Neurons of the brain *(can? cannot?)* store glucose or glycogen. During the period when Mr. Jenkins's blood supply is interrupted, how can his brain receive nutrients?

_____

_____

(c) Is it likely that Mr. Jenkins has had brain cells die as a result of his episode?

_____

(d) If Mr. Jenkins has an insulin reaction, how is this likely to affect his brain?

_____

B. NERVE CELL COMMUNICATION

B1. A nerve impulse is also known as an _____. Refer to Figure 33-5 in *Essentials of Pathophysiology* and answer the following questions about an action potential.

(a) A "resting" neuron is polarized so that the inside of the membrane is more *(positive? negative?)* than the outside.

(b) A stimulus leads to the entrance of *(sodium? potassium?)* into the membrane channels. As a result, membrane potential on the inner side of the membrane becomes less *(positive? negative?)*. If threshold is reached, an action potential *(is? is not?)* initiated. As more sodium enters the neuron, the membrane potential approaches 0 mV; the process of _____ is occurring.

(c) Repolarization takes place as sodium stops entering the neuron and *(sodium? potassium?)* exits through the membrane channels; the membrane potential becomes more *(positive? negative?)* and the cell may even become *(hyper? hypo?)*polarized before it returns to a normal resting potential.

B2. Fill in the blanks within each statement about two types of synapses.

(a) _____ synapses involve gap junctions.

(b) _____ synapses are the more common type of synapses.

B3. Arrange in correct sequence the events in which the neurotransmitter acetylcholine (ACh) functions in synaptic transmission.

(a) Acetylcholine binds to a cholinergic receptor on the postsynaptic cell membrane.

(b) A presynaptic neuron synthesizes and stores ACh within the axon terminal.

(c) The presynaptic neuron is stimulated and releases ACh from vesicles into the synaptic cleft.

(d) Acetylcholine is broken down by acetylcholinesterase (AChE), and choline is recycled into the presynaptic neuron.

(e) Excitation or inhibition of the postsynaptic neuron occurs (depending on the nature of the receptor and postsynaptic cell).

____ → ____ → ____ → ____ → ____

B4. Answer the following questions about the complexity of neural networks.

(a) Explain how neurons serve as integrators.

_____

_____

(b) Describe the split-second timing involved.

_____

(c) List examples of types of stimuli to neurons.

_____

_____

B5. Identify these neurotransmitters and other messenger molecules that fit the characteristics below.

Acetylcholine   Dopamine
Norepinephrine   Endorphins and enkephalins
Serotonin   Substance P

(a) Chemically classified as monoamines:

_____, _____, _____

(b) Peptides involved in pain perception:

_____, _____

(c) Excitatory to skeletal muscle but inhibitory to cardiac muscle: _____

B6. Name a type of chemical that fits each of the following descriptions.

(a) A hormone that can function as a neurotransmitter:_____

(b) A category of chemical that can alter the effect of a neurotransmitter:

_____

(c) A type of chemical that is necessary for long-term survival of postsynaptic cells:

_____

C. DEVELOPMENT AND ORGANIZATION OF THE NERVOUS SYSTEM

C1. Fill in the blanks or circle the correct answers within each statement about development of the nervous system.

(a) Severe brain damage to the rostral (front) end of the brain leads to loss of *(cognition? regulation of breathing?)*, whereas severe trauma to the brain stem results in loss of _____.

(b) During embryonic development, the neural tube develops into the *(central? peripheral?)* nervous system. The notochord develops into *(nervous? skeletal?)* system structures, specifically the _____.

(c) Most congenital disorders known as neural tube defects result from errors in development of the *(spinal cord? meninges, vertebrae, muscles, and skin?)*. Which neural tube defect involves protrusion of the spinal cord? *(Spina bifida with meningocele? Spina bifida with meningomyelocele?)*

(d) Swellings or primary vesicles of the embryonic neural tube form the brain. The first two segments form the prosencephalon or *(forebrain? midbrain? hindbrain?)*.

(e) Write the name of the embryonic layer next to the structure formed from that layer. Follow the first completed example.

  (e1) Brain and spinal cord: <u>Ectoderm</u>

  (e2) Epidermis of skin: _____

  (e3) Dermis of skin: _____

  (e4) Skeletal muscles: _____

  (e5) Skeleton: _____

  (e6) Urogenital structures: _____

  (e7) Lungs: _____

  (e8) Liver and pancreas: _____

(f) Of the 43 longitudinal segments in the developing person, ____ form spinal cord and spinal nerves and ____ form the brain and cranial nerves.

(g) As shown in Figure 33-8 in *Essentials of Pathophysiology*, each spinal segment is connected by *(2? 3? 4?)* pairs of spinal nerve roots. The *(dorsal? ventral?)* root carries afferent or *(sensory? motor?)* neurons, which then synapse with ____ neurons (or input association) neurons in the *(dorsal? ventral?)* horns of the spinal cord.

(h) The cell columns of ventral horns of the spinal cord are known as *(input? output?)* cell columns because they contain *(sensory? motor?)* neurons. These include both *(upper? lower?)* motor neurons and OA (_____ _____) neurons. Axons of these neurons exit the spinal cord in *(dorsal? ventral?)* roots of spinal nerves.

(i) Most of the billions of neurons in the central nervous system are *(afferent? efferent? internuncial?)* neurons.

C2. Identify the type of neuron that enables Matt to enjoy each particular aspect of a hot summer day at a theme park.

General somatic afferent (GSA)
General somatic efferent (GSE)
General visceral afferent (GVA)
General visceral efferent (GVE)
Pharyngeal efferent (PE)
Special somatic afferent (SSA)
Special visceral afferent (SVA)

(a) Matt is aware that he is moving in circles and that his muscles are tense (proprioception) as he spins on a ride at the park: _____

(b) Walking around the park involves Matt's use of his lower motor neurons (LMNs), which are _____ pathways. As he walks around, Matt feels the heat of the sun on his skin: _____.

(c) Matt smells and tastes the lunch that he buys: _____. He chews and swallows the lunch: _____. Then his parasympathetic (vagus) nerves begin the process of digestion: _____. Soon Matt becomes aware of a full stomach and bladder: _____.

C3. Different levels of the spinal cord tracts consist of *(gray? white?)* matter located in the *(inner or "butterfly-shaped"? outer?)* portion of the cord. Answer the following questions about these vertical (or longitudinal) communication pathways.

(a) The *(archi? paleo? neo?)* layer is considered the oldest layer in evolutionary development. This layer consists of the *(longest? shortest?)* pathways.

(b) Spinothalamic tracts (for pain and temperature) lie in the *(archi? paleo? neo?)* layer, which is the *(inner? middle? outer?)* layer of white tracts.

(c) The *(archi? paleo? neo?)* layer extends the entire length of the nervous system and is even "suprasegmental," meaning that it extends into the _____. Myelination of this part of the spinal cord usually is complete at *(birth? about 6 years of age?)*. State the significance of this fact.

D. THE SPINAL CORD AND BRAIN

D1. Circle the correct answers or fill in the blanks within each statement about the spinal cord.

(a) The spinal cord is *(longer? shorter?)* than the vertebral column. In adults, the cord ends as a cone-shaped structure (the conus medullaris) at about vertebral level *(L1 or L2? L3 to L4?)*. The spinal nerve roots that extend below the inferior end of the spinal cord are known as the _____.

(b) At what level is a spinal tap typically performed? Between vertebrae _____ and _____. Explain.

_____

(c) Review Figure 33-9 in *Essentials of Pathophysiology* and Question C1(h). A cross-section of the cord reveals an inner *H*- or butterfly-shaped region of *(gray? white?)* matter. The *(dorsal? ventral?)* gray horns contain cell bodies of *(motor? sensory?)* neurons. These are known as *(lower? upper?)* motor neurons; they innervate *(skeletal? smooth?)* muscle.

(d) Which regions of the spinal cord contain relatively large amounts of gray matter? (See Figure 33-12 in *Essentials of Pathophysiology.*) _____, _____ Explain.

_____

(e) List three anatomic structures that anchor the spinal cord in place.

_____

_____

D2. Answer the following questions about spinal nerves and spinal reflexes.

(a) The human body has a total of _____ pairs of spinal nerves. How many pairs in each location?

Cervical: _____

Thoracic: _____

Lumbar: _____

Sacral: _____

Coccygeal: _____

(b) Spinal nerves are attached by a *(motor? sensory?)* dorsal root and a *(motor? sensory?)* ventral root. Spinal nerves are *(mixed? motor? sensory?)*.

(c) What are "rami" of spinal nerves?

_____

_____

Which are larger: dorsal or ventral rami? Explain.

_____

(d) What do white "rami communicantes" supply?

_____

(e) Plexuses are complex nerve network that include *(sensory? motor? both sensory and motor?)* nerves. Fill in the blanks to arrange the following plexuses from most superior to most inferior:

____ ____ ____ ____

(1) Brachial

(2) Cervical

(3) Lumbar

(4) Sacral

D3. Match the spinal nerves with the following functions.

C1–C4: Cervical nerves no. 1–4
C5–C8: Cervical nerves no. 5–8
L2–S1: Lumbar–upper sacral nerves
S2–S4: Lower sacral nerves

(a) Supply most nerves to lower extremities: _____

(b) Supply nerves to upper extremities: _____

(c) Supply nerves to most neck and shoulder muscles: _____

D4. Identify components of the three major regions of the brain. Write one brain part on each line provided.

Cerebellum	Cerebrum	Hypothalamus
Medulla	Midbrain	Pons
Thalamus		

(a) Forebrain: _____, _____, _____

(b) Midbrain: _____

(c) Hindbrain: _____, _____, _____

D5. Which of the three major regions of the brain makes up the rostral end of the brain? _____brain. This part of the brain is most *(ancient? recent?)* in evolution and is *(more? less?)* vulnerable to injury than other brain parts.

D6. Use words from the list in Question D4 to identify which brain part fits each of the following descriptions.

(a) The name means a "bridge" connecting midbrain with medulla as well as right to left cerebellar hemispheres: _____

(b) The portion of the brain stem immediately anterosuperior to the spinal cord: _____

(c) The cerebral aqueduct carries CSF through this brain part: _____

(d) The fourth ventricle lies anterior to the _____ and posterior to the _____ and _____.

(e) Contains the four colliculi: _____

(f) Form the major structures in the diencephalon: _____ and _____

D7. Refer to Table 33-1 in *Essentials of Pathophysiology* and identify which cranial nerves (I–XII) are attached to each part of the brain stem or cervical spinal cord.

(a) Medulla: _____

(b) Pons: _____

(c) Midbrain: _____

(d) Upper cervical spinal cord: _____

D8. Identify by name and number the cranial nerve that is likely to be impaired in each case. Where indicated, circle whether the right or left nerve is damaged.

(a) Gail has lost most movements of her left eye; she has ptosis (drooping) of her left eyelid: _____, _____ R L

(b) Sean cannot raise his right shoulder, and his head is turned toward the left: _____, _____ R L

(c) Gus lacks facial expression on the left side of his face (Bell palsy): _____ R L

(d) Phoebe's tongue muscles are weak: _____, _____

(e) Dawn has a cranial nerve disorder that causes dry mouth and dry eye: _____, _____

(f) Mark cannot feel touch, pain, or temperature on the right side of his lower jaw, including his lower right teeth; his chewing muscles also are affected: _____, _____

D9. Identify the functions of each major part of the diencephalon by writing *H* (hypothalamus) or *T* (thalamus) next to the related descriptions.

(a) Major regulatory center for hormones, thirst, appetite, and body temperature regulation, as well as autonomic responses: _____

(b) Major relay center for sensations; also involved with selected motor activities and

with the limbic system for emotional responses: _____

(c) Two egg-shaped masses connected by a cross bar that passes through the third ventricle: _____

(d) The posterior pituitary is an extension of this brain part: _____

D10. Answer the following questions about the cerebrum.

(a) Match the cerebral structures with the descriptions below. Then circle *G* or *W* to indicate whether each structure consists of gray or white matter.

Basal ganglia   Corpus callosum
Internal capsule

(a1) A bridge of tracts connecting the two cerebral hemispheres; located immediately superior to lateral ventricles: _____ G W

(a2) The caudate and lentiform nuclei; regulate association movements, such as arm movements that accompany walking: _____ G W

(a3) Major site of tracts between the cerebral cortex and other parts of the CNS; located between basal ganglia and thalamus: _____ G W

(b) Match the cerebral lobes with the descriptions that follow.

Frontal   Occipital
Parietal   Temporal

(b1) Primary reception areas for hearing (area 41): _____

(b2) Primary reception areas for vision (area 17): _____

(b3) Primary somatosensory areas (areas 3, 1, and 2) for the sense of touch on fingers or face; located in the postcentral gyrus: _____

(b4) Primary motor cortex (area 4) located in the precentral gyrus, just anterior to the central sulcus: _____

D11. Identify the area most likely to be dysfunctional in each neural disorder.

Auditory association area (area 22)
Limbic system
Premotor area (6)
Primary auditory cortex (area 41)
Somatosensory association cortex (5 and 7)

(a) Violent behavior with explosive speech:

_____

(b) Apraxia, such as ability to handle scissors but inability to use them to cut paper:

_____

(c) Inability to hear the sounds of music:

_____

(d) Inability to identify a musical sequence as a commonly recognizable song:

_____

(e) Agnosia, such as inability to distinguish whether an object held in the hand is a key or a paperclip: _____

D12. Answer the following questions about meninges.

(a) Arrange meninges from most external to most internal:

Arachnoid   Dura mater   Pia mater

_____, _____, _____

(b) Which is a delicate layer that encases blood vessels to the brain? _____

(c) Its name means "tough mother"; it forms the falx cerebri and tentorium cerebelli:

_____

D13. Jacob experiences a mild blow on the side of his head. List structures that protect his brain during the trauma.

_____

_____

D14. Answer the following questions about cerebrospinal fluid (CSF).

(a) Where is CSF formed?

_____

(b) A total of approximately *(3 to 4? 1.5 to 2.0? 0.5 to 0.75?)* cup(s) of CSF are found within or around the CNS.

(c) Fill in the blanks that follow to arrange these structures in the pathway of CSF from first to last:

Arachnoid villi

Cerebral aqueduct

Fourth ventricle

Lateral ventricles

Subarachnoid space

Superior sagittal sinus

Third ventricle

_____ → Interventricular foramina of Monro → _____

→ _____ →

_____ → Foramina of Luschka and Magendie

→_____ → _____

→ _____

D15. Answer the following questions about the "barriers" that protect the brain.

(a) List structures that form the blood-brain barrier.

_____

(b) Circle each of the following substances that can cross the blood-brain barrier.

Alcohol   Bilirubin in newborns
Epinephrine   Heroin   Nicotine

(c) The CSF-brain barrier is formed by tight junctions of _____ cells of choroid plexuses.

(d) Circle each of the following chemicals that can readily diffuse or osmose across the membrane.

CO_2 H_2O O_2
Protein   Some vitamins

E. THE AUTONOMIC NERVOUS SYSTEM

E1. Briefly summarize the functions of the autonomic nervous system (ANS).

_____

E2. Write *P* (parasympathetic) or *S* (sympathetic) to indicate which division of the ANS better fits each description.

(a) Works with the adrenal medullae to prepare the body for stress or "fight or flight":

_____

(b) Functions when the body is "peaceful" (nonstressed) to help it conserve energy:

_____

(c) Exerts a more widespread effect:

_____

(d) Acts like a brake, slowing heart rate:

_____

(e) Increases salivation and motility of the stomach: _____

(f) The vagus nerve makes up 75% of the efferent nerves of this division of the ANS: _____

(g) Dilates airways and also pupils for better breathing and vision: _____

(h) More involved with anabolism than catabolism: _____

(i) Vasoconstricts blood vessels in areas such as skin and gastrointestinal tract, thereby increasing blood pressure: _____

E3. Choose the two true statements. (Pay particular attention to whether the **bold-faced** word or phrase makes the statement true or false.)

(a) Autonomic pathways from CNS to effector consist of **two** neurons, whereas somatic pathways consist of only one.

(b) In general, sympathetic and parasympathetic nerves have **similar** effects.

(c) Enteric plexuses in the wall of the gastrointestinal tract are **sympathetic** neurons.

(d) Visceral afferent neurons sensitive to changes in blood pressure (BP) pass from **carotid arteries via cranial nerve IX** to cardiovascular centers in the brain stem.

E4. Refer to Figure 33-24 in *Essentials of Pathophysiology* and circle the correct answers or fill in the blanks within each of the following statements about ANS pathways.

(a) Parasympathetic nerves are found in cranial nerves _____, _____, _____, and _____.

(b) Axons of preganglionic neurons are shown by *(solid? broken?)* lines in Figure 33-24. Most *(P? S?)* preganglionic axons reach all the way to viscera.

(c) Known as the "thoracolumbar" outflow, preganglionic neurons of this division begin at levels T1 through L2 of the spinal cord: _____

(d) The *(P? S?)* division has relatively short preganglionic neurons with branches that synapse with *(few? many?)* postganglionic neurons.

(e) The ganglia situated by major abdominal arteries (celiac, superior and inferior mesenteric) are sites where *(P? S?)* neurons synapse. The chains of ganglia that parallel vertebrae are sites where *(P? S?)* neurons synapse.

(f) White and gray rami both contain axons of *(P? S?)* neurons.

(g) Segments S2 through S4 of the spinal cord give rise to *(P? S?)* preganglionic neurons, which then travel in pelvic nerves.

(h) Circle the viscera that receive sympathetic but not parasympathetic innervation.

Adrenal medulla	Blood vessels of skin
Heart	Hair muscles of skin
Stomach	Sweat glands

E5. Describe the roles of the following structures in mediating autonomic activities.

(a) Hypothalamus

_____

_____

(b) Visceral afferent neurons

_____

_____

E6. Write the correct neurotransmitter next to each type of cell that releases it.

Acetylcholine
Norepinephrine (or other catecholamines)

(a) All postganglionic parasympathetic neurons: _____

(b) All somatic neurons (for example, to the gastrocnemius muscle): _____

(c) Most postganglionic sympathetic neurons: _____

(d) A few postganglionic sympathetic neurons (to sweat glands and vasodilator neurons in skeletal muscles): _____

(e) Adrenal medulla cells: _____

E7. Answer the following questions about ANS neurotransmitters and their receptors.

(a) Write the two chemicals that combine to form the neurotransmitter ACh: _____ + _____ → ACh. Name the two types of receptors for ACh: _____, _____. On which of these receptors does the anticholinergic drug atropine exert its effect? _____

(b) Circle the enzyme(s) that destroy(s) ACh.

Acetylcholinesterase (AChE)   Catechol O-methyltransferase (COMT) Monoamine oxidase (MAO)

(c) List in correct sequence the chemicals involved in the formation of the catecholamine norepinephrine (NE):

Dopamine   DOPA
Tyrosine (an amino acid)

_____ → _____ →
_____ → NE

(d) In the adrenal medulla, most *(epinephrine? norepinephrine?)* is converted to *(epinephrine? norepinephrine?)*. The latter chemical makes up about 80% of the hormonal secretion of this gland.

(e) List three mechanisms by which catecholamines can be removed from synapses or neuromuscular junctions.

_____

_____

(f) Receptors for NE are known as *(adrenergic? cholinergic?)*. Answer the following questions about roles of several of these receptors.

(f1) β_1-Adrenergic receptors are located on ___ cells. (Choose the correct answer from the list below.)

(1) Smooth muscle of blood vessels

(2) Smooth muscle of airways

(3) Cardiac muscle

(f2) When NE stimulates a β_1-adrenergic receptor, heart rate *(decreases? increases?)*. A β_1-adrenergic-blocking drug such as propranolol (Inderal) will *(decrease? increase?)* heart rate.

(f3) When NE stimulates a β_2-adrenergic receptor, smooth muscle of airways will *(contract? relax?)* so that airways *(constrict? dilate?)*.

(f4) When NE stimulates an α_1-adrenergic receptor, smooth muscle of blood vessels in skin and GI tract will *(contract? relax?)*, causing vaso*(constriction? dilation?)* and a(n) *(decrease? increase?)* in BP.

CHAPTER 34

Disorders of Somatosensory Function and Pain

■ Review Questions

A. ORGANIZATION AND CONTROL OF SOMATOSENSORY FUNCTION

A1. With her right hand, April attempts to pick up an extremely hot cup of tea from the microwave. Circle the correct answers or fill in the blanks within each statement about April's sensory pathway.

(a) At least *(two? three?)* orders of neurons form the pathway for burning pain. The first-order neuron has its cell body in April's *(central? peripheral?)* nervous system, specifically in a _____ ganglion just lateral to the right side of her spinal cord. Refer to the dermatome map in Figure 34-2 of *Essentials of Pathophysiology*. At which level of the spinal cord do first-order neurons from April's hand enter her spinal cord? *(C6-8? T6-8?)*

(b) April's second-order neurons *(do? do not?)* cross to the left side of her spinal cord and ascend her spinal cord in *(anterolateral? posterior?)* pathways that reach to the *(right? left?)* side of her thalamus.

(c) The third-order neuron axons terminate in April's _____, specifically in the *(right? left?) (frontal? parietal?)* lobe. Refer to Figure 34-6 in *Essentials of Pathophysiology* and determine the exact location of the cortex that receives impulses from April's hand. The map of these sensory neurons is known as the _____ pattern because it roughly parallels a "little man" laid across a cerebral hemisphere. The exact parietal lobe location for reception of sensations from April's fingers is:

(1) Lateral

(2) Medial

(3) Between medial and lateral

(d) Figure 34-6 in *Essentials of Pathophysiology* indicates that most of April's primary sensory cortex would be devoted to perception of sensations from ___ because these areas have a high density of sensory receptors. (Choose the correct answer below.)

(1) Fingers and face

(2) Trunk, hips, and feet

A2. Identify which of the two major somatosensory pathways—anterolateral pathway or dorsal column-medial lemniscal pathway—is described below.

(a) Includes tracts for pain, hot, cold, and "crude touch": _____

(b) Carries impulses that allow distinction between a paperclip and a key (stereognosis): _____

(c) Permits proprioception (awareness of body position and muscle tension) as well as two-point discriminative touch: _____

(d) The second-order neuron crosses to the opposite side of the cord to ascend in neospinothalamic or paleospinothalamic tracts: _____

(e) First-order neurons ascend in dorsal columns (or enter via cranial nerves) to the medulla where they synapse: _____

(f) Second-order neurons convey impulses through the medial lemniscus tract of the brain: _____

(g) Destruction of the left side of the spinal cord would result in loss of these pathways from the right arm and leg: _____

A3. Refer to Figure 34-2 in *Essentials of Pathophysiology* and circle the correct answer within each statement about dermatomes.

(a) Dermatome patterns are most horizontal and segmental in regions supplied by *(cervical? thoracic? lumbosacral?)* nerves.

(b) Injury to *(C5 to C7? T5 to T7?)* would deprive most of the arms of nerve supply.

(c) Inability to sense touch in the anterior thigh region indicates injury to spinal nerves *(L2 and L3? S2 and S3?)*.

A4. Answer the following questions about aspects of sensation.

(a) List three or more modalities of sensation.

_____

_____

(b) Explain what accounts for such modalities.

_____

_____

A5. Identify the type of tactile receptor that fits each description.

Free nerve endings   Hair follicle end-organs
Meissner corpuscles   Merkel disks
Pacinian corpuscles   Ruffini end organs

(a) Abundant in your fingertips and lips where your sense of touch is well developed:

_____

(b) Deep to your skin, these receptors allow sensation for vibration: _____

(c) Lacking a capsule, these account for sensitivity of your skin and the anterior of your eyes (corneas) to touch: _____

(d) Detect slight movement over skin surface:

_____

(e) Detect continuous pressure of a heavy weight on your skin or joints: _____

A6. Answer the following questions about other sensations.

(a) *(Lips? Fingers?)* are more sensitive to cold? *(Lips? Fingers?)* are more sensitive to heat?

(b) Cold and warmth receptors *(do? do not?)* completely adapt. Explain the clinical significance.

_____

(c) Define *proprioception.*

_____

(d) Kinesthesia refers to *(static? dynamic?)* position sense.

B. PAIN

B1. Describe the "good news" and "bad news" of pain.

_____

_____

B2. Circle the correct answers within each statement about pain.

(a) Pain is a *(rare? common?)* reason for people to seek professional help.

(b) Intense stimulation of *(only specific? virtually all?)* types of sensory receptors can lead to pain. This is a statement of the *(pattern? specificity?)* theory of pain.

B3. Answer the following questions about theories of pain.

(a) The "gate control theory" of pain states that tactile sensations that travel over *(fast? slow?)* fibers can block pain pathways that travel over *(fast? slow?)* pathways, thereby blocking pain. This theory was proposed by _____ and _____ in 1965.

(b) Describe Melzack's neuromatrix theory of pain.

_____

_____

_____

B4. Nociception means _____ sense. Answer the following questions about nociceptive mechanisms and pathways.

(a) List several sites in the body where nociceptors are located.

_____

_____

(b) List three categories of stimuli that can be nociceptive and give examples for each.

(b1) _____

_____

(b2) _____

(b3) _____

_____

(c) Acute mechanical and thermal painful stimuli typically are transmitted along:

Fast nerve fibers (Aδ)

Slow nerve fibers (C)

(d) Neurogenic inflammation involves release of chemical mediators by *(Aδ? C?)* nerve fibers, and these chemicals cause *(vasoconstriction? vasodilation?)* of blood vessels and lead to a vicious cycle of *(acute? chronic?)* pain.

(e) Bright, sharp, or stabbing pain is more likely to be transmitted through *(neo? paleo?)*spinothalamic tracts, which are *(fast? slow?)* conduits to the brain. *(Neo? Paleo?)*spinothalamic tracts transmit dull, aching pain, such as chronic visceral pain.

(f) Explain the mechanism by which rubbing the skin near a painful area or acupuncture may provide pain relief: _____

B5. Joe Green trips and falls over something in the middle of the driveway. Match these parts of Joe's brain with their functions related to his pain:

Association areas of parietal cortex
Limbic cortex
Somatosensory area of parietal cortex
Thalamus

(a) Provides Joe with a generalized awareness of hurt or pain: _____

(b) Pinpoints the specific location of the pain to his right foot: _____

(c) Ascribes meaning to the pain: Joe realizes that his son Timmy has left his bicycle out *again*:_____

(d) Provides an emotional response to pain, such as anger and frustration at Timmy: _____

B6. Choose the three true statements related to pain. (Pay particular attention to whether the **bold-faced** word or phrase makes the statement true or false.)

(a) Prostaglandins tend to **enhance** pain.

(b) Glutamate and substance P **both inhibit** pain.

(c) The periaqueductal gray (PAG) region is located in the **thalamus** and it **causes pain**.

(d) The nucleus raphe magnus (NRM) is located in the **medulla** of the brain and is thought to inhibit pain.

(e) The tricyclic antidepressant amitriptyline has the side effect of **producing analgesia**.

B7. Define and describe the effects of endogenous opioids.

_____

List three categories of endogenous opioids.

_____

B8. Which refers to the "amount of pain a person is willing to endure before the person wants some relief"? Pain *(threshold? tolerance?)*. Which is more constant from person to person? Pain *(threshold? tolerance?)*.

B9. Answer the following questions about types of pain.

(a) A sprained ankle is likely to cause *(cutaneous? deep somatic? visceral?)* pain. Cutaneous pain is considered *(diffuse? sharp, bright?)* pain.

(b) Appendicitis, gallstones, and kidney stones cause *(cutaneous? deep somatic? visceral?)* pain. This type of pain also is known as _____ pain. Explain why visceral pain is likely to be accompanied by sweating, pallor, nausea, and vomiting.

_____

(c) Visceral pain is more likely to occur from:

(1) Abnormal contractions, distention, or ischemia of the intestinal wall

(2) Burning (cauterizing) or cutting the wall of the intestine

(d) Visceral pain *(is? is not?)* readily localized. Explain why.

_____

_____

_____

(e) Mr. Jefferson experiences pain of a heart attack in his left arm and the left side of the chest (see Figure 34-11 in *Essentials of Pathophysiology*). This phenomenon is known as *(phantom? referred?)* pain. Explain the mechanism.

_____

_____

(f) Liver and gallbladder pain "refer" to the *(right? left?)* side of the *(chest? neck?)*. Explain.

_____

_____

(g) *(Acute? Chronic?)* pain is defined as pain caused by tissue damage (such as from surgery) that ends when tissues heal. This pain has a duration of less than ___ months. List three factors other than the actual pain stimuli that can exacerbate acute pain.

_____

_____

(h) *(Acute? Chronic?)* pain serves a useful function. Explain.

_____

_____

_____

(i) *(Acute? Chronic?)* pain is more associated with depression, loss of appetite, and sleep disturbances.

B10. Ms. Templeton, age 42, has metastatic ovarian cancer; she is being evaluated for pain and possible treatment. Answer the following questions related to her case.

(a) The single most reliable indicator of the existence and intensity of acute pain is:

(1) The patient's self-report

(2) Patient blood pressure and heart rate

(3) Names of pain medications the patient is taking

(b) Describe methods that the nurse is likely to use to assess Ms. Templeton's pain.

_____

_____

_____

B11. Choose the two true statements about treatment of pain. (Pay particular attention to whether the **bold-faced** word or phrase makes the statement true or false.)

(a) A **pain history** is an important component of an assessment of pain.

(b) Treatment of acute pain is likely to be **more** complex than treatment of chronic pain.

(c) Pain management is considered to be **more** effective if it is initiated **after** pain becomes severe.

(d) Cancer is a **common cause** of chronic pain.

(e) Analgesic drugs are **all** narcotics.

B12. Circle all answers that describe AHCPR guidelines for addressing pain caused by surgery, medical procedures, and trauma.

(a) A generalized plan developed after surgery takes place

(b) Treatment plan that integrates input by health care providers with that from clients and family

(c) The patient's pain frequently reassessed and documented on a pain log

(d) Use of only nondrug or non-narcotic therapies

B13. Circle each of the following that is a mechanism by which aspirin and other nonsteroidal anti-inflammatory drugs (NSAIDs) decrease pain.

(a) **Inhibit** production of prostaglandins through inhibition of cyclooxygenase

(b) **Desensitize** nociceptors to bradykinin and histamine

(c) **Cause** vasodilation of blood vessels

(d) **Decrease** release of inflammatory chemicals from mast cells and lymphokines from T cells

B14. Analgesics are medications that decrease pain *(with? without?)* loss of consciousness. Match these analgesics with the descriptions that follow:

Acetaminophen   Aspirin
Codeine   Nonsteroidal
Morphine   anti-inflammatory
Serotonin reuptake   drugs (NSAIDs)
  inhibitors

(a) Classified as opioid analgesics:

_____, _____

(b) Non-narcotic analgesics that also are antipyretic and anti-inflammatory:

_____, _____

(c) A non-narcotic analgesic that is antipyretic but not anti-inflammatory: _____

(d) Adjuvant analgesics such as the tricyclic antidepressant amitriptyline: _____

B15. Choose the two true statements about pain treatments. (Pay particular attention to whether the **bold-faced** word or phrase makes the statement true or false.)

(a) Morphine causes **euphoria** and **an increase** in respiratory rate.

(b) Opioids can be appropriate therapy management of acute pain **but not for** chronic pain.

(c) The World Health Organization (WHO) **does** recommend morphine use for persons with chronic cancer pain.

(d) Interdisciplinary approaches to pain management are **more likely** to be successful than are approaches with a single focus.

C. ALTERATIONS IN PAIN SENSITIVITY AND SPECIAL TYPES OF PAIN

C1. Select the term that fits each description.

Allodynia	Analgesia	Athermia
Hyperalgesia	Hyperpathia	Paresthesia

(a) Celia's foot "fell asleep" as her nerves were compressed by her crossed legs; now she feels "pins and needles" as her foot "wakes up": _____

(b) Anthony experiences increased sensitivity to pain: _____

(c) Joan has an exaggerated response to painful stimuli; her pain feels "explosive": _____

(d) Elizabeth experiences intense pain initiated by light touch that should not normally induce pain: _____

(e) Dave has lost all ability to feel changes in temperature in his right leg: _____

C2. List several conditions that can cause neuropathy and neuropathic pain that is:

(a) Localized

_____

_____

(b) Widespread

_____

_____

C3. Describe two major categories of treatments for neuropathy by writing sentences using the following key words:

(a) Cause

_____

_____

(b) Palliative

_____

_____

C4. Neuralgia refers to _____. Answer the following questions about neuralgias.

(a) Tic douloureux is another name for _____ neuralgia, which is pain along *(cranial nerve V? spinal nerve C5?)*. This condition typically is *(bilateral? unilateral?)* and involves *(mild, aching? severe, lightning-like?)* pain in the face. State one trigger for tic douloureux: _____. List several treatment approaches.

_____

_____

_____

(b) Postherpetic neuralgia refers to pain more than 1 month after onset of herpes *(simplex? zoster?)*, also known as *(cold sores? shingles?)*. This virus is the same one that causes *(chickenpox? measles? mumps?)*. This condition is *(more? less?)* common among elderly persons. Explain.

_____

(c) Explain why complex regional pain syndrome (formerly known as reflex sympathetic dystrophy) may be exacerbated by emotional upsets and possibly involve pallor, rubor, edema, sweating, or dryness.

_____

C5. Phantom limb pain occurs in about *(17%? 70%?)* of patients who undergo amputation. Use the key words below to describe possible causative mechanisms.

(a) Scar tissue

_____

(b) Spinal cord

_____

(c) Brain

_____

_____

D. HEADACHE

D1. Choose the two true statements about headaches. (Pay particular attention to whether the **bold-faced** word or phrase makes the statement true or false.)

(a) **Approximately 75%** of women experience at least one headache a month.

(b) Migraines and tension-type headaches are **both** considered primary or chronic headaches.

(c) **Most** secondary headaches indicate serious intracranial disorders.

(d) Almost all migraines occur **with** an aura.

D2. List characteristics of headaches that should be investigated for possibly serious causes.

_____

_____

_____

D3. Mari, age 16, has developed chronic headaches. What information should she include in her headache diary?

_____

_____

D4. Match the major types of headaches or head pain with their characteristics.

Cluster   Temporomandibular joint
              (TMJ) syndrome
Migraine   Tension-type

(a) The most common type of headache; does not typically interfere with daily activities or involve nausea or vomiting:

_____

(b) May be caused by caffeine withdrawal, temporomandibular joint pain, or prolonged neck muscle work such as computer activity: _____

(c) More common in women and may be associated with estrogen levels; tend to be familial: _____

(d) Headaches that are pulsatile, throbbing, often accompanied by nausea and vomiting; often disabling: _____

(e) Relatively rare type of headache; occur most often in men at midlife; typically unilateral, affecting one side of the forehead, temple, or nose, or one eye; occur in groups over weeks or months separated by headache-free intervals: _____

(f) Involves dull, aching pain occurring in a hatband distribution around the head:

_____

(g) Likely to be caused by bruxism (grinding of teeth) or poor bite; pain is likely to be referred, for example, causing earache or headache: _____

(h) Increased blood flow into arteries of the hypothalamus may play a key role; typically rapid onset and relatively short duration:

_____

D5. Answer the following questions about migraines.

(a) What is the typical duration of the aura that occurs with some migraines?

_____

(b) Describe the signs or symptoms that accompany these types of migraines:

(b1) Ophthalmoplegic migraine

_____

(b2) Transformed migraine

_____

(c) Migraines _(can? do not?)_ occur in children. Circle each of the following that is a characteristic typical of childhood migraines:

(1) Continuous headaches without pain-free periods

(2) Bilateral head throbbing

(3) Intense nausea and vomiting

(4) Positive family history

(5) Seeking relief in dark environments

(d) Pathophysiologic mechanisms of migraines _(are? are not?)_ well understood. It is known that the _(facial? trigeminal?)_ nerves become activated during migraines. Inflammation of meninges _(does? does not?)_ appear to occur, and meningeal blood vessels vaso_(constrict? dilate?)_.

(e) Describe methods (nonpharmacologic and pharmacologic) of prevention of migraines.

_____

_____

_____

E. PAIN IN CHILDREN AND OLDER ADULTS

E1. Defend or dispute this statement: "Young children and elderly persons do not feel pain."

_____

_____

_____

E2. Describe tools for assessing pain in:

(a) Jewel, age 4

_____

_____

(b) Jade, age 12

_____

_____

E3. Jade (age 12) is scheduled for a painful surgery. It is preferable to teach pain interventions *(before? after?)* the surgery. List several methods of doing so.

_____

_____

_____

E4. Explain the benefit of having a child in pain receive pain medications on a regular schedule rather than "as needed."

_____

_____

E5. Write two reasons elderly persons may be reluctant to report pain.

_____

_____

E6. List reasons why dosages of pain medications for elderly persons may need to be:

(a) Greater than in younger persons

_____

_____

_____

(b) Less than in younger persons

_____

_____

_____

E7. Define the following terms related to pain interventions in the elderly.

(a) Polypharmacy

_____

_____

(b) Noncompliance

_____

_____

CHAPTER 35

Disorders of Neuromuscular Function

■ Review Questions

A. THE ORGANIZATION AND CONTROL OF MOTOR FUNCTION

A1. Arrange the following levels of motor control in correct sequence from highest (purposeful, planned movements) to lowest (reflexes).

A. Spinal cord
B. Basal ganglia and cerebellum
C. Cerebral cortex of frontal lobe

____ → ____ → ____

A2. Define a motor unit.

_____
_____

Large motor units may have *(several? thousands?)* of muscle cells innervated by a single lower motor neuron (LMN). *(Large? Small?)* motor units regulate precise movements of tongue, eyes, or hands.

A3. Refer to Figures 35-3 and 35-4 in *Essentials of Pathophysiology* and match the parts of the cerebrum with each function.

Premotor cortex
Primary motor cortex
Supplementary motor cortex

(a) On medial aspects of area 6 and 8; involved with skillful movements on both sides of the body: _____

(b) Also called the "motor strip" or area 4; this thick area in the left side controls delicate movement sequences on the right side of the body: _____

(c) Programs complex activity patterns, such as picking up a spoon: _____

(d) Neurons are arranged in a person-shaped map known as the "motor homunculus": _____

A4. Refer to Figure 35-2 in *Essentials of Pathophysiology* and arrange these structures

in pyramidal pathways in correct sequence from first to last.

(a) Tracts in the internal capsule

(b) Cell bodies of upper motoneurons (UMNs) in motor cortex in the posterior region of the frontal lobe

(c) Corticospinal tract in the spinal cord

(d) Decussation (crossing) of axons in pyramids of the medulla

(e) Ventral roots and then spinal nerves

(f) Cell bodies of LMNs in ventral horn of the spinal cord

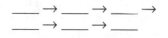

A5. Choose the two true statements about control of movements. (Pay particular attention to whether the **bold-faced** word or phrase makes the statement true or false.)

(a) The homunculus map demonstrates that about half of the primary motor cortex controls movements of **arms and legs.**

(b) Neurons on the lateral aspect of the primary motor cortex regulate **foot** movements.

(c) Most of the neurons in the right primary cortex control movements on the **right** side of the body.

(d) Axons of the lateral corticospinal tract are parts of **UMNs.**

(e) About **half** of the axons in the lateral corticospinal tract synapse with LMNs in cervical regions of the spinal cord and supply upper extremities.

A6. Write *pyramidal* or *extrapyramidal* next to descriptions that fit each of these types of pathways.

(a) Formed of axons of neurons that originate in the primary motor cortex of the cerebrum and continue through corticobulbar lateral or corticospinal tracts: _____

(b) Originate in the cortex of basal ganglia and pass through reticular formation; these pathways do not cross in the medulla: _____

(c) These pathways are altered in Parkinson disease and are likely to lead to muscle rigidity or tremor: _____.

A7. Answer the following questions about spinal reflexes.

(a) List the three components of a spinal reflex.

_____ → _____ → _____

(b) How is a stretch reflex initiated? _____ Give one example of a stretch reflex: _____

(c) Circle the correct answer or fill in the blanks within each statement about what happens in a knee-jerk reflex.

(c1) Muscle spindle receptors are located in the *(belly? tendon?)* of a muscle such as the quadriceps. These consist of *(intrafusal? extrafusal?)* muscle fibers encased in connective tissue and a spiral afferent neuron. These type _____ nerve fibers transmit nerve impulses extremely *(rapidly? slowly?)*.

(c2) Stretching of the muscle triggers the afferent neurons (the first component of a reflex) whose 1a nerve fibers enter the *(dorsal? ventral?)* route of the spinal cord.

(c3) Such sensory neuron synapse with *(alpha? gamma?)* motor neurons in the spinal cord, causing *(intrafusal? extrafusal?)* muscle fibers to contract and shorten the quadriceps. The resulting *(flexion? extension)* of the leg indicates normal function of this stretch reflex arc pathway.

(c4) Other branches of the same 1a nerve fibers (A7[c2]) synapse indirectly to inhibit muscles in the left thigh that are antagonists to the quadriceps, namely the _____ muscles. Describe the effect. _____

_____

(c5) State the role of gamma motor neurons in reflexes. _____

(d) Branches from the afferent neuron can transmit impulses to the cerebral cortex. The resulting awareness of position and movement of the knee during this reflex is called _____.

(e) While Roma is standing, she picks up her right foot. As she uses flexor muscles (hamstrings) for this action, the antagonistic extensor muscles (quadriceps) of her right thigh will be *(stimulated? inhibited?)*. Simultaneously, a reflex will cause her to straighten her left leg (extend it by contracting the left quadriceps) to support her weight while she is on one foot. This is an example of a _____ reflex. (Stand up and try this action or analyze it as a friend demonstrates.)

A8. Circle the correct answers within each statement about muscle disorders.

(a) Hypotonia refers to *(absent? less than normal? spastic?)* muscle tone.

(b) Rigidity, a classic sign of Parkinson disease, involves *(increased? decreased?)* resistance to movements. In this condition the brain fails to *(stimulate? inhibit?)* alpha LMNs. (See Question A7[c3].) As a result, simultaneous stimulation of prime movers and antagonists leads to concurrent flexion and extension of joints.

(c) *(Paralysis? Paresis?)* refers to weakness of muscles. Paralysis of both legs is an example of *(mono? di? para? hemi? quadri?)*plegia. Paralysis of the left arm and left leg is *(mono? di? para? hemi? quadri?)*plegia.

(d) Injury to *(UMNs? LMNs?)* is more likely to lead to flaccid paralysis. *(Clonus? Hypertonia or spasticity?)* is an abnormal increase in muscle tone.

A9. Chad suffered a gunshot wound that severed his spinal cord at vertebra T6.

(a) From level T7 inferiorly, Chad has lost:

(1) Communication with the brain

(2) Spinal cord reflexes

(b) Chad's spinal cord injury (SCI) destroys pathways of *(UMNs? LMNs?)* *(above? below?)* his midthoracic area.

(c) Chad is likely to have *(complete use? spasticity? flaccidity?)* of his arms and *(complete use? spasticity? flaccidity?)* of his legs. Explain.

_____

_____

(d) Chad *(is? is not?)* likely to have bowel and bladder incontinence. He *(may? will not?)* have erections that could permit sexual intercourse. Explain.

_____

_____

A10. Circle the correct answers or fill in the blank within each statement about infections that can injure nerves.

(a) Dan steps on a rusty nail and develops tetanus in his right leg. *Clostridium tetani* toxin travels to Dan's spinal cord and irritates the cell bodies of *(UMNs? LMNs?)*. As a result, muscles innervated by these nerves become *(hyper? hypo?)*excited and develop sustained contractions known as _____.

(b) The polio virus is likely to destroy *(UMNs? LMNs?)*, causing *(spastic? flaccid?)* paralysis and *(atrophy? hypertrophy?)* of muscles.

A11. Injury to Mr. Ross's right *(C7? T3? L4?)* spinal nerve by a herniated disk is most likely to lead to leg weakness and pain, specifically of his *(right? left?)* leg.

B. SKELETAL MUSCLE, NEUROMUSCULAR FUNCTION, AND PERIPHERAL NERVE DISORDERS

B1. Identify the motor disorder of each patient below.

Denervation atrophy	Disuse atrophy
Duchenne muscular dystrophy	Myasthenia gravis
	Mononeuropathy
Polyneuropathy	

(a) Matt, age 10, is wheelchair-bound because of a progressive genetic disorder: _____

(b) Mrs. Meyer, age 48, has been in a coma and paralyzed following traumatic brain injury in an automobile accident 10 years ago: _____

(c) Ms. Allen, age 27, has experienced muscle weakness and fatigue; tests indicate a diagnosis of an autoimmune disease that destroys acetylcholine (ACh) receptors at her neuromuscular junctions: _____

(d) Mrs. Schmidt, age 77, has been wearing an immobilizer of her right leg since she

fractured her tibia 2 months ago; as a result, she has lost 25% of her calf muscle tissue: _____

(e) Lisette, age 37, received a diagnosis of Guillain-Barré syndrome a short time after she recovered from a viral infection; she experienced paralysis in her legs that ascended to her upper body; her recovery is now complete: _____

(f) Brandy, age 29, has worked an assembly line for 11 years; she has carpal tunnel syndrome of both wrists: _____

B2. Answer the following questions about Matt's disorder (Question B1[a]).

(a) His condition occurs in *(females? males? both females and males?)*. Explain.

_____

(b) Matt's condition is a *(muscular? neural?)* disorder. Duchenne muscular dystrophy (DMD) involves formation of a faulty protein, _____, which normally connects muscle cell membranes with actin and myosin filaments.

(c) Circle each of the following that is a typical early manifestation of DMD:

(1) Hip muscle weakness, abnormal postures, and falls

(2) Inability to use utensils to eat

(3) Incontinence

(4) Weakness of thoracic muscles with respiratory infections and scoliosis

(d) Matt's serum levels of creatine kinase are likely to be *(high? normal? low?)*. Explain.

_____

(e) Prenatal diagnosis of DMD is available as early as 12 weeks' gestation by *(amniocentesis? chorionic villi sampling?)*.

(f) With early treatment, DMD *(is? is not?)* curable. Death is likely to occur by failure of muscle tissue in _____ and _____ systems.

B3. Match these chemicals with their effects at neuromuscular junctions or synapses as described below:

Acetylcholinesterase	*Clostridium botulinum* toxin
Curare	
Malathion	Physostigmine and neostigmine

(a) Breaks down the neurotransmitter ACh (review Chapter 33, Question E7[b]):

_____

(b) Inhibits acetylcholinesterase (AChE), causing ACh to linger longer in neuromuscular junctions:

_____

(c) Acts as a muscle relaxant by blocking ACh action on muscles: _____

(d) Produced by microbes from soil, it can cause a serious food poisoning from improperly canned foods. Because it blocks release of ACh, it can be used clinically (Botox) to reduce spasms of extrinsic eye muscles, eyelids, neck, or larynx:

_____

(e) Chemical in some insecticides that binds AChE so ACh lingers longer in neuromuscular junctions:

_____

B4. Answer the following questions about Ms. Allen's disorder (Question B1[c]).

(a) Myasthenia gravis is more common in *(women? men?)*.

(b) Circle Ms. Allen's activities that are most likely to be affected by myasthenia gravis:

(1) Speaking

(2) Lifting her eyelids

(3) Chewing

(4) Writing

(5) Sensation in her feet

(c) Which category of drug listed in Question B3 is most likely to help Ms. Allen?

_____

(d) Plasmapheresis is a treatment that removes _____ from Ms. Allen's blood.

(e) Identify the most serious problem associated with myasthenia crisis.

_____

B5. Answer the following questions about peripheral nerve injury and repair.

(a) Circle all structures that are parts of the peripheral nervous system.

(a1) Cell bodies located within the brain or spinal cord

(a2) Axons located in pyramidal tracts (between motor cortex of the brain and anterior gray horn of the spinal cord)

(a3) Dendrites of afferent (sensory) neurons that carry nerve impulses from skin or muscles to cell bodies in dorsal root ganglia

(a4) Axons of alpha motor neurons that carry nerve impulses from the anterior gray horn of the spinal cord to the quadriceps muscle

(b) Identify which of the two main types of peripheral nerve injury is involved in each disorder. Choose from these answers:

Axonal degeneration   Segmental demyelination

(b1) Guillain-Barré syndrome: _____

(b2) A crushing injury to spinal nerves:

_____

(c) Neurons are more likely to regenerate if the nerve fibers are destroyed *(close to? far away from?)* the cell body.

(d) Which structure(s) must be intact for regrowth of an injured axon? *(Endoneurial tube? Schwann cells?)* Which structure(s) produce new myelin as the axon grows?

_____

(e) Injuries involving neuronal cell bodies are *(more? less?)* common than those affecting axons. Which is more readily repaired? Injuries involving *(cell bodies? axons?)*.

B6. Answer the following questions about Brandy's carpal tunnel syndrome (Question B1[f]).

(a) In addition to the repetitive wrist movements of her job, what other factors might contribute to Brandy's diagnosis? She:

(1) Has diabetes

(2) Takes oral contraceptives

(3) Has hypothyroidism

(b) Circle each of the following that is a typical manifestation of carpal tunnel syndrome:

(1) Numbness of the little finger and ring finger in each hand

(2) Difficulty gripping between thumb and index finger

(3) Pain in her wrists and hands that is worse at night

(c) Wearing wrist splints *(can be? is not?)* helpful for Brandy.

B7. The effects of diabetes or chronic alcoholism on nerves is an example of a *(mono? poly?)*neuropathy.

B8. Back pain is a *(common? rare?)* health problem. About *(10%? 90%?)* of persons with acute lower back problems for less than 3 months recover spontaneously. Circle each of the following that is a conservative treatment for back pain:

(a) Nonsteroidal anti-inflammatory drugs

(b) Back surgery

(c) Exercises to strengthen the back

(d) Muscle relaxants

B9. Answer the following questions about Mr. Ross's "slipped disk" injury (Question A11).

(a) A "slipped disk" is technically known as a _____ intervertebral disk. The portion of the disk that protrudes out of position is the *(annulus fibrosus? nucleus pulposus?)*. It is most likely to herniate *(anteriorly? posteriorly?)*. Explain why.

_____

(b) Herniation is most likely to occur at vertebrate level *(T6–T7? L1–L2? L4–L5?)*. Trauma is a *(common? rare?)* cause of such herniations.

(c) Typically, the first sign of herniated disk is _____, and major muscle weakness is *(common? rare?)*.

C. BASAL GANGLIA AND CEREBELLUM DISORDERS

C1. Refer to Figure 35-12 in *Essentials of Pathophysiology* and answer the following questions about components of the basal ganglia and associated structures.

(a) Basal ganglia are deep-lying regions known as "nuclei" within the *(cerebrum? cerebellum?)*.

(b) The most lateral portion of the basal ganglia is the *(caudate? putamen?)*. Together with the *(caudate nucleus? globus pallidus?)*, the putamen forms the neostriatum.

(c) The midbrain contains cells rich in the pigment melanin; this section of the midbrain is known as the substantia _____ and it is considered part of the basal ganglia. These cells synthesize the neurotransmitter *(serotonin? dopamine?)* and supply it to the striatum via axons in the nigrostriatal pathway.

(d) Basal ganglia *(do? do not?)* form many connections with the cerebral cortex,

cerebellum, brainstem, and thalamus in reciprocal circuits. State the significance.

_____

_____

C2. Refer to Table 35-1 in *Essentials of Pathophysiology* and match these involuntary movement disorders with the descriptions that follow:

Athetosis	Ballismus
Chorea	Dystonia
Tardive dyskinesia	Tic

(a) Brief, rapid, jerky and irregular movements of head and extremities; the term means "to dance"; may include piano-playing-type movement of fingers, curling and protrusion of tongue, raising eyebrows and shoulders: _____

(b) Continuous, wormlike, twisting movements of extremities, trunk, or face: _____

(c) Violent, flinging movements of limbs; the term means "to jump around": _____

(d) Repetitive, bizarre movements of face, including grimacing, protrusion of tongue, and deviations of the jaw; may occur as reaction to long-term use of antipsychotic drugs: _____

(e) Repetitive winking of eyelids, and brief abnormal movements of other parts of face, or shoulder: _____

(f) "Wry neck" or torticollis, affecting neck and shoulder, is the most common form of this disorder: _____

C3. Mr. Gustafson, age 68, has received a diagnosis of Parkinson disease (PD). Answer the following questions related to Mr. Gustafson's condition.

(a) Parkinson disease is more likely to occur *(before? after?)* age 50. This condition is more likely to have a genetic component when onset occurs *(before? after?)* age 45.

(b) Parkinson disease has no known cause, so is known as _____ parkinsonism. List several other causes of parkinsonism.

_____

_____

(c) Parkinson disease *(is? is not?)* a progressive disorder. Symptoms begin once *(20%? 80%?)* of dopamine production is lost from nigrostriatal pathways (see Question C1[c]). Results are classic signs of Parkinson disease: _____, _____, and _____. Tremor and rigidity are likely to begin as *(unilateral? bilateral?)* manifestations.

(d) Identify the manifestations of PD exhibited by Mr. Gustafson:

Autonomic manifestations   Bradykinesia
Cog-wheel movements   Dysphagia
Masklike face   Tremor

(d1) Slow, shuffling gait related to excessive inhibition of movement; difficulty initiating movements; most disabling of PD manifestations: _____

(d2) Ratchet-like movements of arms; a form of rigidity: _____

(d3) The most visible, but least disabling, sign of PD in patients who are awake and at rest; includes "pill-rolling" movements of thumb and forefinger: _____

(d4) Lack of facial expression: _____

(d5) Difficulty swallowing; one sign is drooling: _____

(d6) Excessive sweating, salivation (with drooling), lacrimation, constipation, and impotence: _____

(e) Mr. Gustafson does not exhibit dementia. About one in _____ patients with PD will experience dementia.

(f) Explain how each type of drug might be helpful to Mr. Gustafson:

(f1) Levodopa

_____

(f2) Anticholinergic (anti-ACh) drugs such as Cogentin or Artane

_____

C4. The cerebellum is located *(superior? inferior?)* to posterior regions of the cerebrum; the *(vermis? tentorium cerebelli?)* separates these two brain structures. Describe two major functions of the cerebellum by expanding on the words provided below:

(a) Smooth, skilled

_____

(b) Compare and evaluate

_____

C5. List possible causes of cerebellar impairment.

_____

C6. Mr. Daugherty is being assessed for possible cerebellar damage. Identify the listed manifestations of cerebellar damage.

Nystagmus   Dysarthria
Dysdiadochokinesia   Dysphagia
Intention tremor   Over- and under-
Truncal ataxia   reaching

(a) Mr. Daugherty is not able to stand with a steady posture; he walks a little, with a staggering gait: _____

(b) In a seated position, he has difficulty starting the movement of tracing the back of his left shin with the toes of his right foot: _____

(c) With hands on his knees, he cannot rapidly pronate and supinate his forearms: _____

(d) When he tries to touch his finger to his nose (with eyes closed), he repeatedly misses: _____

(e) His speech is slow and slurred: _____

(f) His eyes constantly readjust: _____

D. UPPER AND LOWER MOTONEURON DISORDERS AND SPINAL CORD INJURY

D1. Craig, age 40, received a diagnosis of amyotrophic lateral sclerosis (ALS) 2 years ago. Answer the following questions about his condition.

(a) Amyotrophic lateral sclerosis is commonly known as _____ disease. *(Most? Few?)* cases of this disease are hereditary. The disease typically is diagnosed in men *(younger? older?)* than Craig. Survival usually is _____ years from onset of symptoms.

(b) What information does each part of the name ALS provide about this condition?

(b1) Amyotrophic

_____

(b2) Lateral

_____

(b3) Sclerosis

_____

(c) Circle each of the following that is a manifestation likely to develop in Craig:

(1) Loss of sensation in hands and feet

(2) Weakness and then paralysis of his hands and feet

(3) Dementia

(4) Difficulty swallowing, speaking, and making any sounds

(5) Loss of sexual sensation and ability to have an erection

(6) Weakness of respiratory muscles, leading to infections

(7) Elevated glutamine levels in his cerebrospinal fluid

(d) Name one type of drug approved for treatment of ALS. _____

(e) In the final stages of ALS, how may Craig still be able to communicate?

_____

D2. Therese, age 31, received a diagnosis of multiple sclerosis (MS) at the age of 25. Answer the following questions about MS.

(a) This condition typically is diagnosed *(before? after?)* age 40 and is more common in *(women? men?)*. There *(is? is not?)* a genetic predisposition.

(b) MS is a disorder in which areas of the *(CNS? PNS?)* become inflamed. As a result, myelin of axons is broken down, forming lesions known as _____. Velocity of nerve condition then *(decreases? increases?)*. MS is related to a decrease in _____ cells that normally produce myelin in the CNS. MS is likely to affect *(movements? sensations? both?)*.

(c) Explain the meaning of the term *multiple sclerosis*.

_____

_____

(d) This disorder *(is? is not?)* likely to be immune related. Explain.

_____

(e) Circle two manifestations likely for initial presentation of MS:

(1) Forgetfulness

(2) Paralysis of one hand

(3) Numbness and tingling

(4) Double vision

(f) List other signs and symptoms of MS.

_____

_____

_____

(g) Circle the two most definitive diagnostic methods for MS in this list:

(1) MRI

(2) CT scan

(3) Elevated IgG levels in CSF

(4) Decreased protein and lymphocyte levels in CSF

(h) List treatments that may help limit the progression of Therese's MS.

_____

_____

_____

D3. Circle the leading cause of spinal cord injury (SCI):

(a) Alcohol and other drugs

(b) Sports injuries

(c) Violence

(d) Motor vehicle accidents

D4. Contrast causes of vertebral column injuries in each pair:

(a) Flexion injuries – extension injuries

_____

_____

_____

(b) Compression injury – axial rotation injury

_____

_____

_____

(c) Primary SCI – secondary SCI

_____

_____

_____

D5. Contrast tetraplegia with paraplegia.

_____

_____

D6. Identify which SCIs are complete *(C)* or incomplete *(I)*.

(a) Central cord syndrome, conus medullaris syndrome, or cauda equina syndrome: ___

(b) All sensory and motor function is lost below the level of the injury: ___

(c) Cord hemisection (Brown-Séquard syndrome): ___

(d) Has a better prognosis: ___

D7. Circle the correct answers within each statement about SCIs.

(a) Anterior spinal artery infarction is more likely to result in loss of ability to sense:

A. Two-point discriminatory touch and proprioception

B. Pain and temperature

(b) Injury to the right spinothalamic tract is more likely to lead to loss of pain and temperature sensation in the *(right? left?)* side of the body. This is a(n) *(contralateral? ipsilateral?)* effect. Injury to a corticospinal (voluntary motor) tract has a(n) *(contralateral? ipsilateral?)* effect.

(c) With central cord syndrome, *(arms? legs?)* are likely to be affected to a greater degree. This condition occurs more commonly in *(children? the elderly?)*.

(d) Conus medullaris syndrome is least likely to affect *(arms? legs? bowel and bladder function?)*. Damage to nerve roots in the lumbosacral area is known as *(Brown-Séquard? cauda equina?)* syndrome. It *(is? is not?)* likely to lead to some paralysis and pain.

(e) *(Primary? Secondary?)* SCI occurs at the time of the mechanical injury; such injury *(is? is not?)* reversible. Edema and vasospasm with ischemia are causes of *(primary? secondary?)* injury and may be reversible.

D8. Give rationales for the following early treatments for SCIs.

(a) Immediate in-line immobilization and "log rolling" onto a rigid backboard

_____

(b) Correcting hypotension and hypoxia

_____

(c) Use of corticosteroids

_____

D9. Ann experiences a complete C3 SCI during a traumatic fall from horseback. Circle the three

true statements about her case. (Pay particular attention to whether the **bold-faced** word or phrase makes the statement true or false.)

(a) A complete SCI at C3 is likely to cause **less** loss of function than a complete SCI at T3.

(b) SCI injuries at C3 level or higher **do** require assistance with ventilation.

(c) Ann is at **increased risk** for serious respiratory infections.

(d) She **is** likely to be able to pick up items as a result of tenodesis.

(e) Ann **is** likely to be able to use an electric wheelchair.

D10. James has a T8 compression SCI resulting from a fall from the roof of a two-story house. Circle the correct answers within each statement about his case.

(a) Because his injury is at T12 or above, James *(is? is not?)* likely to have UMNs affected. UMN destruction with intact LMNs ultimately results in *(flaccid? spastic?)* paralysis.

(b) In the hours immediately after his fall, James goes into a period of spinal shock. This is a time of *(a? hyper?)*reflexia as his spinal reflexes below T12 are *(absent? exaggerated?)*. By the time he is airlifted to the hospital 90 minutes after his fall, spastic reflexes are observed. This fact is a *(positive? negative?)* sign regarding some recovery of function.

D11. The diaphragm receives its innervation from spinal nerves that arise from levels *(C3 to C5? T3 to T5?)* of the cord. Mr. Tenley has a C7 SCI. Explain why his risk of respiratory infections (including pneumonia that may be fatal) is likely to be high.

_____

_____

D12. Both Ann (Question D9) and James (Question D10) are likely to experience *(high? normal? low?)* heart rate, blood pressure, and body temperature after their injuries.

(a) In both cases, vagus nerve function is likely to *(fail? persist?)* and contribute to bradycardia. Explain.

_____

_____

(b) *(Ann? James?)* is more likely to have these conditions persist. Explain.

_____

_____

_____

(c) Ann's heart rate drops when she undergoes suctioning to remove mucus from airways. Explain.

_____

_____

(d) When Ann is raised from a supine to sitting position, she feels dizzy. This condition is known as _____. What can prevent this disorder?

_____

D13. Autonomic dysreflexia leads to distinct contrasts in manifestations above and below the site of an SCI. Answer the following questions about autonomic dysreflexia.

(a) Which two clients are most likely to experience episodes of autonomic dysreflexia after spinal shock has resolved? *(Ann? James? Mr. Tenley?)*. Explain why they are at risk for this disorder.

_____

_____

(b) List common triggers for autonomic dysreflexia.

_____

_____

(c) As a result of these triggers, unregulated sympathetic responses become *(absent? exaggerated?)* below the site of injury. Vasospasm leads to skin *(flushing? pallor?)*, goose bumps, and extremely *(high? low?)* blood pressure with headaches.

(d) Baroreceptor reflexes then call for decreased sympathetic activity above the injury site (where sympathetic structures

still communicate with the brainstem). In the upper body, *(flushing? pallor?)* of skin is evident, along with nasal stuffiness (due to vaso-_____); _____cardia also develops.

(e) Summarizing: In autonomic dysreflexia, sympathetic signs are present in the *(upper? lower?)* body and are absent in the *(upper? lower?)* body. This condition *(is? is not?)* a clinical emergency.

D14. Briefly explain why each of the following conditions is likely to accompany SCIs.

(a) Edema and deep venous thrombosis

_____

_____

(b) Safety and skin integrity issues associated with spasticity (see James, Question D10[a]) and sensory loss

_____

_____

(c) Bladder incontinence

_____

_____

_____

(d) Bowel incontinence

_____

_____

(e) Sexual dysfunction

_____

_____

_____

(f) Poikilothermy

_____

_____

_____

CHAPTER 36

Disorders of Brain Function

■ Review Questions

A. BRAIN INJURY

A1. Answer the following questions about the brain and its blood supply.

(a) The brain makes up approximately _____ % of body weight, yet receives approximately _____% of the blood pumped out of the heart each minute.

(b) Cerebral *(hypoxia? ischemia?)* deprives the brain of blood flow, whereas _____ involves adequate blood flow but reduced oxygen level.

(c) Explain how hypoxic neurons can survive.

_____

(d) A stroke is more likely to lead to *(focal? global?)* ischemia. List two causes of global ischemia.

_____

(e) Ischemia can lead to depletion of the brain's energy resources within *(2 to 4? 5 to 10? 20 to 30?)* minutes. List several mechanisms by which cerebral perfusion might be reduced even after ischemia is reversed.

_____

_____

(f) Most of the ATP used by brain cells goes toward maintenance of _____ within neurons. State two consequences of failure of these pumps.

_____

_____

(g) Circle the three parts of the brain that are especially vulnerable to ischemia:

(1) Pons

(2) Midbrain

(3) Cerebellum

(4) Hippocampus

(5) Basal ganglia

(h) "Watershed areas" of the brain are supplied with blood from *(central? distal?)* regions of cerebral arteries. Explain why these areas are vulnerable to ischemia.

A2. Answer the following questions about injury of the brain caused by excitatory amino acids.

(a) Name the principal excitatory neurotransmitter in the brain.

_____

(b) For what brain functions is this neurotransmitter required?

_____

(c) List four or more conditions that can lead to injury or death of neurons due to excessive glutamate activity in the brain.

_____

_____

(d) Explain how NMDA receptors and excessive glutamate can injure brain cells.

_____

_____

(e) Describe how drugs known as neuroprotectants can reduce brain injury.

_____

A3. Identify which category of brain edema—cytotoxic or vasogenic—is described below.

(a) Caused by impaired blood-brain barrier function resulting from brain injury, infections, tumors, or ischemia; leads to increased extracellular fluid (ECF) between brain cells: _____

(b) Neurons and neuroglia swell and may rupture as excessive fluid moves into them; causes include water intoxication or severe ischemia that disables the sodium pump; more likely to affect gray matter: _____

A4. Mrs. Smith has been transported to a clinic. Her intracranial pressure (ICP) is increasing as a result of a severe head trauma in a domestic violence incident yesterday. Her blood pressure is 200/110 mm Hg, and her pulse is 50 bpm. She appears lethargic and confused. Answer the following questions related to her case.

(a) List the three major components within Mrs. Smith's cranium. Then give one or more mechanisms by which each of these cranial components might increase in volume, thereby elevating ICP.

(a1) _____

_____

(a2) _____

_____

(a3) _____

_____

(b) Which of these volumes is likely to be increased in Mrs. Smith's cranium?

_____

_____

_____

(c) Mrs. Smith's ICP is likely to rise *(minimally? dramatically?)* when her intracranial volume increases significantly.

(d) List the manifestations that are reliable early indicators of increased ICP in Mrs. Smith.

_____

_____

(e) If Mrs. Smith's ICP is 55 mm Hg, her cerebral perfusion pressure (CPP) is _____ mm Hg. This value is *(high? normal? low?)*.

(f) Mrs. Smith's blood pressure is significantly *(decreased? increased?)*, especially the *(systolic? diastolic?)* value because decreased cerebral perfusion leads to systemic vaso*(constriction? dilation?)*. As a result, pulse pressure is *(widened? narrowed?)*.

(g) Mrs. Smith's pulse indicates *(brady? tachy?)*cardia. This manifestation and those listed above in A4(f) are signs of the CNS _____ response (or Cushing _____). These manifest as *(early? late?)* signs of high ICP.

A5. By circling the correct answers or filling in the blanks in the following questions, describe factors that typically compartmentalize the

brain and explain how these may be altered by increased ICP.

(a) The falx cerebri consists of tough *(dura? pia?)* mater that extends *(horizontally? vertically?)* to compartmentalize the *(two cerebral hemispheres? cerebrum from the cerebellum?)*. *(Cingulate? Uncal?)* herniations can pass under the falx cerebri and press on the *(anterior? middle? posterior?)* cerebral artery. Reduced flow through this vessel affects *(medial? lateral)* aspects of a cerebral hemisphere that controls *(arm? leg?)* muscles.

(b) Describe the normal functions of the following structures and name a type of herniation associated with each structure.

(b1) Tentorium cerebelli

_____

_____

(b2) Incisura

_____

_____

(c) Circle each of the following that is a manifestation associated with uncal (lateral) herniation:

Arm weakness	Respiratory arrest
Blindness	Leg weakness
"Clouding" of consciousness	Posturing (decorticate or decerebrate)
Death by compression of vital structures in the medulla	Dilated pupil

(d) Elbows are flexed in *(decerebrate? decorticate?)* posturing.

(e) Circle the correct answer within each statement about conditions related to increased ICP.

(e1) *(Cingulate? Infratentorial?)* herniation is more likely to compress the brainstem.

(e2) *(Brainstem? Cerebral? Diencephalon?)* compression is most life-threatening.

A6. Answer the following questions about hydrocephalus.

(a) Hydrocephalus involves an excessive volume of _____.

(b) Identify whether the hydrocephalus caused by reduced reabsorption of CSF is communicating *(C)* or noncommunicating *(NC)*:

(b1) Narrowing of the (cerebral) aqueduct of Silvius connecting the third and fourth ventricles related to embryonic viral infection or midbrain tumor:

_____

(b2) Arachnoid villi are injured by scarring or infectious debris: _____

(c) Enlargement of the head is likely to occur when hydrocephalus occurs in *(infants? older children or adults?)*. Explain.

_____

(d) Circle each of the following that is likely to be a manifestation present in a 10-month-old infant with hydrocephalus.

(1) Vomiting

(2) Bulging fontanels

(3) Visual disorders

(4) Ventricular enlargement observed by imaging

(e) Papilledema is a sign of high ICP and hydrocephalus. How is papilledema assessed?

_____

A7. Discuss the "good news" and the "bad news" about the skull and CSF as protectors of the brain.

_____

_____

_____

A8. Circle the correct answers or fill in the blank within each statement about head injuries.

(a) Most fatal head injuries result from *(falls? accidents involving vehicles and pedestrians?)*. A skull fracture involving a multiple fracture line is known as a *(basilar? comminuted? laminar?)* fracture.

(b) Which of the following are primary head injuries?

Ischemia	Diffuse axonal injury
Brain herniation	Edema
Concussion	Infection
Contusion	Subdural hematoma

(c) A *(concussion? contusion?)* refers to a brief interruption in brain function with recovery likely within 24 hours; typically, there is no residual damage. A *(concussion? contusion?)* involves a longer period of unconsciousness with bruising of the brain; contusions *(do? do not?)* cause permanent brain injury.

(d) Which type of primary head injury is the most common cause of post-traumatic dementia and can lead to the persistent vegetative state? _____

(e) When the skull is hit on the anterior, a contrecoup trauma involves injury to the *(anterior? posterior?)* of the brain.

(f) _____ is the most common cause of secondary brain injury.

A9. Circle the correct answers within each statement about hematomas.

(a) Alex, age 20, was riding his bike without a helmet when his bike swerved and he fell on the right side of his head. He immediately became unconscious, then conscious and able to speak clearly for a brief period; he then became unconscious again.

(a1) This pattern suggests a(n) *(epidural? intracranial? subdural?)* hematoma. Tearing of Alex's right middle meningeal artery during the accident is likely to lead to *(rapid? slow?)* compression of his brain.

(a2) Neurologic assessment of Alex is likely to reveal a fixed, dilated *(right? left?)* pupil and *(right? left?)*-sided hemiplegia of his arm and face.

(a3) With rapid treatment, Alex *(is? is not?)* likely to have a good prognosis.

(b) Miranda experienced jarring of her head as it snapped backward in an automobile accident on Saturday. At the accident site, Miranda stated that she felt "fine" and refused medical help. On Thursday, the onset of severe headache, lethargy, and confusion prompted her to see a physician.

(b1) Miranda receives a diagnosis of a subdural hematoma; its classification is *(acute? subacute? chronic?)*.

(b2) A subdural hematoma is located between the dura mater and the *(arachnoid membrane? cranial bones?)*. The torn vessels are likely to be *(arteries? veins?)*, which bleed relatively *(rapidly? slowly?)*.

A10. Answer the following questions about Missy's altered consciousness as her brother splashes her in the swimming pool.

(a) Circle the structures that comprise Missy's reticular formation.

Cerebral cortex   Medulla   Midbrain
Hypothalamus   Pons   Thalamus

(b) Arousal and wakefulness (for example, Missy's startled reaction as water splashes on her face) are functions most associated with the *(ascending reticular activating system [ARAS]? cerebral cortex?)*. The content and cognitive aspects of consciousness (for example, her awareness that it was water that was splashed on her face and that it was her brother who initiated that action) are regulated by the

_____.

(c) The ARAS relay to the *(hypothalamus? limbic system?)* is most likely to make Missy's heart race, whereas the ARAS relay to her _____ is most associated with Missy's determination to splash her brother in return.

A11. Circle all of the following statements that are true concerning levels of consciousness (LOC). (Pay particular attention to whether the **bold-faced** word or phrase makes the statement true or false.)

(a) Injury to a single region of the brain is known as **global** injury.

(b) Problems with breathing and altered blood pressure are **more likely** to be signs of injury to brainstem rather than to cerebral hemispheres.

(c) A stroke involving one cerebral hemisphere **is** likely to lead to altered level of consciousness (ALC).

(d) Shearing injury that traumatizes white matter of the RAS and cerebral hemispheres **can** lead to ALC.

(e) Hallucinations and delusions are most associated with a state of **confusion.**

(f) An obtunded person **may respond** to significant shaking.

(g) A state of stupor indicates a **lower** LOC than a state of obtundation.

(h) A client with doll's-head eye response will have eyes stay fixed in the head (**and not** rotate) as the head is moved.

A12. Ms. Delgado scores a 14 on the Glasgow Coma Scale assessment. This is a relatively *(high? low?)* score. List the three aspects of neurologic functioning measured by this scale:

_____, _____, _____

A13. Answer the following questions. Severity of altered LOC depends on the site of brain injury, progressing from most anterior/superior or *(caudal? rostral?)* to most posterior/inferior or *(caudal? rostral?)*. Determine which level of brain injury is indicated in each of the following cases.

Diencephalon   Medulla
Midbrain   Pons

(a) Mrs. Ellington lies rigid in full extension; her pupils are midsize and fixed (do not constrict to light); she exhibits doll's-head eye response; her respirations are 42 per minute: _____

(b) Ms. Rutenschrorer is comatose with flaccidity; her sporadic respirations require ventilatory assistance: _____

(c) Mr. Lopez lies in full extension except for flexor posturing of elbows, wrists, and hands; his pupils react to light, and his gaze follows a moving finger; he exhibits Cheyne-Stokes breathing: _____

A14. Explain why the definition of "brain death" has changed during the past several decades.

_____

_____

List six clinical factors that should be documented to confirm brain death: _____

_____

_____

A15. Mrs. Meyer is in a persistent vegetative state (PVS). List six or more criteria used to determine PVS.

_____

_____

_____

B. CEREBROVASCULAR DISEASE

B1. Select from the list of arteries to fill in the blanks within each statement below.

Anterior cerebral arteries
Basilar artery
Internal carotid arteries
Middle cerebral arteries
Posterior cerebral arteries
Posterior communicating arteries
Vertebral arteries

(a) Right and left _____ ascend in the posterior of the neck, enter the skull, and then form the _____ that lies at the base of the brain. These arteries are vital to survival because they perfuse the brainstem.

_____

_____

(b) The right and left _____ supply the anterior of the circle of Willis. Emboli from these arteries pass directly into the _____, which are the most common sites of embolic strokes.

List two or more examples of possible effects of such strokes.

_____

_____

(c) Located on the medial aspect of frontal and parietal lobes, the _____ supply motor neurons to the lower extremities.

(d) _____ connect middle cerebral arteries with _____ to complete the posterior portion of the circle of Willis.

B2. Answer the following questions about the veins that drain the brain.

(a) Which are more vulnerable: *(deep? superficial?)* cerebral veins? Explain.

_____

(b) Venous blood from the brain empties into venous sinuses composed of *(dura? pia?)* mater. These structures empty into _____ veins that carry blood back toward the heart.

B3. Fill in the blanks or circle the correct answers within each statement about factors that regulate cerebral blood flow.

(a) At rest, about _____ % of the total cardiac output supplies the brain. Cerebral blood flow—especially *(deep? superficial?)* flow—normally is regulated by *(local?*

sympathetic nerve?) control. These mechanisms are known as _____ regulation, and they work as long as mean arterial pressure (MABP) is maintained within a range of _____ to _____ mm Hg.

(b) Circle three local factors that dilate cerebral vessels.

(1) Acidosis

(2) Alkalosis

(3) Hypercarbia

(4) Hypocarbia

(5) Hypoxia

(c) Acidosis *(stimulates? depresses?)* CNS function. Explain how cerebral artery vasodilation helps to correct cerebral acidosis.

_____

B4. Compare the terms in each pair.

(a) Heart attack (MI) – brain attack stroke

_____

_____

(b) Angina – transient ischemic attack (TIA)

_____

_____

(c) Ischemic stroke – hemorrhagic stroke

_____

_____

_____

B5. Circle the factors that increase risk of stroke.

(a) *(African American? White?)* race

(b) Age *(65 years? 75 years?)*

(c) *Chronic* (hypotension? hypertension?)

(d) *(History? No history?)* of previous stroke

B6. Explain why each of the following patients may be at increased risk for stroke.

(a) Angeline, age 8, has a sickle cell crisis.

_____

(b) Mr. Polk, age 61, has atrial fibrillation.

_____

(c) Gustav has been "blood doping" and has a hematocrit of 64%.

_____

B7. List five or more lifestyle modifications that can decrease the risk for stroke.

_____

_____

_____

B8. Mrs. Everly, age 66, manifests early signs of a stroke. Answer the following questions related to her case.

(a) Define the penumbra of a stroke.

_____

_____

(b) Explain how penumbral cells can survive.

_____

_____

B9. Circle the two true statements about strokes. (Pay particular attention to whether the **bold-faced** word or phrase makes the statement true or false.)

(a) Ischemic strokes are **more** likely to occur at sites of bifurcation of arteries with atherosclerotic plaques.

(b) Thrombotic strokes **are** associated with increased activity in older adults.

(c) The name "lacunar infarcts" refers to the **small cavities** or **lacunae** in the brain that remain after such strokes.

(d) Lacunar infarcts cause **global cortical deficits,** such as the inability to **speak or to accomplish tasks performed before the stroke.**

B10. Which type of stroke is most frequently fatal?

(a) Cardiogenic embolic

(b) Hemorrhagic

(c) Lacunar

(d) Thrombotic

These strokes usually occur when the person is _(active? sedentary?)_. List several causes of this type of stroke.

_____

B11. Review Question B1 and Table 36-5 in _Essentials of Pathophysiology,_ and then identify the cerebral artery involved in each case of stroke. Where possible, indicate whether the affected artery is on the right or left side of the brain.

Anterior cerebral artery
Middle cerebral artery
Posterior cerebral artery

(a) Ms. Weldon has paralysis and sensory loss of her right arm and the right side of her face; she cannot turn her eyes toward her right, and she is confused and sometimes appears delirious: _(L? R?)_ _____

(b) Mr. Knowlton's left leg and foot are paralyzed with sensory loss resulting in impaired gait; his wife states that "his mind is slower, and he's distracted all the time": _(L? R?)_ _____

(c) Mrs. Penn's daughter reports that her mother "just keeps repeating the same couple of phrases all day long, she's been having trouble remembering things, and her senses just aren't what they were—her vision, hearing, taste . . . .":

_____

B12. Ms. Weldon has been transported to the emergency department and then to intensive care. A history and physical examination have identified manifestations described in Question B11(a); onset was 36 hours ago and symptoms have persisted. Answer the following questions related to her case.

(a) The duration of her symptoms indicates that her condition _(is? is not?)_ a TIA. Explain.

_____

(b) Ms. Weldon's symptoms of stroke are largely unilateral with sudden onset. This _(is? is not?)_ a typical pattern for strokes. Her neurologic examination also reveals dysarthria, which means _____; ataxia, which means _____; and restlessness and some brief periods of delirium.

(c) Explain why it is critical to determine quickly the cause of her stroke.

_____

_____

(d) _(Computed tomography? Magnetic resonance imaging?)_ is the diagnostic imaging considered superior for differentiating ischemic from hemorrhagic lesions.

(e) Thrombolytic agents are most helpful for salvaging penumbral areas around _____ strokes.

(f) List five contraindications for taking thrombolytic medications.

_____

_____

_____

B13. Describe common manifestations of strokes by matching terms with related clinical descriptions below.

Agnosia   Dysarthria
Anomic aphasia   Hemineglect
Apraxia   Nonfluent aphasia
Babinski sign   Wernicke aphasia

(a) Stanley knows what he wants to say but cannot articulate the words:_____

(b) Suzanne is unable to convert a thought into a spoken or written sentence:

_____

(c) Jonathan cannot understand what his partner has said or written:

_____

(d) Emily has lost the ability to name common words such as "trouble," "snow," or "nephew": _____

(e) Mark's big toes move upward (not downward) when the nurse lightly traces the lateral plantar surface of Mark's foot:_____

(f) Tracy Ann is unable to open a jar, squeeze toothpaste out of a tube, or button her clothing:_____

(g) After Bud's right-sided stroke, he forgets to use left arm and leg:_____

(h) Meg can no longer recognize images of birds as birds or distinguish a dog from a tiger:_____

B14. Choose the two true statements about aneurysmal subarachnoid hemorrhages. (Pay particular attention to whether the **bold-faced** word or phrase makes the statement true or false.)

(a) These aneurysms are thought to result from a **congenital defect** in a cerebral artery.

(b) **Most** aneurysms of the brain are berry aneurysms.

(c) The larger the aneurysm, the **less** likely it is that the aneurysm will rupture.

(d) There **is no** evidence of hereditary predisposition for these aneurysms.

B15. Circle each of the following that is a manifestation of a ruptured subarachnoid aneurysm.

(a) Nuchal rigidity

(b) Mild headache

(c) Photophobia

(d) Altered extraocular muscle function

(e) Loss of consciousness

B16. Briefly describe the three following possible and serious complications of ruptured subarachnoid aneurysm.

(a) Vasospasm

_____

(b) Rebleeding

_____

(c) Hydrocephalus

_____

B17. Answer the following questions about arteriovenous (A-V) malformations.

(a) What is unique about blood flow through these vascular systems?

_____

_____

_____

(b) Arteriovenous malformations *(are? are not?)* thought to be congenital and *(do? do not?)* appear to increase risk for neurologic deficits and learning disorders.

C. INFECTIONS AND BRAIN TUMORS

C1. Answer the following questions about infections of the central nervous system (CNS).

(a) Infection of the brain is known as _____, whereas infection of the spinal cord is _____. (Select from the following three options.)

Encephalitis   Meningitis   Myelitis

(b) Circle the two major routes by which CNS infections occur:

(1) Via a lumbar puncture

(2) By spread of infection via fractured skull bones

(3) Via a blood-borne infection that crosses the blood-brain barrier

(4) Through surgery

(c) Meningitis typically spreads *(rapidly? slowly?)*. Explain.

_____

(d) Write *B* for bacterial or *V* for viral next to characteristics of each form of meningitis.

  (d1) Likely to be more severe and possibly fatal: _____

  (d2) A lumbar puncture will reveal presence of lymphocytes and normal glucose in CSF: _____

  (d3) CSF is cloudy and contains enormous numbers of neutrophils, elevated protein, and low glucose: _____

  (d4) Causes include the meningococcus and *Hemophilus influenzae*: _____

(e) Identify the signs of acute bacterial meningitis that fit the following descriptions.

  Petechiae   Nuchal rigidity
  Fever and chills

  (e1) Neck stiffness: _____

  (e2) Rash found on most persons with meningococcal meningitis: _____

(f) In addition to antibiotics, which other class of drugs is used to combat the effects of meningitis? _____ Give a rationale for this treatment.

_____

(g) Most cases of encephalitis are *(bacterial? viral?)*. Signs and symptoms typically *(do? do not?)* include fever and nuchal rigidity.

C2. Name the types of cells in each category that can develop into brain tumors.

Breast cancer cells   Meningeal cells
Neurons   Neuroglia: astrocytes
Neuroglia: Pineal cells
  oligodendroglia   Pituitary cells
Prostate cancer cells

(a) Primary tumors of CNS tissue:

  _____ , _____ , _____

(b) Primary tumors of non-CNS tissue:

  _____ , _____ , _____

(c) Secondary (metastatic) tumors:

  _____ , _____

C3. Choose the three true statements about brain tumors. (Pay particular attention to whether the bold-faced word or phrase makes the statement true or false.)

(a) Benign brain tumors **cannot** cause death.

(b) Most primary brain tumors in adults are **astrogliomas.**

(c) Many manifestations of brain tumors are **similar to** those of head injuries or infections.

(d) Meningiomas typically are **malignant** with **rapid** growth.

(e) Primary brain tumors are **more** common than metastatic brain tumors.

(f) The most common subgroup of seizures in children is **febrile** seizures.

C4. Defend or dispute this statement: "Because the brain has no pain receptors, pain is not a symptom of a brain tumor."

_____

_____

C5. Choose the three true statements about diagnosis and treatment of brain tumors. (Pay particular attention to whether the **bold-faced** word or phrase makes the statement true or false.)

(a) A funduscopic examination checks for the presence of **papilledema.**

(b) Computed tomographies **are more sensitive** in detecting brain tumors than are MRIs.

(c) Skull x-rays and cerebral angiography are **likely** to be helpful diagnostic tools for brain tumors.

(d) Surgery is **rarely** a part of the initial management of brain tumors.

(e) Lymphomas of the central nervous system (CNS) **are** associated with the Epstein-Barr virus (EBV) and are more common in immunosuppressed persons.

D. SEIZURE DISORDERS

D1. Define *seizures*:

_____

Now define *convulsions*:

_____

Seizures are a *(common? rare?)* disorder in pediatric neurology. Typically, first seizures take place *(before? after?)* 20 years of age. Manifestations of seizures *(are identical? vary?)*

among different persons. List several examples of manifestations of seizures.

_____

_____

_____

D2. Circle the three true statements about seizures. (Pay particular attention to whether the **bold-faced** word or phrase makes the statement true or false.)

(a) Seizures are **rare** neurologic disorders in adults.

(b) Idiopathic seizures have **no identifiable cause.**

(c) Seizures may be caused by **decrease of inhibitory neurotransmitters** such as GABA.

(d) A provoked seizure is also known as a **primary** fever.

(e) **Epileptic syndrome** refers to a seizure disorder.

D3. Answer the following questions about seizures.

(a) Kyle, age 18 months, has a seizure preceded by a fever. In children, fever *(is? is not?)* a common antecedent of seizure.

(b) List six systemic or metabolic disorders that can provoke seizure.

_____

_____

_____

(c) A simple partial seizure *(does? does not?)* involve loss of consciousness, and it involves *(one? both?)* hemisphere(s).

(d) Generalized-onset seizures *(do? do not?)* involve unconsciousness with effects on *(one? both?)* hemisphere(s). This type of seizure is a *(common? rare?)* type in young children.

(e) Indicate whether the following manifestations of seizures are autonomic *(A)*, motor *(M)*, or sensory *(S)* alterations:

(e1) Flushing, excessive sweating, and change in blood pressure: ___

(e2) "Crawling" sensations: ____

(e3) "Jacksonian seizure": ____

(e4) Lip-smacking, grimacing, or rubbing clothing: _____

(f) How does an aura or prodrome relate to seizures?

_____

During an aura or prodrome, the person *(is? is not?)* conscious.

(g) The *(clonic? tonic?)* component of tonic-clonic seizures involves alternating rhythmic contractions and relaxations of muscles.

D4. Match the type of generalized-onset seizure with the appropriate description.

Absence   Atonic   Myoclonic   Tonic-clonic

(a) Formerly called grand mal seizures; unconsciousness, incontinence, and impaired respirations may accompany dramatic muscle movements: _____

(b) Called "drop attacks" related to a brief loss of muscle tone: _____

(c) Brief blank stare and unresponsiveness along with lip smacking are signs; occur only in children; formerly called petit mal seizures: _____

D5. Answer the following questions about diagnosis and treatment of seizure disorders.

(a) Electroencephalograms *(are? are not?)* helpful in diagnosing seizures.

(b) State the first rule of treatment during a seizure.

_____

_____

(c) Explain how monotherapy can help patients with seizures.

_____

D6. Define *status epilepticus.*

_____

E. DEMENTIAS

E1. Explain why depression must be ruled out in diagnosing dementia.

_____

_____

_____

E2. Select the term that fits the correct description related to Alzheimer disease (AD).

Acetylcholine   Amyloid precursor protein
Cortical atrophy   Neurofibrillary tangles
Senile plaques   Sundown syndrome

(a) Loss of neurons indicated by narrowing of gyri and enlargement of ventricles; particularly affects parietal and temporal lobes of the cerebrum: _____

(b) Tendency of patients with second-stage AD to wander, particularly in the early evening: _____

(c) Fibrous proteins arranged in helical fashion within abnormal neurons of patients with AD: _____

(d) Patches of parts of degenerating neurons wrapped around β-amyloid; found in the hippocampus and other brain areas of persons with AD: _____

(e) A neurotransmitter required for memory; decreased in AD: _____

(f) A large protein that appears to be required for normal cytoskeleton; mutation of the gene for this chemical is associated with a hereditary form of early-onset AD: _____

E3. The incidence of Alzheimer disease is *(high? low?)* in people with Down syndrome. Explain.

_____

_____

_____

E4. Identify whether the following descriptions are characteristics of the first, second, or third stage of Alzheimer disease.

(a) Confusional stage likely to last for several years; client may become hostile and abusive: _____

(b) Short-term memory loss with inability to remember names; mild changes in personality: _____

(c) Inability to recognize family members or to communicate; incontinence of bowel and bladder: _____

E5. Briefly describe diagnosis of Alzheimer disease.

_____

_____

_____

E6. Match each type of dementia with its major characteristics.

Creutzfeldt-Jakob disease
Vascular dementia
Pick disease
Huntington disease
Wernicke-Korsakoff syndrome

(a) Related to atrophy of frontal and temporal lobes; may involve echolalia, apathy, and hypotonia: _____

(b) Associated with vitamin B deficiency in alcoholics; severely affects recent memory and eye muscles; confabulation is a distinctive feature: _____

(c) A rare autosomal dominant disorder transmitted by a gene on chromosome 4; causes movement disorders (chorea and later rigidity), personality changes, and dementia: _____

(d) A rapidly progressing, rare dementia transmitted by infective proteins known as prions; affects personality and motor coordination; similar to mad cow disease in cows: _____

(e) Second most common type of dementia; risk is greater among smokers and persons with hypertension: _____

CHAPTER 37

Disorders of Special Sensory Function: Vision, Hearing, and Vestibular Function

■ Review Questions

A. THE EYE AND DISORDERS OF VISION

A1. Refer to Figures 37-1 and 37-3 in *Essentials of Pathophysiology* and answer the following questions about the eye.

(a) Arrange the following structures in correct sequence from outside to inside of the eyeball:

Retina   Sclera
Uveal tract (or vascular layer)

_____ → _____ → _____

(b) Arrange the following structures in correct sequence from anterior to posterior:

Anterior cavity   Cornea
Lens   Posterior cavity

_____ → _____ → _____ → _____

(c) List three or more protective structures of the eye.

_____

_____

_____

A2. On Monday evening, Leslea's eyes feel irritated and appear red; her lids are swollen and tender. By Tuesday morning, Leslea has a yellow-green discharge from both eyes. Answer the following questions related to her case.

(a) Leslea sees her physician on Tuesday and reports that (to her knowledge) she has experienced no eye injuries. It is likely that her conjunctivitis is *(bacterial? viral? caused by a foreign body?)*. Explain.

_____

_____

(b) Conjunctivitis is commonly known as _____. A Gram stain and culture indicates infection with *Neisseria*

gonorrhoeae. Her conjunctivitis is likely to be *(acute? chronic? hyperacute?)*. Leslea's condition *(is? is not?)* sight-threatening. She *(is? is not?)* likely to have antibiotics prescribed.

(c) Describe appropriate treatments for Leslea's conjunctivitis.

_____

_____

A3. Circle the correct answers or fill in the blanks to answer the following questions about several other types of conjunctivitis.

(a) Viral conjunctivitis typically manifests with *(copious? minimal?)* production of tears and minimal exudate that is *(pus filled? watery?)*.

(b) List conditions or environments linked with viral conjunctivitis.

_____

_____

_____

(c) Herpes infections of the conjunctiva typically are *(bilateral? unilateral?)*. Circle medications helpful for herpetic conjunctivitis:

Antibiotics   Antivirals
Corticosteroids

(d) Conjunctivitis caused by *(Chlamydia trachomatis A to C? Herpes simplex? Neisseria gonorrhoeae?)* is the leading cause of preventable blindness in the world. This form of conjunctivitis has a higher prevalence in newborns born by *(cesarean section? vaginal delivery?)*. This form of eye infection occurs in approximately 1 in *(12? 1,200?)* newborns in the United States.

(e) Conjunctival redness and swelling of eyelids that occurs 7 days after birth most likely is caused by ophthalmia neonatorum in newborns caused by:

(1) Silver nitrate treatment

(2) *N. gonorrhoeae*

(3) *C. trachomatis*

A4. Abigail has hay fever. Describe the cause, symptoms, and treatment of hay fever.

_____

_____

_____

_____

A5. Answer the following questions about the cornea and its disorders.

(a) The cornea *(is? is not?)* penetrated by blood vessels. State the significance of this.

_____

_____

_____

(b) The cornea is *(highly? minimally?)* sensitive to pain. List several examples of causes of corneal pain.

_____

_____

(c) Explain how corneal trauma can affect the eye.

_____

_____

_____

(d) Inflammation of the cornea is known as _____. List three causes of each type of keratitis:

(1) Nonulcerative

_____

_____

(2) Ulcerative

_____

_____

(e) Herpes simplex virus is a *(common? rare?)* cause of corneal ulceration. In adults most cases involve HSV *(1? 2?)*. Neonatal keratitis involves HSV *(1? 2?)* infection during the birth process.

(f) List early symptoms of keratitis.

_____

(g) Herpes zoster ophthalmicus is a corneal disorder resulting from infection by the virus that causes _____.

(h) Transplantation of corneas from cadavers *(does? does not?)* involve a high rate of tissue rejection.

A6. Arrange in correct sequence the pathway of aqueous humor in the eye:

Anterior chamber (of anterior cavity)
Ciliary processes
Trabeculae and canal of Schlemm
Posterior chamber (of anterior cavity)

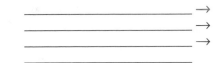

A7. Mr. Fuller, who is 33 years old, has received a diagnosis of glaucoma. Answer the following questions related to his case.

(a) In glaucoma, the volume of *(aqueous humor? vitreous body?)* is excessive. In most cases glaucoma results from *(overproduction? obstructed outflow?)* of aqueous humor.

(b) It is more likely that Mr. Fuller's diagnosis was made *(on an eye screening provided at his work site? as a result of severe pain?)*. Explain.

_____

(c) Circle the normal intraocular pressure(s): *(10? 17? 28?)* mm Hg. Glaucoma involves a(n) *(increase? decrease?)* in intraocular pressure.

(d) Mr. Fuller's glaucoma is "open-angle," also known as *(wide? narrow?)*-angle glaucoma. Circle factors that increased his risk for this type of glaucoma.

(1) His age

(2) Having a father with glaucoma

(3) Having diabetes mellitus

(4) Being near-sighted

(5) Being African American

(e) What causes open-angle glaucoma?

_____

_____

(f) Glaucoma is *(rare? a leading cause of blindness?)* in the United States. Explain how untreated glaucoma could result in blindness for Mr. Fuller.

_____

(g) Most treatment of open-angle glaucoma is *(surgical? pharmacologic?)*. Medications for glaucoma work either by increasing *(production? outflow?)* of aqueous fluid or by decreasing *(production? outflow?)* of aqueous fluid.

A8. Circle the correct answers or fill in the blanks about another form of glaucoma.

(a) Angle-closure glaucoma results from obstruction of the aqueous humor pathway by the iris. This form of glaucoma occurs in a *(large? small?)* percentage of patients with glaucoma.

(b) Also known as *(narrow? wide?)*-angle glaucoma, this condition is exacerbated by *(constriction? dilation?)* of the iris, which then "bulges" and narrows the angle between the iris and the cornea (see Figure 37-4 in *Essentials of Pathophysiology*). List several factors that can trigger episodes of closed-angle glaucoma.

_____

_____

_____

(c) Circle typical manifestations of closed-angle glaucoma.
   (1) Eye pain
   (2) Blurred vision
   (3) Halos around lights
   (4) Nausea and vomiting
   (5) Excruciating unilateral headache

(d) Describe typical treatment for acute closed-angle glaucoma.

_____

_____

A9. Answer the following questions about processes involved as you look at a bird in a distant tree and then to the bird feeder just outside your window.

(a) Focusing images on the retina requires bending (or changing direction) of light rays, a process known as _____.

Explain how light rays are refracted as they pass though the eye.

_____

(b) As you focus from far to near, the anterior of your lens must be made more *(flat? rounded or convex?)*. *(Ciliary? Iris?)* muscles perform this process, which is known as _____.

(c) If your eyeball is too long, the image of the bird (or feeder) will be focused *(anterior? posterior?)* to your retina. You would have the condition known as *(myopia? hyperopia?)*, also known as ___-sightedness because you can see near items but not those far away. *(Biconcave? Biconvex?)* lenses or radial keratotomy can correct this disorder.

(d) Other processes that increase your visual acuity as you focus on a nearby object are *(constriction or miosis? dilation or mydriasis?)* of the pupil (by contraction of _____ muscles) and *(widening? narrowing?)* of the slit between the eyelids to control light entering your eye.

(e) As you age, your lens will become *(thicker? thinner?)* and less able to accommodate; this condition is known as _____opia.

A10. Answer the following questions about cataracts.

(a) A cataract is a disorder of the *(aqueous humor? cornea? lens? retina?)*. It is much more common in *(younger? older?)* persons. Cataract surgery is very *(common? rare?)*.

(b) List several factors that contribute to development of cataracts.

_____

_____

_____

A11. Cataracts typically develop *(rapidly? slowly?)*. Describe aging-related changes in the lens that lead to cataracts.

_____

_____

_____

A12. List typical manifestations of senile cataracts.

_____

_____

A13. Discuss treatments of cataracts.

(a) Medical

_____

(b) Surgical

_____

A14. Write C next to descriptions of cones and R next to descriptions of rods.

(a) Three types (for red, green, and blue) allow for color vision: ___

(b) Decomposition of the visual pigment rhodopsin occurs when light strikes these cells: ___

(c) Vitamin A deficiency impairs function of these cells: ___

(d) Involved with night (or low-illumination or scotopic) vision in black-gray-white:

___

A15. The fovea centralis is located in the (anterior? posterior?) of the eye near the origin of the optic nerve. The fovea is positioned in the center of the "yellow spot," known as the _____. This area (does? does not?) contain bipolar and ganglia cells and consists of (cones? rods? both rods and cones?). The fovea is the (blind spot? point of sharpest vision?).

A16. Select the source of blood supply that perfuses the retinal structures that follow.

Choriocapillaris of the choroid
Central retinal artery branches

(a) Most posterior portions of the retina, such as pigment cells, rods and cones of the photoreceptor layer, and the all-important fovea: _____

(b) Anterior two layers of the retina (bipolar and ganglion layers):

_____

A17. Explain the clinical significance of the following.

(a) Why can funduscopic examination of retinal blood vessels provide clues about more generalized blood vessel health?

_____

_____

_____

(b) What is indicated by a "choked disk" seen funduscopically?

_____

_____

_____

A18. Mrs. Giovanni, age 34, has type 2 diabetes and sees her physician about "changes in my vision, especially glare." Circle the correct answer or fill in the blank within each statement related to her condition.

(a) She receives a diagnosis of background retinopathy. This disorder involves:

(1) Formation of fragile blood vessels that may grow into the vitreous and obscure vision

(2) Thickening of retinal capillary walls with small hemorrhages confined to the retina and also macular edema

(b) Control of her blood cholesterol and glucose levels and blood pressure (is? is not?) likely to reduce visual impairment in Mrs. Giovanni.

(c) Name the major treatment for diabetic retinopathy. _____

A19. (Background? Proliferative?) retinopathy that may accompany diabetes is more sight-threatening. Describe two mechanisms of this disorder that can cause blindness.

_____

_____

_____

_____

A20. Select from this list to identify the retinal disorders that fit each description.

Cotton-wool spots or exudates on the fundus
Detached retina
Hypertensive retinopathy
Macular degeneration
Papilledema

(a) Retinal arteries thicken and appear more pale than do normal arteries:

_____

(b) Caused by accumulation of exudates on arteriolar walls in atherosclerotic vessels:

_____

(c) Swelling of the optic disk; can occur with malignant hypertension or high intracranial pressure: _____

(d) May result from shrinking of the vitreous or cataract surgery that exerts traction on the retina; robs photoreceptors of their only blood supply and can lead to blindness; typically painless:

_____

(e) Can be "wet" or "dry"; causes bilateral loss of central vision; large pale yellow spots ("drusen") suggest greater severity of the disorder; more common in elderly:

_____

A21. Contrast functions of the primary visual cortex (area 17 in Figure 37-12 in *Essentials of Pathophysiology*) and the visual association areas (areas 18 and 19 in Figure 37-12).

_____

_____

A22. Refer to Figure 37-11 in *Essentials of Pathophysiology* and circle the correct answers within each of the following statements about visual pathways.

(a) An optic nerve transmits nerve impulses from (one? both?) eye(s), whereas an optic tract carries nerve impulses from (one? both?) eye(s).

(b) In the optic chiasma, axons from the ganglion layer of both retinas (do? do not?) synapse. The term *chiasma* indicates that axons cross here, specifically those from the (nasal? temporal?) portions of the retinas.

(c) A lesion that destroys the entire left optic tract will result in loss of the (right? left?) visual field of (the right? the left? both?) eye(s).

A23. Match the terms related to visual defects with their descriptions.

Anopia   Hemianopia
Heteronymous   Homonymous
Quadrantanopia

(a) The same type of visual loss (such as loss of the right visual field) in both eyes:

_____

(b) The opposite type of visual loss in the two eyes: _____

(c) Total blindness in an eye, for example by destruction of an optic nerve:

_____

(d) Loss of one quarter of a visual field, such as occurs with partial lesions of an optic radiation or the primary visual cortex:

_____

(e) "Tunnel vision" caused by a pituitary tumor; involves bilateral loss of temporal fields of view or: _____

A24. Explain how coordinated eye movements of both eyes help you read the words on this page.

_____

_____

_____

A25. Select the extraocular eye muscles that fit the descriptions that follow.

Inferior oblique   Inferior rectus
Levator palpebrae superioris   Medial rectus
Lateral rectus   Superior rectus
Superior oblique

(a) Moves the eyeball so that you can look directly up to the sky: _____

(b) When the lateral rectus of your right eye contracts (abducting your right eye), which muscle of your left eye is likely to contract (so that both eyes will be directed toward your right)? Your left _____

(c) Innervated by the right cranial nerve VI (abducens); damage to this nerve results in medial strabismus of the right eye:

_____

(d) Raises the upper eyelid; innervated by the oculomotor nerve: _____

(e) Innervated by cranial nerve III (oculomotor):

_____

A26. Refer to Figure 37-15 in *Essentials of Pathophysiology* and identify the name of the disorder of eye movements that fits each description.

Amblyopia   Esotropia
Exotropia   Cyclotropia
Diplopia   Hypertropia
Hypotropia   Strabismus

(a) Double vision: _____

(b) Uncoordinated eye movements that result in diplopia: _____

(c) Sometimes called "lazy eye," it involves diminished vision that is uncorrectable by lenses but has no detectable organic cause: _____

(d) Upward deviation of the eye: _____

(e) Torsional deviation of the eye: _____

(f) Weakness of the right lateral rectus muscle (or damage to cranial nerve VI) is likely to lead to medial deviation of that eye, a condition known as: _____.

A27. Circle the correct answers within each statement related to strabismus.

(a) In which type of strabismus is there no primary muscle impairment? (*Concomitant [nonparalytic]? Nonconcomitant [paralytic]?*)

(b) In which type of strabismus is deviation equal in all directions of gaze? (*Concomitant [nonparalytic]? Nonconcomitant [paralytic]?*)

(c) The onset of strabismus, particularly the (*paralytic? nonparalytic?*) type, typically is in (*childhood? adulthood?*). By the age of 5 to 6 (*days? weeks? months?*), infants should have synchronized eye movements, with eyes in alignment during all of their waking hours.

(d) Almost all adult strabismus is of the (*paralytic? nonparalytic?*) type. List several causes.

_____

_____

A28. Write a common term for amblyopia. _____ By what age should children begin treatment for amblyopia? _____

B. THE EAR AND DISORDERS OF AUDITORY FUNCTION

B1. Select the part of the ear that fits each description.

External ear   Inner ear   Middle ear

(a) The eardrum (tympanic membrane) is located between the _____ and the _____.

(b) Includes the pinna and the external ear canal that is lined with ceruminous glands: _____

(c) Location of ossicles (ear bones), stapedius, and tensor tympani muscles: _____

(d) Site of entry of the eustachian (auditory) tube from the nasopharynx: _____

(e) Location of the cochlea, semicircular canals, and vestibular apparatus, which are collectively called the labyrinth: _____

(f) Location of perilymph, endolymph, and the organ of Corti: _____

(g) Infection of the _____ ear is most likely to lead to mastoiditis.

B2. List several causes of external ear infection (otitis externa).

_____

_____

B3. Choose the three true statements about the external and middle ear. (Pay particular attention to whether the **bold-faced** word or phrase makes the statement true or false.)

(a) Most otitis externa infections are caused by gram-**positive** bacteria or fungi.

(b) Swimmer's ear is **otitis externa.**

(c) Removal of cerumen should be carried out by gentle irrigation using a bulb syringe and **cold** tap water.

(d) Impacted cerumen usually produces no symptoms until the canal is **completely occluded.**

(e) The **malleus** ("hammer") is the ossicle partially fixed to the tympanic membrane.

B4. Answer the following questions about the eustachian tubes.

(a) List three functions of the eustachian tubes.

_____

_____

_____

(b) Explain how eustachian tubes help your ears "pop" when you experience a change in altitude.

_____

_____

_____

_____

(c) The opening of each of these tubes into the nasopharynx normally is *(open? closed?)*. How can this tube be opened?

_____

_____

(d) Describe two reasons the eustachian tubes of young children may collapse.

_____

_____

_____

(e) Collapse of the eustachian tube because of lack of tubal stiffness is an example of a *(functional? mechanical?)* obstruction of the tube.

(f) State two reasons infants are more likely to experience otitis media (OM) than are older persons.

_____

_____

B5. Circle the risk factors for otitis media (OM) in Evan, who is 8 months old and bottle fed: He and his 3-year-old brother Devon attend a large suburban day-care center. Devon has a history of three episodes of OM within the past 4 months. Evan had acute otitis media (AOM) with antibiotic treatment earlier this month. Neither their parents nor other close relatives smoke.

B6. Circle the correct answers within each statement about acute otitis media (AOM).

(a) The most common causative agent of AOM is:

(1) *Escherichia coli*

(2) *Moraxella catarrhalis*

(3) *Respiratory syncytial virus*

(4) *Streptococcus pneumoniae*

(b) Most cases of AOM *(do? do not?)* follow respiratory infections. Describe the likely pathway of the microbes in this infection?

_____

(c) If Evan (Question B5) experiences AOM, which three manifestations are most likely?

(1) Diarrhea

(2) Being fussy at feeding time

(3) Tugging on his affected ear

(4) Rhinitis (runny nose)

(5) Bulging yellow or red eardrum seen by otoscopy

B7. Give a rationale for the following treatments of OM.

(a) Antibiotics—including those given prophylactically—are used judiciously.

_____

_____

(b) Immunization with pneumococcal and influenza vaccines

_____

(c) Myringotomy

_____

_____

(d) Tympanostomy with the directive that the child keeps his or her head out of water

_____

_____

_____

B8. Circle the two true statements about OM. (Pay particular attention to whether the **bold-faced** word or phrase makes the statement true or false.)

(a) Recurrent OM is defined as three new AOM episodes within **1 year,** and these accompany almost every upper respiratory infection.

(b) In otitis media with effusion (OME), signs of infection are **severe.**

(c) In both AOM and OME, **hearing loss** may occur.

(d) **Most** cases of OME resolve without treatment within 3 months of onset.

B9. Answer the following questions about the complications experienced by Phillip, who has a history of recurrent OM.

(a) Explain how OM may be related to Phillip's delayed language development.

_____

(b) List three complications of OM that may contribute to Phillip's hearing loss.

_____

_____

_____

(c) Briefly describe two complications that can lead to destruction of some of Phillip's cranial bone tissue.

_____

_____

_____

B10. Stephanie is a junior in college and is experiencing gradual hearing loss diagnosed as otosclerosis. Answer the following questions related to her case.

(a) Both her mother and grandfather have this condition, which is an *(autosomal dominant? autosomal recessive? sex-linked?)* disorder.

(b) Arrange in correct sequence the typical events in the progression of this condition.

Bone becomes spongy and soft
Overgrowth of hard bone develops
Resorption of bone

_____ → _____

→ _____

(c) Eventually, Stephanie is likely to experience immobilization of her *(malleus? stapes? tympanic membrane?)*. What type of surgery could correct this condition?

_____

(d) Stephanie *(is? is not?)* likely to be able to hear on the telephone. A hearing aid *(is? is not?)* likely to help Stephanie.

B11. Circle the correct answers within each statement about the ear.

(a) The parts of the ear that are inside the skull are located within the *(parietal? temporal?)* bone.

(b) The stapes exerts a piston-like action against the *(oval? round?)* window.

(c) The *(cochlea? vestibule?)* is a snail shell–shaped structure that winds around the bony modiolus.

B12. Refer to Figures 37-19 and 37-20 in *Essentials of Pathophysiology* and arrange the following structures in the correct sequence.

(a) From first to last in the pathway of sound waves and mechanical action:

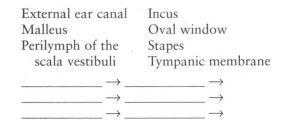

External ear canal   Incus
Malleus   Oval window
Perilymph of the   Stapes
  scala vestibuli   Tympanic membrane

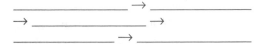

_____ → _____ →
_____ → _____ →
_____ → _____ →
_____

(b) From superior to inferior within the cochlea:

Basilar membrane
Cochlear duct containing the organ of Corti and endolymph
Scala tympani containing perilymph
Scala vestibuli containing perilymph
Vestibular membrane

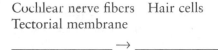

_____ → _____
→ _____ →
_____ → _____

(c) From superior to inferior within the organ of Corti:

Cochlear nerve fibers   Hair cells
Tectorial membrane

_____ → _____ →
_____

B13. Choose the three true statements about nerve pathways involved with hearing. (Pay particular attention to whether the **bold-faced** word or phrase makes the statement true or false.)

(a) The **organ of Corti** within the cochlear duct is the starting point of nerve pathways for hearing.

(b) Cranial nerve **VII** conducts impulses from the ear to the brainstem.

(c) **Both** sides of the brain receive nerve impulses from **both** ears.

(d) Nerves of hearing pathways are conveyed to the **medial geniculate** nucleus in the **thalamus.**

(e) Primary auditory area (41) and association auditory area (42) are located in the **occipital** lobes of the cerebral cortex.

B14. Choose the two true statements about hearing disorders. (Pay particular attention to whether the **bold-faced** word or phrase makes the statement true or false.)

(a) Tinnitus is a **rare** disorder in the United States.

(b) **Objective** tinnitus refers to a **rare** form of ringing in the ears in which the sound **can** be heard by an observer.

(c) Nicotine and caffeine **can** cause tinnitus.

(d) **Profound hearing loss** is defined as a loss greater than 20 to 25 decibels (dB) in adults.

B15. Answer the following questions about Wernicke's area of the brain.

(a) This area is located in the dominant hemisphere, usually the *(right? left?)* side, in the *(primary auditory? auditory association?)* cortex.

(b) Circle the manifestations of damage to Wernicke's area:

(1) Inability to speak intelligibly

(2) Inability to read normally

(3) Inability to understand what is spoken or read

(c) In other words, patients with damage to Wernicke's area have *(expressive? receptive?)* aphasia and agnosia of speech.

B16. Refer to Chart 37-1 in *Essentials of Pathophysiology* and match the inner ear disorders in this list with the descriptions that follow:

Conduction deafness   Presbycusis
Mixed conductive and   Sensorineural deafness
   sensorineural hearing
   loss

(a) Repeated exposure to sound intensities greater than 100 to 120 dB: _____

(b) External or middle ear conditions: _____

(c) Disorders affecting the inner ear, auditory pathways, or the primary cortical hearing area: _____

(d) Hearing loss caused by ototoxic drugs: _____

(e) Ménière disease: _____

(f) Hearing loss that accompanies aging: _____

(g) Cytomegalovirus (CMV) infection is the most common cause of this type of hearing loss: _____

B17. Circle the known ototoxic drugs in this list:

Aminoglycoside antibiotics such as kanamycin
Aspirin
Chemotherapeutic drugs
Loop diuretics such as furosemide (Lasix)

B18. Mr. Franklyn, age 79, has presbycusis. Answer the following questions related to his case.

(a) His condition is *(common? rare?)* among older adults. Explain why it is underdiagnosed.

_____

(b) He is more likely to have difficulty distinguishing:

(1) Vowels (low-pitched sounds), as in "bard," "bird," "bored"

(2) Consonants (high-pitched sounds), as in "sin," "thin," "fin"

(c) In conducting a patient history, the nurse needs to question Mr. Franklyn and also _____. List several questions to be included in a patient history.

_____

_____

_____

(d) _____ are used to help differentiate conductive and sensorineural loss.

B19. List several communication techniques that you can use to be better understood by hearing-impaired persons.

_____

_____

_____

B20. Explain why early diagnosis of hearing disorders is crucial in these two populations:

(a) Infants

_____

(b) Elderly

_____

C. THE VESTIBULAR SYSTEM AND MAINTENANCE OF EQUILIBRIUM

C1. Answer the following questions about vestibular function.

(a) State two functions of the vestibular receptive organs.

_____

_____

(b) Describe functions of the following neural connections with the vestibular organs.

(b1) Cerebellum

_____

(b2) Cranial nerves (CN) III, IV, VI

_____

(b3) Chemoreceptor trigger zone

_____

C2. Match the components of the vestibular system with their characteristics.

Saccule   Semicircular canals   Utricle

(a) Regulate responses to angular movement, such as riding around curves of a roller coaster: _____

(b) Facilitate awareness of body position, such as lying supine, sitting up, or tilting the head: _____, _____

(c) Function in reflex bracing of the neck and rapid changes in eye movements, such as in response to rapid acceleration of a motor vehicle: _____, _____

(d) Contain crystals (otoliths, see Figure 37-22 in *Essentials of Pathophysiology*) that exert weight caused by gravity upon hair cells of the maculae: _____, _____

(e) Consist of three canals each dilated into an ampulla with stereocilia extending from hair cells into a gelatinous mass that initiates nerve impulses: _____

C3. Match these types of vestibular alteration with the patient cases that follow:

Benign paroxysmal positional vertigo (BPPV)
Ménière disease
Motion sickness
Nystagmus

(a) Elaine exhibits slow-fast-slow eye movements (vestibulo-ocular reflexes) even when her head is held still; this condition is worsened when she is tired: _____

(b) Jenny is on a boat in a violent storm; her blood pressure decreases and pulse increases, and she is sweating; she becomes nauseous and vomits: _____

(c) Marie's disorder is caused by excesses of endolymph fluid and manifests with hearing loss, vertigo, and ringing of the ears: _____

(d) Laurie, a "regular" at the amusement park, feels nauseous as the careening roller coaster curves and dives; she recovers and is ready for more action within a few minutes: _____

C4. Circle all true statements about inner ear disorders. (Pay particular attention to whether the **bold-faced** word or phrase makes the statement true or false.)

(a) Nystagmus is **always** pathologic if it occurs when the head is held still.

(b) Nystagmus typically starts with **unilateral** effects.

(c) Most cases of vertigo involve **brainstem (central)** disorders.

(d) In BPPV, portions of **otoliths** of the utricle break off and form debris that **increases** sensitivity of a semicircular duct.

(e) In the progression of Ménière disease after initial episodes, **hearing** is likely to worsen and **vertigo** tends to improve.

C5. Explain how the following treatments can improve inner ear disorders.

(a) Low-sodium diet and diuretics for Marie (Question C3[c]) or endolymphatic shunt surgery:

_____

(b) Otolith repositioning for Laurie (Question C3[d]):

_____

(c) Avoidance of alcohol for persons with vertigo:

_____

C6. List three possible causes of disorders of central vestibular function.

_____

C7. Match the tests of vestibular function with the descriptions that follow.

Caloric stimulation   Electronystagmography
Romberg test   Rotational tests

(a) A check for balance and postural stability, the person stands with feet together, arms raised forward, and eyes closed: _____

(b) Electrodes placed lateral to eyes evaluate nystagmus eye movements: _____

(c) Ice water instilled into each ear checks for vestibular response: _____

(d) Rotation in a rotatable chair (like a barber's chair) is followed by abrupt stoppage; postrotational reflex nystagmus and related limb movements are measured: _____

C8. Identify mechanisms of action of these drugs used to treat vestibular disorders:

Anticholinergics   Antidopaminergics
Antihistamines

(a) Suppress nausea and vomiting; an example is phenothiazines: _____

(b) Suppress the vestibular system; examples include scopolamine and atropine: _____

(c) Suppress the illusion of motion; examples include meclizine and promethazine: _____

C9. Describe how physical therapists can work with clients to improve vestibular disorders.

_____

_____

_____

CHAPTER 38

Disorders of the Male Genitourinary System

■ Review Questions

A. PHYSIOLOGIC BASIS OF MALE REPRODUCTIVE FUNCTION

A1. List two main functions of the testes.

_____

_____

A2. Contrast these two processes:

(a) Spermatogenesis: _____

(b) Spermiation: _____

A3. Circle all true statements about Sertoli cells.

(a) They form the inner lining of seminiferous tubules within testes.

(b) They produce nourishment for developing sperm.

(c) They secrete estradiol.

(d) They secrete inhibin.

A4. Arrange in correct sequence from first to last these structures in the pathway of sperm:

(a) Ejaculatory duct

(b) Epididymis

(c) Seminiferous tubules

(d) Urethra

(e) Vas deferens

___ → ___ → ___ → ___ → ___

In which of these structures do sperm mature? ___

A5. Circle the correct answers or fill in the blank within each statement about the glands that produce seminal fluid.

(a) There is/are *(one? two?)* seminal vesicle(s) located just *(inferior? posterior?)* to the urinary bladder. *(Fructose? Prostaglandins?)* in seminal vesicle secretions provide energy for sperm, whereas _____ cause

cervical mucus to be ideal for sperm passage.

(b) The *(seminal vesicles? prostate?)* is/are responsible for forming about 70% of semen.

A6. Match the hormones or other chemicals that regulate male reproduction with the related descriptions that follow.

Estradiol	Follicle-stimulating
Gonadotropin-releasing	hormone (FSH)
hormone (GnRH)	Inhibin
Luteinizing hormone	Plasminogen
(LH)	activator
Testosterone	

(a) Hormone produced by the hypothalamus that stimulates production of gonadotropins: _____

(b) Gonadotropins made by the anterior pituitary: _____, _____

(c) Binds to Sertoli cells and stimulates testes to produce sperm: _____

(d) Inhibits production of FSH, which then inhibits spermatogenesis: _____

(e) Also known as interstitial cell-stimulating hormone (ICSH) because it triggers production of testosterone by these cells: _____

(f) Inhibits anterior pituitary production of luteinizing hormone (LH) by negative feedback mechanism: _____

(g) A female reproductive hormone that is required in males for sperm production: _____

(h) The major androgen produced in testes; small amounts also produced in the adrenal cortex: _____

A7. Describe the effects of testosterone at each of these different stages of life:

(a) In embryo

_____

(b) At puberty

_____

(c) Throughout the life of the male

_____

A8. Answer the following questions about the penis.

(a) The enlarged end of the penis is known as the (*glans? prepuce? shaft?*); the foreskin is known as the _____. The foreskin is removed in the surgery known as a _____.

(b) Bodies composed of erectile tissue are known as _____. The urethra passes through the corpus (*cavernosa? spongiosum?*).

A9. Circle the correct answers or fill in the blank within each statement about male sexual response.

(a) The (*sympathetic? parasympathetic?*) division of the autonomic nervous system is responsible for erection. These nerves travel from (*lumbar? sacral?*) levels of the spinal cord through (*pelvic? pudendal?*) nerves to the penis.

(b) Erection is a result primarily of:

(1) Filling of the penis with blood by relaxation of vascular smooth muscle and compression of penile veins.

(2) Contractions of ischiocavernosus and bulbocavernosus muscles of the penis.

In which areas of the penis does blood accumulate during erection?

_____

(c) The (*sympathetic? parasympathetic?*) division of the autonomic nervous system is responsible for ejaculation and also the return of the penis to the relaxed (flaccid) state, a process known as _____.

(d) Nitric oxide released within the penis leads to the formation of _____, which causes (*contraction? relaxation?*) of smooth muscles in blood vessels, contributing to the (*erect? flaccid?*) state of the penis.

(e) Ischiocavernosus and bulbocavernosus muscles are located (*in the glans? at the base?*) of the penis. What is their function?

_____

A10. Mr. Rathwell is 62 years old, is divorced, and has erectile dysfunction (ED). He has been a smoker for 48 years and recently celebrated 4 years of sobriety. His type 1 diabetes mellitus is under poor control. In addition to his oral hypoglycemic, he also takes medications for hypertension, a cholesterol-lowering agent, and an antidepressant. Answer the following questions related to his case.

(a) In which category of ED is Mr. Rathwell's condition classified?

Mixed   Organic   Psychogenic

Which type of ED is most common?

Mixed   Organic   Psychogenic

(b) What factor included in his patient history indicates a neurogenic origin of his disorder?

_____

(c) Which factors contribute to decreased vascular flow to his external genitalia?

_____

_____

(d) List any other factors in Mr. Rathwell's history that may contribute to his ED.

_____

_____

(e) Mr. Rathwell (*does? does not?*) have risk factors for metabolic syndrome.

(f) Mr. Rathwell has his blood levels of hormones evaluated. Which of his hormone levels are likely to be decreased? _____ and _____

(g) He begins taking Viagra (sildenafil). How does this help patients with ED?

_____

By what mechanism could prostaglandin-E analogs help Mr. Rathwell?

_____

B. DISORDERS OF THE PENIS, THE SCROTUM AND TESTES, AND THE PROSTATE

B1. Circle the correct answer within each statement about disorders of the penis.

(a) In phimosis, the foreskin of the penis is so tight that it cannot (*cover? be retracted over?*) the glans?

(b) Which condition is inflammation of the glans and the foreskin, possibly caused by *(Chlamydia? Balanitis? Balanoposthitis?)*

B2. Select the name of the disorder that best fits each description.

Balanitis xerotica obliterans   Peyronie disease
Priapism   Smegma

(a) Stiffening of the fibrous covering around the corpora cavernosa; may cause upward bowing of the penis and pain during intercourse: _____

(b) Epithelial cellular debris that can lead to infection of the foreskin and phimosis, and possibly penile cancer: _____

(c) White, patchy lesion that originates on the glans; middle-aged diabetic men are at high risk: _____

(d) Prolonged, painful erection, usually without sexual desire: _____

B3. Circle the correct answer or fill in the blank to answer the following questions about priapism.

(a) Priapism is considered a *(mild clinical problem? true urologic emergency?)*. State the major concern about the long-term effects of priapism.

_____

_____

(High-flow? Low-flow [stasis]?) priapism is more likely to lead to ischemia with permanent damage.

(b) List two or more causes of priapism in each category.

(b1) Primary

_____

(b2) Secondary

_____

(c) Explain how sickle cell disease can lead to priapism.

_____

_____

B4. Complete this exercise about penile cancer by circling or filling in the correct answer.

(a) This condition is most common among *(young? middle-aged?)* men. It is *(highly? rarely?)* curable if diagnosed early. What factor do you think is most likely to hinder early diagnosis? _____

(b) List four risk factors for cancer of the penis.

_____

_____

(c) Almost all penile cancers are *(carcinomas? sarcomas?)*. Two types of lesions that can evolve into invasive carcinomas are red lesions known as *(Bowen disease? erythroplasia of Queyrat?)* and thickened, gray-white lesions known as _____.

B5. Answer the following questions about several clinical applications of male reproductive anatomy.

(a) Dennis is born at 29 weeks of gestation. Palpation of his scrotum indicates absence of testes. What is the likely explanation?

_____

Where do testes develop during embryologic life? At what point do they typically descend into the scrotum?

_____

_____

Explain why eventual descent of testes is important.

_____

_____

(b) Mr. Jamison, age 66, has testicular cancer that has metastasized to lymph nodes surrounding his abdominal aorta. Explain.

_____

_____

_____

(c) Patrick and Jane both lift heavy machinery as part of their jobs. Patrick has had bilateral inguinal hernias develop; Jane has not. Explain.

_____

_____

_____

B6. Circle the correct answers or fill in the blanks within each statement about structures associated with the testes or scrotum.

(a) The tunica *(albuginea? vaginalis?)* is a double-layered covering derived from abdominal peritoneum and immediately surrounds the testes. The tunica _____ also protects the testes. A hydrocele forms when fluid accumulates

between the layers of the tunica
_____.

(b) Name the two sets of muscles that contract to pull the testes and scrotum closer to the body during cold temperatures:
_____ muscles and _____ muscles

(c) The pampiniform plexus consists of *(arteries? veins?)* that supply the testes. These vessels *(do? do not?)* help to maintain testicular temperature consistent with sperm production.

B7. Match the condition with the correct description.

Hematocele   Hydrocele
Spermatocele   Varicocele

(a) Accumulation of blood around the testes:
_____

(b) Accumulation of fluid within the tunica vaginalis around the testes: _____

(c) Varicose veins of the testes: _____

(d) Sperm-containing cyst at the end of the epididymis; rarely causes problems:
_____

B8. Circle the three true statements. (Pay particular attention to whether the **bold-faced** word or phrase makes the statement true or false.)

(a) Most hydroceles of infancy **do** resolve spontaneously before the age of 1 year.

(b) A dense hydrocele that does not transilluminate is **more** likely to be cancerous than a soft mass that does illuminate.

(c) In adults, hydroceles typically **do** require treatment.

(d) Incidence of varicoceles is greatest **after age 60.**

(e) Varicocele is more likely to occur on the **right** side than on the **left.**

(f) "Heaviness" of the scrotum is a sign of **both** hydrocele and varicocele.

B9. List four or more causes of hydrocele.

_____

_____

_____

_____

B10. Discuss each of these phrases related to variocele.

(a) "Bag of worms"

_____

(b) Examination in standing and recumbent positions

_____

_____

B11. Circle the correct answers or fill in the blanks to answer the following questions about testicular torsion.

(a) Testicular torsion involves twisting of the spermatic cord; this structure includes

_____

(b) Extravaginal testicular torsion occurs more often in *(neonates? boys 8 to 18 years?).*

(c) Intravaginal testicular torsion is *(more? less?)* common than extravaginal torsion and is a true surgical emergency in which patients are in acute distress; the condition *(can? does not?)* lead to destruction of the involved testis.

B12. Claude, age 20, has epididymitis. Answer the following questions related to his case.

(a) Describe the location and functions of the two epididymides.

_____

_____

(b) Claude's epididymitis is caused by *Chlamydia trachomatis.* Name another sexually transmitted disease (STD) that commonly leads to epididymitis:
_____. Identify the population most likely to experience this form of epididymitis. _____

(c) Explain how urethritis or prostatitis could spread to cause epididymitis.

_____

_____

(d) List two other sources of infection that can cause epididymitis.

_____

(e) Claude's infection was typical in that it led to pain and swelling by 1 or 2 *(hours? days? weeks?)* after onset of epididymitis. His fever and painful urination are *(common? rare?)* signs. Is he likely to have a urethral discharge? _____

(f) *(Bed rest? Exercise?)* is likely to be recommended for Claude. Explain why his scrotum is elevated on a pillow or rolled towel as he rests.

_____

Name three types of medications that he will receive: _____, _____, _____. During this recovery period, sexual activity is *(encouraged? discouraged?)*.

(g) Claude's condition spreads to cause orchitis, which is an infection of _____.

B13. What childhood infection is most likely to lead to orchitis? _____

(a) Compare and contrast signs and symptoms of orchitis with those of epididymitis.

_____

_____

(b) What percentage of bilateral orchitis cases caused by mumps result in sterility? _____

B14. Circle the correct answers or fill in the blanks to answer the following questions about neoplasms of the scrotum or testes.

(a) *(Scrotal? Testicular?)* carcinoma is more common.

(b) Explain what is distinctive about scrotal cancer in the history of medicine.

_____

_____

In addition to exposure to these occupational carcinogens, what other factors can lead to scrotal cancer?

_____

(c) Testicular cancer is the leading cause of cancer in males ages *(15 to 35? 35 to 55?)* years old. If diagnosed early, it *(is? is not?)* highly curable.

(d) Name the disorder that has the strongest association with cancer of the testes: _____. Seminomas are testicular tumors that develop from _____ tubules, and these develop most commonly in *(children? men in their 20s? men in their 30s?)*. Seminomas are *(highly? rarely?)* curable tumors.

(e) Which is the most common first sign of testicular cancer?

(1) Slight enlargement of the testis with feeling of heaviness with or without pain

(2) Swelling of legs and back pain

(3) Cough and blood in sputum (hemoptysis)

(f) Circle the tumor markers used to evaluate testicular cancer.

Alpha-fetoprotein
Alkaline phosphatase
Human chorionic gonadotropin
Lactic dehydrogenase
Prostate serum antigen

(g) Treatment of *(some? all?)* testicular cancers involves surgical removal of the affected testis, a procedure known as an _____.

B15. Answer the following questions about the prostate gland.

(a) One function of the prostate is production of secretions. The *(mucosal? submucosal? main?)* prostatic glands are enlarged in benign prostatic hyperplasia (BPH). The _____ prostatic glands secrete the fluid that contributes to semen. This *(acidic? alkaline?)* secretion neutralizes fluid from the vas deferens that is strongly acidic. The pH of semen must be about _____ for sperm to be motile.

(b) A second function of the prostate is based on its _____ tissue, which helps in the process of _____. State one other function of the muscle of the prostate.

_____

B16. Match the types of prostatitis in this list with the related descriptions that follow:

Acute bacterial prostatitis
Chronic bacterial prostatitis
Chronic prostatitis/chronic pelvic pain syndrome

(a) Mr. Harrell has a prostate condition with no known cause; urine cultures reveal no bacteria in urine, but his prostatic fluid shows evidence of leukocytes (a sign of inflammation). Mr. Harrell has a decreased libido and impotence: _____

(b) Mr. Tomlinson presents with dull, aching pain in the perineal area, frequent and urgent urination of cloudy and malodorous urine, fever and chills; most commonly caused by *E. coli*; treatment includes antibiotic therapy for up to 4 weeks: _____

(c) Rev. Peter has recurrent urinary tract infections (UTIs) with *Pseudomonas*. Like Mr. Tomlinson, he has frequent and urgent urination and perineal discomfort; his condition is more difficult to treat than acute bacterial prostatitis because antibiotics do not readily penetrate his chronically inflamed prostate:

_____

B17. Choose the two true statements related to benign prostatic hyperplasia (BPH). (Pay particular attention to whether the **bold-faced** word or phrase makes the statement true or false.)

(a) The prostate gland lies **posterior** to the urinary bladder.

(b) BPH typically affects the **outer** regions of the prostate gland.

(c) This condition affects at least **half** of men older than 60 years.

(d) In the prostate gland, **almost all** testosterone is normally converted to dihydroxytestosterone (DHT) by action of 5α-reductase.

(e) The enzyme 5α-reductase is likely to **improve** BPH.

B18. Circle risk factors for BPH.

African American descent
High levels of dihydroxytestosterone (DHT)
Elevated estrogen levels
Family history of BPH
Japanese descent
Older men

B19. Answer the following questions about manifestations and diagnoses of BPH.

(a) State the major clinically significant effect of BPH.

_____

(b) List three or more significant sequelae of BPH.

_____

_____

_____

(c) Circle correct answers about three factors that contribute to manifestations of BPH:

(c1) The position of the prostate *(posterior to? surrounding?)* the urethra

(c2) Prostatic smooth muscle with *(greater? less?)* than normal tone that narrows the urethra

(c3) *(Increased? Decreased?)* detrusor muscle contractility that might lead to urinary stasis

(d) Explain the diagnostic information indicated by these clinical findings:

(d1) Presence of bacteria and leukocytes in urine

_____

(d2) Normal PSA

_____

(d3) Elevated postvoided residual volume (PRV) of urine detected by catheterization

_____

(d4) Serum creatinine level of 2.5 mg/100 mL

_____

B20. American Urological Society Symptom Index scores in the range of 12 to 18 indicate *(mild? moderate? severe?)* BPH.

B21. Answer the following questions about treatments for BPH.

(a) Prostatectomy surgery *(is? is not?)* currently the primary treatment for BPH. What does the acronym TURP stand for?

_____ _____ _____ of the _____

(b) Mr. Davidson, age 89, has congestive heart failure (CHF) and advanced emphysema. How can a stent help his BPH?

_____

B22. Choose the two true statements about prostate cancer. (Pay particular attention to whether the **bold-faced** word or phrase makes the statement true or false.)

(a) This form of cancer is **rare** in the United States.

(b) More than 80% of all prostate cancers are diagnosed in men **older than** 65 years.

(c) Incidence of prostate cancer is **greater** in men with a family history and also with high dietary fat content.

(d) Prostate cancer typically presents with symptoms **early** in the course of the disease.

B23. Explain what the following signs or symptoms suggest in patients with prostate cancer.

(a) Voiding pattern similar to that of BPH

_____

(b) Dyspnea (shortness of breath)

_____

(c) Low back pain and pathological fracture of a lumbar vertebra

_____

B24. List three methods of screening for prostate cancer.

_____

_____

_____

B25. Mr. van den Ende, age 51, has been in apparently good health but recently was diagnosed with prostate cancer that is grade 4. The grading indicates that his tumor is *(highly? poorly?)* differentiated. Given his age and otherwise good health, what treatment is likely? _____

C. DISORDERS IN CHILDHOOD AND AGING CHANGES

C1. Circle the correct answers or fill in the blanks within each statement about disorders of the penis.

(a) In *(epi? hypo?)*spadias, the urethral opening lies on the under (ventral) surface of the penis. This disorder occurs in about 1 in *(300? 30,000? 3 million?)* male infants born each year. Name another condition that is common in boys born with hypospadias: _____ Explain why boys with both of these disorders should have chromosomal studies performed.

_____

Surgery to correct this condition is more likely to be performed at age *(9 months? 5 years?)*.

(b) Epispadias is much *(more? less?)* common than hypospadias. Name another condition often associated with epispadias.

_____

C2. Choose the two true statements about disorders of the penis. (Pay particular attention to whether the **bold-faced** word or phrase makes the statement true or false.)

(a) Circumcision **is** the treatment of choice for hypospadias.

(b) Most newborns **do not** have a fully retractable foreskin.

(c) The foreskin of all 2-year-old boys **should** be forcibly retracted for thorough cleaning of the area.

(d) **Paraphimosis** is a condition in which the foreskin is so tight that it cannot cover the glans.

C3. Zachariah (see Chapter 21, Question C4) was born at 26 weeks of gestation. In addition to his respiratory distress syndrome, he has cryptorchidism of the left testis. Answer the following questions related to his case.

(a) Define cryptorchidism.

_____

(b) Cryptorchidism is *(common? rare?)* among premature boys and relatively *(common? rare?)* in full-term infants. Most cases of cryptorchidism are *(unilateral? bilateral?)*. The testes normally descend during the _____ months of fetal life.

(c) Spontaneous descent of the testis is more likely to occur when Zachariah is *(birth to 3? 6 to 9?)* months old.

(d) Contrast a retractable testis with one that is undescended.

_____

_____

(e) State three reasons why early diagnosis and treatment of Zachariah's condition are important.

_____

_____

(f) Treatments for this condition should take place before the child is 2 *(months? years?)* of age. Hormonal therapy *(is? is not?)* likely to help babies with cryptorchidism. Surgical placement and fixation of Zachariah's undescended testis into his scrotal sac is a procedure known as _____. This surgery can produce a ____% fertility rate for unilateral undescended testis.

C4. Choose the three true statements about the aging reproductive system. (Pay particular attention to whether the **bold-faced** word or phrase makes the statement true or false.)

(a) Aging-related changes in the reproductive system are **more** profound and rapid in women than in men.

(b) The force of ejaculation is likely to **decrease** with aging.

(c) Blood vessels in the penis are likely to become **more** sclerosed with aging.

(d) Testes become **larger** with aging.

(e) Seminal vesicles **become larger** with aging.

(f) The prostate gland becomes **larger** with aging.

C5. Describe effects of:

(a) Andropause

_____

(b) Androgen replacement in males

_____

_____

CHAPTER 39

Disorders of the Female Genitourinary System

■ Review Questions

A. STRUCTURE AND FUNCTION OF THE FEMALE REPRODUCTIVE SYSTEM

A1. Arrange these female external genitalia from anterior to posterior in location.

Anus   Clitoris
Urinary opening   Vaginal orifice

_____, _____,

_____, _____

A2. Match the structure to the related description.

Clitoris   Introitus
Labia majora   Labia minora
Mons pubis   Urinary meatus
Vaginal orifice   Vestibule

(a) Vaginal opening; may be surrounded by hymen: _____

(b) Prepuce is the "hood" of this structure:

_____

(c) Surrounded by the Skene glands:

_____

(d) Located between labia minora; site of urethral and vaginal openings:

_____

(e) Structures that are developmentally analogous to the male scrotum:

_____

A3. Choose the two true statements about female genitalia. (Pay particular attention to whether **the bold-faced** word or phrase makes the statement true or false.)

(a) The **vaginal lining** contains receptors for sexual sensations.

(b) The term *fornices* refers to the **uterine cervix.**

(c) Vascular tissue within **labia minora** becomes engorged during sexual excitement.

(d) The internal os and endocervical canal are openings in the **vagina.**

(e) The endocervical canal produces a **mucoid plug** during pregnancy.

A4. Circle the correct answers or fill in the blanks to answer the following questions about the uterus.

(a) Arrange the parts of the uterus from most superior to most inferior in location:

Body   Cervix   Fundus

_____, _____, _____

(b) Arrange these structures from most posterior to most anterior in location:

Bladder   Rectum   Uterus

_____, _____, _____

(c) Which is more anterior in location?

(1) Rectouterine pouch

(2) Vesicouterine pouch

(d) Arrange the layers of the uterine wall from most deep to most superficial:

Endometrium   Myometrium   Perimetrium

_____, _____, _____

(e) Which layer of the uterus is the thickest? _____ metrium.

A5. Match the phases of the menstrual cycle with the correct descriptions below. Choose from these answers:

Menstrual   Proliferative   Secretory

(a) The endometrium thickens in response to estrogen stimulation: _____

(b) Progesterone (made by the corpus luteum) is most active during this postovulatory (or luteal) phase: _____

(c) Superficial tissue from the endometrium sloughs off: _____

A6. Select the female reproductive organ that fits each description.

Fallopian tubes   Ovaries   Uterus

(a) Fingerlike fimbriae draw in ova:

_____

(b) Part of the lining is shed as menses:

_____

(c) Usual site where fertilization occurs:

_____

(d) Sites where ova and the hormones estrogen and progesterone are produced:

_____

A7. Indicate where each hormone related to female reproduction is made.

Estrogen
Follicle-stimulating hormone (FSH)
Gonadotropin-releasing hormone (GnRH)
Luteinizing hormone (LH)
Prolactin
Progesterone
(a) Hypothalamus: _____
(b) Anterior pituitary: _____,

_____, _____

(c) Ovaries: _____, _____

A8. Which hormones listed in Question A7 are gonadotropic?

_____, _____

A9. Circle the two true statements about female reproductive hormones. (Pay particular attention to whether the **bold-faced** word or phrase makes the statement true or false.)
(a) During pregnancy, estrogens, progesterone, insulin, and cortisol **all** help prepare breasts for lactation.
(b) **Estrogens** are needed for normal female physical maturation.
(c) Estrogen levels increase **during menstruation.**
(d) The most abundant and potent form of estrogen is **estriol.**

A10. Circle each of the following that is an action of estrogens.
(a) Stimulate development of pubic hair and other secondary sexual characteristics
(b) Increase blood levels of the "good cholesterol" (HDLs)
(c) Increase risk of osteoporosis
(d) Help to maintain memory by promoting cerebral blood flow
(e) Cause retention of Na^+ and H_2O
(f) Stimulate development of reproductive organs in the developing embryo and fetus
(g) Stimulate glandular development of breasts at puberty

A11. Explain how progesterone is "pro gestation."

_____

A12. Women normally *(do? do not?)* produce androgens. Where are these made?

_____

A13. Fill in the blanks that follow with the correct abbreviation to arrange in sequence these events in the ovarian cycle:

Corpus albicans, a white scar on the ovary, formed postovulation (CA)
Corpus luteum formed postovulation (CL)
High estrogen inhibits FSH, inhibits follicle development, and increases LH (IF)
A surge of LH triggers ovulation of the oocyte with its corona radiata (LH)
One dominant follicle (ODF) forms, producing estrogen
Primary follicle develops under FSH stimulation (PF)
Secondary follicles (6 to 12) develop (SF)

_____ → _____ → _____ →
_____ → _____ → _____ →
_____

A14. Choose the two true statements about the menstrual cycle. (Pay particular attention to whether the **bold-faced** word or phrase makes the statement true or false.)

(a) **Ovaries** are primarily responsible for changes within the menstrual cycle.
(b) **Theca externa** cells are ovarian cells that produce hormones.
(c) Mittelschmerz is a term that refers to **menstrual pain.**
(d) The average length of the female menstrual cycle is **28 days.**

B. DISORDERS OF THE FEMALE REPRODUCTIVE ORGANS

B1. The vulva refers to *(internal? external?)* genitalia. Select the condition from the list below that fits each description of a vulvar disorder.

Bartholin gland cyst   Cyclic vulvovaginitis
Essential vulvodynia   Leukoplakia

(a) Syndrome of vulvar pain sufficient to interfere with daily activities:

_____

(b) Episodes of vulvodynia that coincide only with premenstrual phase or after sexual activity:

_____

(c) Benign, white lesions of the vulva that may cause pain during sexual activity:

_____

(d) Fluid-filled sac lateral to the vagina that can reach the size of an orange:

_____

B2. Choose the two true statements about vulvar lesions. (Pay particular attention to whether the **bold-faced** word or phrase makes the statement true or false.)

(a) The risk for invasive vulvar carcinoma is **greater** in women in their 30s than for women in their 60s.

(b) Vulvar intraepithelial neoplasia (VIN) is **a diagnosis** that always means vulvar cancer.

(c) Human papillomavirus (HPV) infection **increases** risk for VIN and cancer of the vulva.

(d) Metastatic vulvar cancer is **likely** to spread first into inguinal, femoral, and iliac lymph nodes.

B3. Circle the correct answers within each statement about vaginal disorders.

(a) Döderlein bacteria are *(pathogens? normal flora?)* of the vagina. They break down *(glycogen? proteins?)* in the lining of the vagina. Products of this breakdown normally cause the vaginal lining to have a pH below *(4.5? 7.0? 9.5?)*.

(b) Postmenopausal women are likely to have a(n) *(decreased? increased?)* number of Döderlein bacteria and a more *(acidic? alkaline?)* vaginal pH. This environment *(decreases? increases?)* risk of vaginal infections. Describe two primary preventions to help avoid vaginal infections.

_____

_____

B4. Sally, age 27, is recovering from 3 weeks of bronchitis for which she took antibiotics. She is highly stressed as semester exams approach. Answer the following questions related to her case.

(a) Sally has been producing a malodorous vaginal discharge; her vagina is red,

burning, and itching. Are these simply normal changes within the menstrual cycle?

_____

(b) Sally is diagnosed with a *Candida* yeast infection. How does this diagnosis relate to Sally's recent history?

_____

B5. Answer the following questions about vaginal cancer.

(a) This form of cancer is *(common? rare?)*, and occurs mostly in women age ___ years or older. Write two causes of vaginal cancer in women about 40 years of age.

_____

(b) DES (diethylstilbestrol) was taken by women *(for nausea? to prevent miscarriage?)* primarily during the years *(1940–1971? 1972–2002?)*. Daughters of these women have a greatly increased risk for *(benign? malignant?)* extension of cervical tissue into the vagina, which predisposes to cancer.

(c) The most common sign of cancer of the vagina is _____.

(d) List four types of treatment that may be used depending on the nature of the malignancy.

_____

_____

B6. Circle the correct answers or fill in the blanks within each statement about disorders of the cervix of the uterus.

(a) The cervix is normally lined with _____ epithelium, whereas the vagina is lined with _____ epithelium. Select from these answers:
    (1) Simple columnar
    (2) Stratified squamous

(b) Which of the tissues in B6(a) undergoes a change to form the other? Some of *(1 becomes 2? 2 becomes 1?)*. The region where such change occurs is known as the _____ zone.

(c) This change results in *(dysplasia? metaplasia?)*, which means growth of tissue that is *(abnormal? normal for the body but not for this region?)*. Such change *(can? cannot?)* lead to dysplasia and neoplasia (such as cancer).

(d) List factors that can increase such transformation.

_____

(e) _____ cysts may develop in the transformed tissue. Are these malignant? _____

(f) Soft, red, velvety lesions known as _____ are the most common lesions of the cervix. Most are *(benign? malignant?)*.

B7. Contrast acute *(A)* and chronic *(C)* cervicitis.

(a) Often results from minute tears in the cervix that develop during childbirth: _____

(b) The cervix becomes red and edematous with large amounts of white mucopurulent discharge: _____

B8. Karla, age 30, has been diagnosed with cervical intraepithelial neoplasia CIN2. Answer the following questions about her disorder.

(a) It is likely this condition has been developing for *(days? weeks? years?)*. Explain.

_____

(b) Karla's cervical disorder is graded as "LSIL," which indicates a *(better? poorer?)* prognosis than a grading of "HSIL."

(c) Defend or dispute this statement: "Cervical cancer is a sexually transmitted disease."

_____

_____

(d) List several other risk factors for cervical cancer.

_____

_____

(e) Cervical cancer is a *(common? rare?)* cause of death. If detected early, it *(is? is not?)* readily curable. The incidence of cervical cancer has *(decreased? increased?)* in the last half century, largely related to early diagnosis. Explain.

_____

(f) The Pap smear is a *(diagnostic? screening?)* method. A follow-up procedure permitting a well-lit stereoscopic view of the cervix is likely to be performed; this procedure is known as _____.

B9. Answer the following questions about pelvic inflammatory disease (PID).

(a) List the three major organs most involved in PID. Then add the term for inflammation of each of these organs.

_____

_____

_____

(b) Name the two microbes that most often cause PID.

_____

_____

What is the origin of these microbes?

_____

_____

(c) Circle risk factors for PID.

(1) Age 25 to 35 years
(2) Married, multiparous woman
(3) Previous history of PID
(4) History of multiple sex partners

(d) What signs or symptoms of PID distinguish this condition from other pelvic disorders?

_____

_____

In addition, with PID white blood cell count and erythrocyte sedimentation rate both *(decrease? increase?)*. Because this is a widespread infection, fever *(is? is not?)* likely to occur.

(e) Name one category of medication typically administered to patients with PID.

_____

B10. Emily, age 27, has been diagnosed with endometriosis. Answer the following questions related to her case.

(a) Circle the factors that increased Emily's risk for endometriosis.

(1) She started menstrual periods at age 16.
(2) Her periods have been heavy with intense cramping.
(3) Her mother and older sister both have endometriosis.
(4) She has not been able to become pregnant after 5 years of trying to conceive.

(b) Emily has "chocolate cysts." Describe these in terms of location, composition, and possible complications.

_____

_____

(c) List two possible mechanisms by which endometrial tissue reached Emily's ovaries.

_____

_____

(d) Why does this tissue continue to grow?

_____

(e) In addition to her dysmenorrhea, what other symptoms are likely for Emily?

_____

(f) The most accurate diagnostic method for endometriosis is _____. The most definitive treatment is _____. Incidence of recurrence after surgery is _(high? low?)_.

B11. Match each uterine disorder with the correct description.

Adenomyosis	Endometritis
Endometriosis	Leiomyoma

(a) "Fibroids" that grow within the myometrium; the most common form of pelvic tumor; often asymptomatic; typically do not interfere with pregnancy and most regress with menopause:

_____

(b) Endometrial tissue is present within the myometrium; likely to occur in middleaged, multiparous women and resolve with menopause:

_____

(c) Infection of the endometrial lining with a variable clinical picture but often marked by a foul-smelling vaginal discharge:

_____

(d) Presence of endometrium in ectopic sites usually within the pelvic cavity; likely to occur in young women who are infertile or who have chronic pelvic pain:

_____

B12. Circle the correct answers about endometrial cancer.

(a) Endometrial cancer is much _(more? less?)_ common than cervical cancer. It almost always occurs in women _(younger than? older than?)_ 40 years of age.

(b) Circle risk factors for endometrial cancer:
  (1) Obesity
  (2) Hormone replacement therapy that combines estrogen and progesterone
  (3) Tamoxifen therapy for breast cancer
  (4) Diabetes mellitus
  (5) Hypertension

(c) Circle typical early manifestations of endometrial cancer:
  (1) Vaginal bleeding between menstrual periods in a 40-year-old woman
  (2) Vaginal bleeding in a 65-year-old woman
  (3) Pain that accompanies abnormal bleeding
  (4) Enlarged inguinal lymph nodes

(d) Circle the most definitive tool for diagnosing this type of cancer:
  (1) Papanicolaou smear
  (2) Biopsy
  (3) Transvaginal ultrasonography
  (4) Dilation and curettage (D&C)

(e) With early diagnosis and treatment, the 5-year survival rate for endometrial cancer is _(20%? 50%? 90%?)_.

B13. Answer the following questions about supportive structures of the pelvis and uterus and related disorders.

(a) Which ligaments secure the cervix laterally to the pelvis to help prevent uterine prolapse?
  (1) Round
  (2) Broad
  (3) Cardinal
  (4) Uterosacral

(b) Which structure provides the most support for pelvic viscera?
  (1) Pelvic diaphragm
  (2) Bony pelvis
  (3) Peritoneum

(c) List several factors that lead to relaxation of pelvic support structures.

_____

_____

(d) Which condition involves sagging of the urinary bladder into the anterior wall of the vagina?
  (1) Rectocele
  (2) Uterine prolapse
  (3) Cystocele
  (4) Enterocele

(e) Evelyn's cervix has prolapsed so that it protrudes outside of her vaginal opening. This is a _____-degree uterine prolapse.
  (1) First
  (2) Second
  (3) Third

(f) The most common variation in uterine position is:
  (1) Acute anteflexion
  (2) Retroflexion
  (3) Simple retroversion

B14. Most disorders of pelvic relaxation *(do? do not?)* require surgery. List nonsurgical interventions for these disorders.

_____

_____

B15. Choose the three true statements. (Pay particular attention to whether the **bold-faced** word or phrase makes the statement true or false.)

(a) Cysts are a **rare** form of ovarian tumor.

(b) Chronic **failure to ovulate** is thought to be the cause of polycystic ovary syndrome (PCOS).

(c) Women with polycystic ovary syndrome (PCOS) are likely to experience **high** blood levels of LH and androgens and relatively **low** levels of FSH.

(d) Weight loss in obese women has been found to **increase** ovulation in women with PCOS.

(e) Dermoid cysts are **malignant** ovarian tumors.

(f) **Androgen-secreting** ovarian cysts are likely to increase growth of hair and deepen the voice in women.

B16. Answer the following questions about ovarian cancer.

(a) Circle women at increased risk for this type of cancer:
  (1) Stacy is 27 years old.
  (2) Tanya's mother died of ovarian cancer.
  (3) Joan bottle-fed both of her infants.
  (4) Yvonne has given birth to five children.
  (5) Patrice has used oral contraceptives for 8 years.

(b) Ovarian cancer is *(frequently? rarely?)* fatal. It usually is diagnosed *(before? after?)* metastasis because early symptoms are *(severe? vague?)*. Which system most commonly manifests early symptoms?

_____

(c) There *(are? are no?)* good screening tests for ovarian cancer. Name a serum marker

that can be used to monitor ovarian cancer after it is diagnosed and is being treated: _____. Surgery *(is? is not?)* required for diagnosis and staging.

C. MENSTRUAL DISORDERS

C1. Choose the two true statements about the menstrual cycle. (Pay particular attention to whether the **bold-faced** word or phrase makes the statement true or false.)

(a) **Ovaries** are primarily responsible for changes within the menstrual cycle.

(b) Menarche refers to the **first menstrual bleeding**.

(c) For a woman to menstruate, it is necessary for her to ovulate.

(d) The average length of the female menstrual cycle is **38 days**.

C2. The ability to maintain a regular menstrual cycle *(is? is not?)* related to body fat. Explain.

_____

Circle women who are likely to experience amenorrhea:

(a) Karen, age 20, who is 5'6" tall, weighs 95 lb, and has a diagnosis of anorexia

(b) Eileen, age 30, who weighs 340 lb

(c) Sandra, who runs 70 miles a week

(d) Geraldine, age 38, with end-stage cancer

C3. Identify the type of dysfunctional menstrual cycle in each case.

Amenorrhea   Hypomenorrhea
Menorrhagia   Metrorrhagia
Oligomenorrhea

(a) Bleeding between periods: _____

(b) Excessive menstruation: _____

(c) Absence of menstruation: _____

(d) Periods more than 35 days apart: _____

C4. Answer the following questions about abnormal menstrual cycles.

(a) Estrogen inadequacy causes a *(thinner? thicker?)* than normal endometrium.

(b) Estrogen without progesterone leads to a *(thinner? thicker?)* than normal endometrium. Progesterone is reduced when a follicle *(does? fails to?)* mature, ovulate, and form a corpus luteum.

(c) *(High? Low?)* levels of both estrogen and progesterone lead to anovulatory bleeding with *(light? heavy?)* flow that *(is? is not?)* typically accompanied by cramps. List two populations of women likely to experience such cycles.

_____

(d) List two components of a minimal evaluation of menstrual cycle disorders.

_____

(e) Indicate whether each of the following patient's amenorrhea is primary *(P)* or secondary *(S)*.

(e1) Juliette, age 25, runs 6 to 10 miles a day and has a diagnosis of bulimia; she has not had a period since she was 21.

_____

(e2) Roberta, age 18, has never menstruated. _____

C5. Menstruation with cramping and possibly diarrhea and headache is known as _____menorrhea. Severe dysmenorrhea caused by endometriosis or pelvic adhesions is classified as *(primary? secondary?)*.

C6. Choose the three true statements related to premenstrual syndrome (PMS). (Pay particular attention to whether the **bold-faced** word or phrase makes the statement true or false.)

(a) Premenstrual syndrome (PMS) **is** a psychosomatic disorder.

(b) The incidence of PMS is greatest among women in their **early 20s**.

(c) The cause of PMS is **estrogen deficiency**.

(d) Fluid retention, headache, and swollen breasts are **typical manifestations** of PMS.

(e) PMS **usually** is relieved by menstruation.

(f) Premenstrual dysphoric disorder is a **psychiatric** diagnosis in which symptoms **are not** relieved by onset of menses.

C7. Describe an integrated treatment approach for PMS.

_____

_____

_____

C8. Answer the following questions about Ms. Grayling, who is 51 years old.

(a) Ms. Grayling has experienced menstrual irregularity for 3 years; her last menstrual period was 4 months ago. She is said to be _____menopausal.

(b) Her estrogen levels are likely to be *(zero? diminished?)*. Explain.

_____

(c) Ms. Grayling experiences "vasomotor instability," commonly manifested as _____.

(d) She has some sleep deprivation. Explain.

_____

(e) She is at *(increased? decreased?)* risk for osteoporosis. Explain.

_____

(f) Estrogen *(can? cannot?)* be administered topically as a treatment for vaginal atrophy associated with menopause.

D. DISORDERS OF THE BREAST

D1. Select the term that fits the related description.
Alveoli   Areolar tissue   Cooper ligaments
Lobes   Nipple

(a) Milk-producing glandular cells located in grapelike clusters within lobes of breast:

_____

(b) Fibrous tissue in spoke-like arrangement that supports breasts: _____

(c) Smooth area surrounding the nipple; darkens at puberty and during pregnancy; contains Montgomery tubercles:

_____

D2. Match each breast disorder with the related description.
Ductal ectasia   Mastitis
Fibrocystic disease   Papilloma

(a) Inflammation of the breast starting with nipple irritation, infection, or hormonal changes: _____

(b) Inflammation of the ducts, leading to gray-green discharge from nipples; occurs in older women: _____

(c) Benign tumors of epithelium that can be palpated in the areola area:

_____

(d) The most common breast lesion, especially in women ages 30 to 50: _____

D3. Circle the correct answers within each statement about fibrocystic disease.

(a) Fibrocystic disease is more common in women who are *(30 to 50? 50 to 70?)* years of age. In this condition, breasts *(are? are not?)* lumpy.

(b) A(n) *(mammogram? ultrasound?)* is more helpful in differentiating a breast cyst from a tumor.

(c) Coffee, tea, cola, and chocolate should be *(increased? avoided?)* by women with fibrocystic disease. Explain.

_____

D4. Mrs. Cappel, age 34, with a history of normal menstrual cycles, has received a diagnosis of breast cancer. Answer the following questions related to her case.

(a) Mrs. Cappel's cancer is a *(common? rare?)* form of female cancer. One in *(8? 80? 800?)* women is likely to develop breast cancer in her lifetime. The diagnosis of breast cancer has *(decreased? increased?)* within the last 25 years. Explain.

_____

(b) Circle Mrs. Cappel's risk factors for breast cancer:
   (1) Her age
   (2) Onset of menarche at age 11
   (3) Mrs. Cappel gave birth to her first child 12 years ago.
   (4) Both her mother and her older sister have breast cancer.
   (5) She has the BRCA1 mutation on chromosome 17.

(c) Which type of breast cancer is more common?

(1) Invasive lobular carcinoma
(2) Ductal carcinoma

D5. List the three diagnostic methods that can best diagnose breast cancer.

_____

_____

(a) Mammography can identify lesions as small as _____, whereas palpation *(breast self-examination [BSE])* can identify tumors as small as _____. Palpated malignancies typically are found to be *(painful? painless?)*.

(b) List several other diagnostic methods for identifying and evaluating breast cancer tumors.

_____

_____

D6. Circle the three true statements about treatment for breast cancer. (Pay particular attention to whether the **bold-faced** word or phrase makes the statement true or false.)

(a) Radical mastectomy is **no longer used** as surgical therapy for most breast cancers.

(b) Prognosis depends **more** on the size of the breast tumor than on nodal involvement.

(c) A sentinel node refers to the **farthest** node that cancer cells are likely to reach.

(d) Tamoxifen blocks **estrogen receptors**, so it is likely to decrease growth of breast cancers that are estrogen-receptor positive.

(e) Paget disease, which usually affects bone tissue, **is** a rare form of breast cancer.

CHAPTER 40

Sexually Transmitted Diseases

■ Review Questions

A. INFECTIONS OF THE EXTERNAL GENITALIA

A1. Circle the correct answer within each statement about sexually transmitted diseases (STDs).

(a) STDs are *(more? less?)* common in persons who have more than one sexual partner.

(b) It *(is? is not?)* possible for a person to be infected with more than one STD at a time.

(c) Human papillomavirus infections are *(decreasing? increasing?)* in numbers each year.

A2. List five possible portals of entry for microbes that cause STDs.

_____

_____

_____

A3. Circle the correct answers or fill in the blanks to complete this exercise about human papillomavirus (HPV) infections.

(a) Circle the type of external genital warts most likely to infect moist surfaces such as the vulva.

(1) Flat warts

(2) Planar warts

(3) Common warts

(4) Condyloma acuminata

(b) There are approximately ____ different types of HPV viruses. It *(is? is not?)* possible to be infected with more than one type at a time.

(c) A link between HPV and _____ cancer has been established. List several other factors that increase risk for these cancers.

_____

_____

_____

(d) Amelia is exposed to HPV on January 1. She is likely to exhibit signs or symptoms during the period of February 15 through _____. List typical manifestations that would lead to a diagnosis of HPV.

_____

_____

_____

(e) Describe treatments that can eradicate Amelia's HPV infection.

_____

_____

(f) A vaccine has been developed against *(type 16? type 18? all types of?)* HPV virus(es). The vaccine *(eradicates the HPV virus? helps reduce the risk of cervical cancer?)*.

A4. There are ____ known types of herpesviruses that cause infections in humans. Herpes (or varicella) zoster is known to cause _____ and _____. Genital herpes is caused by the herpes _____ virus (HSV). Circle the correct answers or fill in the blanks to answer the following questions about genital herpes.

(a) HSV-*(1? 2?)* is responsible for more than 90% of cases of recurrent genital herpes. HSV-1 typically causes "cold sores" or _____. HSV-1 *(also can? does not?)* cause genital herpes by orogenital sex.

(b) About *(50,000? 5 million? 50 million?)* Americans have genital herpes. The incidence of genital herpes is greater in *(men? women?)*. Explain why.

_____

(c) HSV viruses on the skin or mucosa travel to _____ of *(sacral? thoracic?)* spinal nerves, where they reside during a latent period of months or years. Because HSV grows in neurons, these viruses are known as *(lymphotropic? neurotropic?)* viruses. Antiviral medications *(are? are not?)* effective against these latent viruses.

(d) Most episodes of HSV-2 are subclinical and *(do? do not?)* have recognizable manifestations, and most spread of HSV-2 occurs from persons who *(do? do not?)* have symptoms, which explains the *(limited incidence? epidemic proportions?)* of herpes globally.

(e) List several areas where herpes lesions are likely to form in women, in men, or in either gender.

_____

_____

(f) Circle common manifestations of genital lesions.

Discomfort with urinating	Discomfort with sexual activity	Pain
Itching	Tingling	Vesicles that rupture

(g) List examples of systemic manifestations of HSV-2.

_____

_____

_____

(h) Diagnosis of genital herpes involves identification of the virus in specimens taken from *(crusted lesions? vesicles or pustules?)*.

A5. Circle the correct answers or fill in the blanks to answer the following questions related to two patients with genital herpes.

(a) Philip states that he has a history of fever blisters but that this is the first episode of genital herpes of which he is aware.

(a1) Philip's genital herpes diagnosis is most likely to be classified as:

A. Initial nonprimary infection

B. Primary infection

C. Recurrent infection

(a2) Signs or symptoms of *(primary? nonprimary?)* episodes of genital herpes typically are more acute. Explain.

_____

_____

(a3) Philip's symptoms are likely to last about *(2 to 4? 7 to 10? 12 to 14?)* days.

(a4) There *(is a? is no known?)* cure for genital herpes. Why does Philip's physician prescribe antiviral drugs for Philip?

_____

_____

(a5) The clinic nurse advises Philip to be extremely careful to wash his hands well, especially before applying his contact lenses. Explain.

_____

(b) Mary Lee has a history of genital herpes outbreaks about once a month; she is 8 months pregnant.

(b1) She is experiencing prodromal manifestations of genital herpes. These include:

A. Burning, tingling (paresthesia), or itching

B. Painful vesicles that rupture, crust over, and heal

(b2) If Mary Lee continues to have active lesions at the time her baby is due, it is likely that she will be advised to have a *(cesarean? vaginal?)* delivery.

A6. Match each microbe in this list with the category to which it belongs.

Bacteria	*Chlamydia*	Fungi
Parasites	Protozoa	Virus

(a) Genital warts (condyloma acuminata): _____

(b) Chancroid: _____

(c) Granuloma inguinale; characterized by buboes: _____

(d) Herpes simplex: _____

A7. Which two STDs listed in A6(a-d) are most common in the United States? _____ _____ Which of these infections involves ulcer formation that increases risk of transmission of HIV? _____

B. VAGINAL INFECTIONS

B1. Circle all the terms that refer to *Candida* infections.

Bacterial vaginosis	Moniliasis	Thrush
Trichomoniasis	Yeast infection	

B2. Circle the three true statements about *Candida* infections. (Pay particular attention to whether the **bold-faced** word or phrase makes the statement true or false.)

(a) **One of four** women in the United States is likely to experience candidiasis within a lifetime.

(b) Candidiasis is **always** transmitted through sexual contact.

(c) Pregnancy, use of oral contraceptives, and antibiotic therapy **increase** the risk of *Candida* infections.

(d) Healthy women **rarely** harbor the *Candida* fungus in moist areas of skin or mucosa.

(e) Vulvar candidiasis typically is accompanied by **pruritus** and a **thick, cheesy** discharge.

(f) Candidiasis **can** be effectively treated by over-the-counter medications.

B3. Where else (other than external genitalia) can *Candida* infections occur?

_____

B4. Mrs. Emerus has a diagnosis of trichomoniasis. Circle the correct answers or fill in the blanks within each statement related to her condition.

(a) She has a copious discharge from her vagina that *(has an? has no?)* odor and has a pH *(under 4.5? over 6.0?)*.

(b) Mrs. Emerus receives a prescription for metronidazole. The nurse advises her that she can expect a *(metallic? putrid? salty?)* taste in her mouth and that alcohol use while taking this drug is *(acceptable? contraindicated?)*. The nurse also describes side effects to the _____ and _____ systems that also may accompany use of this drug.

(c) *Trichomonas (is? is not?)* transmitted through sexual contact. Cessation of sexual activity during the course of the infection *(is? is not?)* recommended for Mrs. Emerus.

B5. Choose the two true statements about bacterial vaginosis. (Pay particular attention to whether the **bold-faced** word or phrase makes the statement true or false.)

(a) This condition involves growth of **anaerobic** bacteria that **raise** vaginal pH.

(b) Bacterial vaginosis **is a highly** inflammatory disorder.

(c) Bacterial vaginosis is a **common** vaginal disorder.

(d) Burning, itching, and redness **are all** manifestations of bacterial vaginosis.

(e) The presence of *Gardnerella vaginalis* in the vagina—even with no other signs—**is** an indication for treatment.

B6. Circle each of the following signs that is diagnostic of bacterial vaginosis.

(a) A fishy- or ammonia-smelling white discharge

(b) Vaginal pH of 4.0

(c) Presence of flat epithelial cells covered coccobacilli

C. VAGINAL-UROGENITAL-SYSTEMIC INFECTIONS

C1. *(Chlamydia? gonorrhea? syphilis?)* is the most prevalent reportable STD in the United States.

Write one characteristic that distinguishes the effects of gonorrhea, syphilis, and *Chlamydia* from the effects of the STDs discussed thus far in this chapter.

_____

_____

_____

C2. Answer the following questions about *Chlamydia*.

(a) In the United States, *Chlamydia* transmission is *(primarily? rarely?)* by sexual contact.

(b) There *(is one type? are many types?)* of *Chlamydia*.

These microbes exist in two forms: _____ bodies and _____ bodies.

(c) Manifestations of *Chlamydia* and gonorrhea are *(quite similar? very dissimilar?)*, although *(Chlamydia? gonorrhea?)* is more likely to be asymptomatic. In fact, more than *(20%? 50%? 90%)* of patients infected with *Chlamydia* have no symptoms. Explain why this lack of symptoms may be problematic.

_____

_____

_____

(d) In addition to infection of the urethra, list other parts of the body affected by Reiter syndrome.

_____

(e) Identify the most common organ affected by neonates who are infected by their mothers' chlamydial infections.

_____

C3. Circle the correct answers or fill in the blanks to complete this exercise about gonorrhea.

(a) It is estimated that there are approximately *(6,000? 600,000?)* new cases of gonorrhea in the United States each year. Infection typically occurs 2 to 5 *(days? months? years?)* after exposure. In addition to the genitourinary tract or anorectum, what areas can serve as portals of entry?

_____

(b) Myra, age 22, has gonorrhea. Describe these symptoms that accompany her condition:

(b1) Dysuria

_____

(b2) Dyspareunia

_____

(b3) Salpingitis

_____

(c) Suzy, age 5, has gonorrhea in her throat. What is the likely cause?

_____

C4. The VDRL test is a classic screening test for the STD _____. Another test for this STD is the fluorescent _____ antibody absorption test. The tertiary stage can involve rubbery, necrotic lesions known as _____ in locations such as liver, testes, or bone. List two other systems likely to have lesions in the tertiary stage: _____ and _____. Name the treatment of choice for this STD: _____.

C5. Contrast major STDs by completing Table 40-1.

Table 40-1 Comparison of Sexually Transmitted Diseases

Name of STD	Causative Microbe	Description
(a)		Genital warts, pruritus; increased risk of cervical cancer; rapidly growing STD in the U.S.; treatments cannot cure but reduce symptoms
(b)	Protozoan: pear-shaped with flagallae	
(c)		The most prevalent reportable STD in the U.S.; often no symptoms in 90% of cases but women may have mucopurulent discharge; spread to fallopian tubes can cause infertility; can cause blindness in infected neonates and Reiter syndrome (of eyes) in adults
(d) Chanchroid		
(e)	*Neisseria* bacteria (gram-negative diplococci)	
(f)		Thin, gray-white discharge with foul, fishy odor; "clue cells" seen on slides; very common; **minimally inflammatory**
(g)	Spirochete bacteria *Treponema pallidum*	
(h) Genital herpes		
(i)		Most women have this infection at least once; thick, cheesy, odorless discharge; antifungals can cure

CHAPTER 41

Structure and Function of the Skeletal System

■ Review Questions

A. CHARACTERISTICS OF SKELETAL TISSUE

A1. Answer the following questions about the skeletal system.

(a) List five or more functions of the skeletal system.

_____

_____

_____

(b) Contrast the axial with the appendicular skeleton.

_____

_____

(c) List types of tissues that form the skeletal system.

_____

A2. Identify the following as collagen *(C)* or elastic *(E)* fibers.

(a) Formed primarily of elastin, which gives these fibers great stretchability: ____

(b) Fibrous protein that provides great tensile strength to tendons: ____

A3. Identify the type of cartilage that fits each description.

Elastic   Fibrous   Hyaline

(a) The most abundant type of cartilage in the body, it forms most of the fetal skeleton:

_____

(b) Found on the ends of bones (articular cartilage) and connecting ribs to sternum:

_____

(c) Found in areas where flexibility is needed, for example in the external ear:

_____

(d) Provides strength and support in intervertebral disks and the pubic symphysis: _____

A4. Answer the following questions about cartilage tissue.

(a) Cartilage cells are known as _____cytes. Most cartilage is covered by a membrane known as the _____.

(b) Blood vessels *(do? do not?)* perfuse cartilage. Explain how cartilage receives its oxygen and nutrients.

_____

A5. Refer to Figures 41-1 and 41-2 in *Essentials of Pathophysiology* and answer the following questions about bone tissue.

(a) *(One? Two?)* third(s) of bone tissue is composed of inorganic salts made primarily of *(calcium? potassium?)*. The remainder of bone includes bone cells, blood vessels, nerves, and _____ fibers.

(b) *(Compact? Cancellous?)* or trabecular bone is relatively lightweight and forms the bulk of rounded ends of long bones. *(Compact? Cancellous?)* bone forms the strong outer portion of the shafts of long bones.

(c) Arrange in correct sequence from first to last in bone formation:

Osteoblasts   Osteocytes
Osteogenic cells

_____ → _____ →

_____

(d) Which cells (in Question A5[c]) synthesize collagen and other proteins that make up osteoid (prebone) tissue? _____

These cells then secrete the enzyme_____, which results in calcification of osteoid.

(e) Which cells (in Question A5[c]) are mature bone cells? _____ These cells lie in microscopic lakes known as *(canaliculi? lacunae?)* and produce bony matrix in concentric layers called _____ .

(f) Each unit of 4 to 20 lamellae forms a unit known as a(n) _____ that surrounds a central canal containing _____ .
Explain how bone cells in lacunae receive nutrients.

_____

_____

(g) Explain how blood vessels reach bone tissue.

_____

_____

(h) Osteo_____ are cells that function in the resorption of bone. These cells are formed from *(osteoblasts? monocytes?)* under the influence of the hormone *(calcitonin? PTH?)*.

A6. Explain why tetracycline is contraindicated during pregnancy and in children younger than 6 years of age.

_____

A7. Describe functions of the following membranes attached to bone.

(a) Fibrous periosteum

_____

_____

(b) Osteogenic periosteum

_____

_____

(c) Endosteum

_____

_____

A8. Circle the correct answers or fill in the blanks within each statement about embryonic development.

(a) The skeleton forms from *(ectoderm? mesoderm?)*.

(b) Arrange the following skeletal structures from first to last according to their development chronologically:

(1) Arms
(2) Legs
(3) Vertebrae

_____ → _____ → _____

(c) Ossification of the skeleton is first apparent during the *(third? sixth? ninth?)* month of fetal development.

(d) Bones grow in length as long as the _____ growth plate is present, typically throughout the first 20 years of life. At this plate, _____ cells are replaced by bone cells when nutritional and hormonal balance is provided. Vitamin *(C? D?)* deficiency will slow down growth at the epiphyseal plate, resulting in scurvy. Impaired calcification of new bone can result in rickets because of deficiency of vitamin ___ .

(e) Bones grow in diameter as new bone is formed from cells in the *(endosteum? periosteum?)*. Cells in the *(endosteum? periosteum?)* assure resorption of bone facing the marrow, so the growing bone is not excessively thick and heavy.

A9. Fill in the blanks below with names of the correct chemicals.

Calcitonin   Parathyroid hormone   Vitamin D

(a) _____ and _____ tend to increase the blood level of calcium, whereas _____ decreases the blood level of calcium.

(b) _____ stimulates osteoclasts and bone resorption, whereas _____ inhibits osteoclasts.

(c) Which of these chemicals increase(s) renal excretion of phosphates? _____

(d) _____ is synthesized by the thyroid gland.

(e) Hypocalcemia serves as a trigger for release of the hormone _____, whereas hypercalcemia stimulates release of the hormone _____ .

A10. PTH raises the blood level of calcium by drawing calcium from which three sources?

_____

_____

A11. Answer the following questions about vitamin D.

(a) Vitamin D is a(n) *(amine? steroid?)* hormone. Name three food sources of vitamin D.

_____

(b) Name a human organ that synthesizes a relatively inactive form of vitamin D. _____ Identify organs that activate vitamin D. _____ _____

(c) Explain why elderly persons may be at higher risk for activated vitamin D deficiency.

_____

_____

(d) Circle the form of vitamin D that is most potent in intestinal absorption of calcium and promoting action of PTH in activating osteoclasts:

(1) 7-dehydrocholesterol

(2) 25-hydroxyvitamin D_3

(3) 1,25-hydroxyvitamin D_3

(4) 24,25-hydroxyvitamin D_3

(e) PTH and prolactin *(stimulate? inhibit?)* formation of 1,25-hydroxyvitamin D_3, whereas calcitonin *(stimulates? inhibits?)* formation of this active form of vitamin D.

(f) In parts of the world or seasons with limited sunlight, human vitamin D production is likely to be *(decreased? increased?)*.

A12. Circle the correct answer or fill in the blanks.

(a) There *(are? are no?)* known syndromes of calcitonin (CT) excesses or deficiencies.

(b) Name one condition for which CT might be prescribed. _____ Explain why.

_____

B. SKELETAL STRUCTURES

B1. Identify the type of bone that fits each description.

Flat   Irregular   Long   Short

(a) Vertebrae, mandible, and maxillae are examples: _____

(b) Wrist bones are examples; falls on the wrist often lead to fractures because carpals are composed mostly of spongy bone: _____

(c) A femur: _____

B2. Refer to Figure 41-5 in *Essentials of Pathophysiology* and match the part of a long bone with the related description.

Diaphysis   Epiphysis   Metaphysis

(a) Broad, rounded end of a long bone that serves as a site for articulation: _____

(b) Shaft of a long bone composed primarily of compact bone surrounding the medullary cavity: _____

(c) Located between the diaphysis and the growth plate in bones of young persons: _____

B3. Circle the correct answers within each statement.

(a) Bones of *(children? adults?)* have relatively more red marrow and less yellow marrow.

(b) *(Ligaments? Tendons?)* connect bone to bone, whereas *(ligaments? tendons?)* connect muscles into periosteum of bones. Aponeuroses are broad *(ligaments? tendons?)*. Ligaments and tendons have a(n) *(abundant? limited?)* blood supply.

(c) *(Diarthroses? Synarthroses?)* are joints with limited or no motion. Which of the following is a joint in which bones are joined by cartilage (as in costosternal joints)?

Synchondrosis   Syndesmosis   Synostosis

(d) Most joints of the body are *(diarthroses? synarthroses?)*; these are also known as *(cartilaginous? synovial?)* or *(freely movable? immovable?)* joints.

B4. Describe the structure of a diarthrodial joint.

_____

_____

_____

B5. Circle the two true statements. (Pay particular attention to whether the **bold-faced** word or phrase makes the statement true or false.)

(a) Articular cartilage **is** covered by synovial membrane.

(b) Normal synovial fluid is **clear or pale yellow** and has the consistency of egg white.

(c) The synovial membrane has a rich blood supply that helps it **heal rapidly** when injured, for example, in joint surgery.

(d) Synovial membranes are **well innervated** by nerve fibers that transmit pain.

B6. Mr. Dennis has an injured right hip, yet he feels pain in his right knee. Explain.

_____

_____

B7. Contrast a bursa with a bunion.

_____

_____

CHAPTER 42

Disorders of the Skeletal System: Trauma, Infection, and Childhood Disorders

■ Review Questions

A. INJURY AND TRAUMA OF MUSCULOSKELETAL STRUCTURES

A1. The musculoskeletal system makes up about ____% of the body. List structures that compose the musculoskeletal system.

_____

_____

A2. Answer the following questions about musculoskeletal injuries.

(a) Trauma is a *(common? rare?)* cause of musculoskeletal injury. Trauma from _____ is the leading cause of death in adults younger than 45 years.

(b) _____ are the most common cause of deaths in individuals older than 35 years, especially among adults who have developed significant osteoporosis. Fractures are *(more? less?)* likely in elderly who have osteoporosis. List two bones most likely to be fractured in such falls.

_____

(c) List two types of acute injuries that are common among athletes:

_____. List one type of chronic overuse injury that is more common among athletes:

_____

A3. Select the soft tissue injury that fits each description.

Contusion   Hematoma
Laceration   Puncture wounds

(a) Involves tearing of skin: _____

(b) An injury that does not result in tearing of the skin, although the area may be bruised:

_____

(c) Of these injuries, most likely to lead to gas gangrene (tetanus): _____

(d) Large accumulation of blood that causes the area to become "black and blue":

_____

A4. Answer the following questions about joint injuries.

(a) Ligaments connect *(bones? muscles?)* to bones, and tendons connect *(bones? muscles?)* to bones.

(b) Strains involve injury or partial tearing of *(ligaments? muscles or muscle-tendon units?)*. *(Sprains? Strains?)* involve no externally evident injury and heal relatively quickly. Circle regions that are likely sites for strains:

Cervical vertebrae   Elbows
Feet   Lumbar vertebrae
Shoulders

(c) After a joint is sprained or strained, *(cold? heat?)* should be applied to reduce pain and swelling.

(d) The joint most often sprained is the _____ and this more commonly involves turning of the foot *(in? out?)*ward. In Grade(s) *(1? 2? 3? 4?)* knee sprains, the medial collateral ligament is totally ruptured.

(e) Explain why affected joints are immobilized for several weeks.

_____

(f) A subluxation is a *(partial? complete?)* dislocation. Once a joint is dislocated, it is *(more? less?)* likely to be dislocated again. Which two joints are most likely to experience congenital dislocations? _____ and _____

(g) List two types of loose bodies that are most commonly found in joints.

_____

A5. Answer the following questions about injuries to specific joints.

(a) Rotator cuff injuries affect the *(elbow? knee? shoulder?)* joints. Such injuries are likely to occur by trauma in _____ or _____ players or by slow onset overuse in elderly persons. Name the muscles and tendons that form the rotator cuff, and circle the one most often affected in rotator cuff injuries.

_____

(b) Menisci are located in *(elbow? knee? shoulder?)* joints. They are composed of C-shaped *(bone? cartilage? fat?)* tissue. List several functions of menisci.

_____

(c) Explain why torn menisci heal slowly.

_____

Why is reconstructive surgery advisable before degeneration of menisci is complete?

_____

(d) Which types of sports tend to cause patellar dislocation? _____ and _____ List treatments for this disorder.

_____

(e) Chondromalacia refers to _____ of articular cartilage.

(f) Hip dislocation *(is? is not?)* an emergency situation. After reduction to prevent reoccurrence of dislocation, weight bearing *(is? is not?)* usually limited.

(g) Hip fracture usually involves fracture of the *(hip bone? proximal femur?)*. Circle all risk factors for hip fracture.

Age 28 years   Male   White   Tall, lean
Dementia   Osteoporosis   stature

A6. Identify the type of fracture likely in each patient.

Fatigue (stress fracture)   Pathologic fracture
Sudden injury fracture

(a) Mrs. Blumstein, age 84, fractures an osteoporotic hip as she rises from her chair: _____

(b) Bonnie, a 34-year-old long-distance runner, experiences a tibial fracture caused by overuse: _____

(c) Mr. Steves fractures his radius by a fall on the ice: _____

A7. Choose the three true statements about fractures. (Pay particular attention to whether the **bold-faced** word or phrase makes the statement true or false.)

(a) **Stress fractures** are the most common type of fracture.

(b) A stress fracture **is not** the same condition as shin splints.

(c) An **open** fracture involves movement of part of the bone through the skin.

(d) A **distal** fracture of the tibia is closer to the knee joint than to the ankle joint.

(e) Comminuted fractures involve a break of a bone into **more than two** pieces.

(f) Greenstick fractures occur more often in **elderly** and involve a **complete** break across the bone.

A8. Answer the following questions about fractures.

(a) Define *reduction* as it relates to fractures.

_____

A *(comminuted? spiral? transverse?)* fracture is not likely to lose its position after it is reduced.

(b) In addition to pain, what other signs and symptoms may accompany fractures?

_____

(c) List three types of deformities that may occur with fractures: _____, _____, _____. Explain what causes these deformities.

_____

(d) Define *crepitus* as it relates to fractures.

_____

(e) Explain how fracture reduction may be accomplished without pain within minutes after the break occurs.

_____

A9. List the three main objectives for treatment of fractures: _____, _____, _____. Circle the one of these that is most critical to achieving union of fracture fragments. Circle the correct answer within each of the following statements about treatment of fractures.

(a) Surgical reduction with internal fixation of bone fragments is known as *(closed? open?)* reduction.

(b) If a fracture is suspected, a splint *(should? should not?)* be applied before the patient is moved.

(c) While a fractured right tibia is in a cast, leg exercises should be performed involving the:

(1) Right leg

(2) Left leg

A10. Arrange the phases of fracture healing in correct sequence, and then match the phases to the descriptions.

Fibrocartilaginous callus   Hematoma
Ossification   Remodeling

(a) Soft tissue from torn blood vessels and other injured soft tissues combine with clotting factors and fibrin to provide a scaffolding for granulation tissue by the end of the first week after the fracture:_____

(b) Granulation tissue formed from fibroblasts, chondrocytes, and osteoblasts that migrate from periosteum and endosteum creates a "collar" that bridges the two broken bone fragments:_____

(c) Calcification begins to harden this tissue by about a month after the fracture:

_____

(d) Osteoclastic removal of excess callus shapes the new bone: _____

A11. Circle each of the following that is a factor that lengthens the time required for fracture healing.

(a) Age:

(1) 76 years

(2) 16 years

(b) Bones with ___ surface areas at fracture sites:

(1) Large

(2) Small

(c) Shape of bones:

(1) Short bones

(2) Long bones

(d) General health:

(1) Diabetic

(2) Nondiabetic

(e) Circulation:

(1) Normal

(2) Compromised

A12. Identify types of impaired healing likely from a tibial fracture that occurred on January 1.

Delayed union   Malunion   Nonunion

(a) Not healed by June 15: _____

(b) Still not healed by November 15:

_____

(c) Abnormal angulation of the fracture is visible on an x-ray: _____

A13. Identify types of complications that may follow fractures or other musculoskeletal injuries. One answer will be used twice.

Compartment syndrome   Fracture blisters
Fat embolism syndrome   Reflex sympathetic
                          dystrophy

(a) May occur from small globules of fat released from bone marrow (especially from a femur or the pelvis) that pass through major veins and lead to potentially fatal pulmonary emboli (PE):

_____

(b) Epidermis and dermis are separated by twisting injuries; localized edema with possible infection resulting: _____

(c) Severe aching or burning pain that is out of proportion to the injury; excessive sweating and pallor also may manifest:

_____

(d) Burning pain, tingling, or loss of sensation occurs that is intense relative to the degree of the injury; fasciotomy may be required for resolution of this condition; most commonly occurs in the leg: _____

(e) Increase in pressure within a femur and subtle changes in behavior are important signs of this complication: _____

A14. Potential causes of compartment syndrome are listed below. Add to the list of causes in each category here.

(a) Decreased compartment size—circumferential eschar in burn area; casts:

_____

_____

(b) Increased compartment volume—bleeding; swelling after thrombosis or burns:

_____

_____

A15. Circle the three true statements about compartment syndrome. (Pay particular attention to whether the **bold-faced** word or phrase makes the statement true or false.)

(a) Compartment syndrome is likely to cause changes in sensation **before** muscle dysfunctions such as contractures occur.

(b) Pain **is not** typically a symptom of this syndrome.

(c) Capillary refill time and peripheral pulses are often **normal** with this syndrome.

(d) Elevation of the extremity **is** part of the typical treatment plan for compartment syndrome.

(e) Skin changes **do** commonly accompany compartment syndrome.

A16. Describe signs or symptoms within a few days of the injury that may point to fat embolism syndrome. Build on these key terms or phrases:

(a) Signs of diminished cerebral blood flow

_____

(b) Chest pain, dyspnea and sympathetic responses, such as

_____

(c) Rash on anterior of chest, neck, shoulders, and axillae

_____

_____

A17. Circle the form of fat embolism syndrome that is most likely to be fatal:

(a) Fulminating

(b) Overt clinical

(c) Subclinical

B. INFECTIONS AND OSTEONECROSIS

B1. Circle or fill in the correct answers about osteomyelitis.

(a) Osteomyelitis involves infection of bone *(cortex? marrow?)*. Typically, bone infections are *(difficult to cure? readily cured?)*.

(b) List three possible origins of such infections.

_____

_____

(c) Osteomyelitis is more likely to result from *(blood-borne infections? bone contamination from an open wound?)*.

(d) The most common microbe causing such infections is the bacterium _____, which normally is present on the skin surface. Describe two mechanisms that account for this infection.

_____

_____

(e) Osteomyelitis from blood-borne infections occurs more commonly among *(children? middle-aged persons?)*. In children, such conditions are likely to occur *(in vertebrae? at growing points of long bones?)*, whereas _____ are the most common sites in adults.

B2. Ruth has osteomyelitis 10 weeks after her hip replacement surgery. Answer the following questions related to her case.

(a) At this point she has *(acute? chronic?)* osteomyelitis. Explain.

_____

(b) The hallmark sign of chronic osteomyelitis is presence of infected, necrosed bone known as *(sequestrum? involcrum?)* that is ensheathed in new bone called _____. These regions of osteomyelitis *(are? are not?)* visible on x-rays or bone scans.

(c) Ruth's hip infection requires additional hip surgery. Explain the possible reasons.

_____

_____

B3. Mr. Vonnahme, who has diabetes mellitus, has a deep ulcer on his foot. Explain what is likely to be the underlying cause of that foot ulcer.

_____

_____

B4. Fill in the blanks about tuberculosis osteomyelitis.

Tuberculosis of a bone or joint is caused by the same microbe that causes tuberculosis of the lung, namely _____ *tuberculosis*. Which bones are most often infected with the tuberculosis organism?

_____

B5. Max, age 58, has been taking corticosteroids for many years for his rheumatoid arthritis. He now has a diagnosis of osteonecrosis. Answer the following questions about his experience.

(a) Osteonecrosis refers to *(damage? injury? death?)* of bone tissue caused by inadequate *(blood? nerve?)* supply.

(b) Which parts of a bone does osteonecrosis commonly affect?

_____

_____

Why not the cortical bone?

_____

(c) Max's necrosis is of the femoral head within the hip joint. Is this a typical site for osteonecrosis? *(Yes? No?)* Explain.

_____

(d) Osteonecrosis is *(often? seldom?)* idiopathic, which means _____. List several factors that can lead to the ischemia that underlies osteonecrosis.

_____

_____

(e) Which of the factors you just listed would increase Max's risk for osteonecrosis?

_____

(f) Identify the prominent symptom Max is most likely to experience:

_____

(g) What treatment will Max most likely need for his osteonecrosis?

_____

Osteonecrosis accounts for about ___ % of hip replacements in the United States.

B6. Explain what causes the "soap" that may create lesions in necrotic bone and be visible on x-rays for a lifetime.

_____

_____

C. NEOPLASMS

C1. Circle the correct answers within each statement about bone tumors.

(a) Most bone cancers are *(primary? metastatic?)*.

(b) *(Benign? Malignant?)* tumors typically grow slowly and do not metastasize.

(c) A chondroma is a *(benign? malignant?)* tumor of cartilage. Osteochondromas are *(common? rare?)* types of benign tumors.

(d) Osteoclastomas are *(benign? malignant?)* tumors that *(do? do not?)* metastasize.

(e) Malignant tumors are likely to have *(well? poorly?)* defined borders.

C2. Most malignant bone tumors are accompanied by pain that *(is? is not?)* relieved by rest. Describe another major manifestation of bone tumors.

_____

C3. Saidee, age 18, has been diagnosed with osteosarcoma of the right proximal tibia. Answer the following questions related to her case.

(a) Arrange the incidence of osteosarcoma in these age groups from greatest to least:

Adolescents   35-year-olds   Elderly

_____, _____,

_____

(b) This is *(the most common? a rare?)* form of bone cancer in children and adolescents. The location of Saidee's tumor *(is? is not?)* a site of rapid bone growth and a common location of osteosarcomas in adolescents.

(c) Saidee experienced pain in her leg as the first sign of her tumor. Tumor pain is more likely to have a(n) *(sudden? insidious?)* onset.

(d) Describe common effects of osteosarcoma on:

(d1) Skin in the region of the tumor

_____

(d2) Muscles in the region of the tumor

(e) Metastases to *(lungs? lymph nodes?)* tends to occur early in the disease.

(f) Saidee will have limb-salvage surgery. Describe this procedure.

C4. Answer the following questions about other primary bone cancers.

(a) Circle the correct answers about Ewing sarcoma.

(a1) The greatest incidence of Ewing sarcoma is among:
(1) African American, late teens
(2) Asian children
(3) White adolescents

(a2) Ewing sarcoma usually is found in:
(1) Shafts of long bones
(2) Epiphyses of long bones
(3) Vertebrae
(4) Pelvis

(a3) Explain why diagnosis of Ewing sarcoma may be difficult.

(b) Circle the correct answers about chondrosarcoma.

(b1) This type of tumor occurs more in:
(1) Children or adolescents
(2) Middle-aged or elderly adults

(b2) Chondrosarcoma tends to be:
(1) Rapid growing and metastasizing early
(2) Slow growing and metastasizing late

(b3) Circle the bones that are most likely to be sites of chondrosarcoma:
(1) Pelvis
(2) Femoral head
(3) Carpals
(4) Distal radius

(b4) Circle the most effective treatment for chondrosarcoma:

(1) Early radical surgical excision
(2) Radiation
(3) Chemotherapy

C5. Answer the following questions about metastasizing bone cancers.

(a) About *(1%? 10%? 50%?)* of all people with cancer will have bone metastases during the course of their disease.

(b) Metastases are likely to occur:
(1) In extremities
(2) Within or close to the trunk

(c) Circle the three most common types of cancers that metastasize to the skeletal system.

| Breast | Colorectal | Lung |
| Prostate | Stomach | Tongue |

(d) What causes the pain of metastasis?

(e) Explain why the following diagnostic or treatment approaches are used.

(e1) Blood tests for alkaline phosphatase and calcium

(e2) Radiation therapy

(e3) Intramedullary rods

D. SKELETAL DISORDERS IN CHILDREN

D1. Answer the following questions about abnormal musculoskeletal development.

(a) The typical fetal position in utero involves *(flexion? extension?)* of shoulders, elbows, hips, and knees. (Refer to Figure 42-11 in *Essentials of Pathophysiology.*) Most *(flexion? extension?)* contractures present at birth normally disappear in newborns by the age of 4 to 6 *(days? weeks? months?).*

(b) List factors that can contribute to torsional deformities, such as intoeing or outtoeing.

(c) Intoeing or metatarsus adductus is a *(common? rare?)* congenital deformity of the foot. The condition *(often? rarely?)* corrects itself spontaneously.

(d) Internal tibial torsion (bowing of the tibia) is a common cause of *(intoeing? outtoeing?)* in children under 2 years of age. External femoral torsion is a common cause of *(intoeing? outtoeing?)* in children. This condition *(is? is not?)* likely to correct itself when the child walks.

(e) When a child lies in the prone position with legs flexed and ankles apart, the degree of *(internal? external?)* rotation of femurs can be measured (Figure 42-14B, left side, in *Essentials of Pathophysiology*). Excessive rotation of this type is also known as femoral _____. Children with this condition are more comfortable sitting in the _____ position, which *(improves? exacerbates?)* the condition.

D2. Answer the following questions about knock-knees and bowlegs.

(a) When Tyler, age 31 months, stands with his inner ankles touching, his knees are at least 2" apart. His condition is *(bowlegs? knock-knees?)*, also known as genu _____. (Note: *genu* = knees.) This disorder is *(very common? uncommon?)* in toddlers. It is *(sometimes? always?)* pathologic.

(b) When Toby, age 6, stands with his knees touching, his inner ankles are several inches apart. This condition is known as _____ or genu _____ and is more associated with laxity of the *(medial? lateral?)* collateral ligament(s). It *(rarely? usually?)* requires treatment.

(c) Explain why severe genu varum or valgum should be diagnosed early.

_____

_____

(d) Tiffany has a diagnosis of Blount disease in her right leg; this is a condition in which the _____ of the tibia fails to form on the medial side. Blount disease is more likely to lead to *(bowlegs? knock-knees?)*. Incidence is greater in *(small? large?)* children and in *(early? late?)* walkers. It is usually *(bi? uni?)*lateral.

D3. Circle the answers that match a term with its correct description.

(a) Syndactyly: webbing of fingers

(b) Polydactyly: presence of an extra bone in a finger

(c) Thalidomide: a teratogenic drug known to cause absence of limbs or limb parts, especially if mothers took the drug during the second month of gestation

D4. Answer the following questions about hereditary and congenital deformities.

(a) Osteogenesis imperfecta (OI) is a condition in which bones are extremely *(fragile? thick and strong?)* because of defective collagen synthesis. OI is more commonly an autosomal *(dominant? recessive?)* disorder. An autosomal *(dominant? recessive?)* form (also known as type __) is more lethal because bones are so fragile they can fracture *in utero*. There *(is? is no?)* known treatment for OI.

(b) In almost all cases of congenital clubfoot, the forefoot is turned *(inward? outward?)* so that the foot resembles a horse's hoof. This condition is known as equino*(valgum? varus?)*. (Note: *equus* = horse.) List one health practice an expectant mother can take to lower risk for congenital clubfoot.

_____

D5. Katelyn is a white 24-month-old who was born breech. She has developmental dysplasia of her left hip (DDH) with generalized joint laxity. Katelyn is her parents' first child, and there is no known family history of this condition.

(a) Circle factors in Katelyn's history above that increase her risk for DDH.

(b) DDH is *(quite common? extremely rare?)*. Katelyn's DDH in her left hip is *(more? less?)* common than right-sided DDH.

(c) Luxation refers to a hip that is *(dislocated? dislocatable?)*, whereas subluxation refers to a _____ hip.

(d) Katelyn exhibits a typical gait associated with DDH. Describe it.

_____

(e) Treatment for DDH involves maintenance of Katelyn's left hip joint in a(n) _____ position.

D6. Select the condition that fits each description.

Blount disease   Congenital clubfoot
Developmental dysplasia   Legg-Calvé-Perthes
    of the hip   disease
Osteogenesis imperfecta   Osgood-Schlatter
    disease   Slipped capital
                                       femoral epiphysis

(a) Three hereditary or congenital disorders:

_____, _____,

_____

(b) Formerly known as congenital hip dislocation; present to some degree in 1% of all newborns; repeated dislocations with limited abduction of thigh and asymmetrical gluteal folds suggest this condition: _____

(c) A deformity known as "talipes":

_____

(d) A disorder in which bones lack collagen and are so brittle that they can fracture; may affect other sites of collagen, such as skin, joints, muscles and teeth; no cure:

_____

(e) Three conditions in which the head of the femur is not properly seated in the hip socket (acetabulum): _____,

_____, _____

(f) Trevor, age 5 years and white, has a disorder in which the bone-forming center in the head of his left femur becomes ischemic; as the femoral head degenerates and necroses, the head develops an abnormally flattened shape. This fact leads to the alternative term for this condition— coxa plana _____

(g) Kathleen has tenderness and swelling in the front of her knee region (tibial tubercle) because there are microfractures at the sites of insertion; cartilage there is abnormally ossified; associated with growth periods and typically resolves afterward:

_____

(h) Onset of signs and symptoms usually is during the teen years, more often in boys with rapid growth periods; although a hip problem, pain may refer to knees; early treatment is critical to prevent lifelong crippling: _____

(i) Two conditions from the list above primarily affecting knee joints: _____

_____

D7. Answer the following questions about Trevor (Question D6[f]) and his Legg-Calvé-Perthes (L-C-P) disease.

(a) Circle each of the following that is a factor that increases risk for L-C-P.

(1) White (Caucasian)

(2) Male

(3) Short stature

(4) Well-nourished

(b) Trevor's L-C-P is *(bi? uni?)*lateral. Is this typical? *(Yes? No?)*

(c) What is likely to be the goal of treatment for Trevor?

_____

He is fitted with a brace that keeps his left hip joint in *(abduction? adduction?)*.

(d) The success of Trevor's treatment is likely to be *(greater? less?)* because he received a diagnosis at the age of 5 years, rather than at 10 years. Explain.

_____

D8. Suzannah, age 12, has right thoracic scoliosis, which is a(n) *(anterior-posterior? lateral?)* deviation of the spinal column; her *(concavity? convexity?)* is on the right side. Answer the following questions related to her condition.

(a) Scoliosis is much more common in *(boys? girls?)* and is severe in about one of *(2? 20? 1,000?)* cases.

(b) *(Postural? Structural?)* scoliosis can be corrected by exercise; *(postural? structural?)* scoliosis cannot.

(c) Suzannah's scoliosis is structural; the cause of most cases of structural scoliosis is _____; it has been associated with joint *(laxity? tightness?)*. The most common age group for onset of idiopathic scoliosis is:

(1) Adolescent

(2) Infantile

(3) Juvenile

(d) Suzannah's mother first questioned if her daughter might have scoliosis. What indicators may she have noticed?

_____

_____

(e) *(Bracing? Surgery?)* halts the progression of scoliosis, whereas *(bracing? surgery?)* decreases the curvature.

CHAPTER 43

Disorders of the Skeletal System: Metabolic and Rheumatic Disorders

■ Review Questions

A. METABOLIC BONE DISEASE

A1. Answer the following questions about processes involved in bone remodeling.

(a) Osteo*(blasts? clasts?)* tear down or resorb old bone, and osteo*(blasts? clasts?)* lay down new bone. These cells are derived from _____ cells in marrow and periosteum.

(b) One cycle of bone resorption and formation requires about 4 *(days? weeks? months? years?)*. With aging, which process occurs more? Bone *(formation? resorption?)*.

(c) Mechanical stress stimulates osteo*(blasts? clasts?)*. List one or more factors that would decrease mechanical stress so that new bone would not be laid down.

_____

(d) Which vitamin is required for laying down organic matter (collagen) in bone? Vitamin *(C? D?)*. Which vitamin is needed for calcium absorption from foods? Vitamin

_____

(e) Which hormone stimulates osteoclasts to tear down bone and release Ca^{2+} into blood? _____ This hormone triggers production of interleukin-_____, which plays a key role in this process. Too much of this chemical can cause excessive bone breakdown, as in _____ disease.

(f) Name a hormone that helps to build bones.

_____

(g) Briefly describe roles of the RANK ligand (RANKL) and RANK receptors in bone resorption.

_____

_____

(h) Explain how osteoprotegerin (OPG) can oppose osteoporosis.

_____

_____

(i) Osteo_____ means bone mass is less than normal for a person of a particular age, race, or gender. List several causes of this condition.

_____

_____

A2. *Osteoporosis* literally means _____ bone—the bone resembles a _____; in this condition the rate of bone resorption *(increases? decreases?)* relative to the rate of bone formation. Answer the following questions about osteoporosis (OP).

(a) This is a *(common? rare?)* condition affecting about *(44,000? 44 million?)* Americans.

(b) OP in postmenopausal women is classified as *(primary? secondary?)* osteoporosis. Bone mass reaches its maximum at about age 30. By age 50, a typical age for menopause, a woman is likely to have lost ____% of her bone mass; by age 70, her loss probably will be about ____%.

(c) Circle the factors that increase risk for OP.

(1) African American

(2) Asian

(3) A child

(4) Female

(5) A woman whose mother and sister had fractured hips

(6) A woman receiving hormone replacement therapy (HRT)

(7) Low calcium dietary intake

(d) The rate of bone loss is greater *(early? late?)* in menopause because osteoclastic activity is *(increased? decreased?)*. The greatest losses are in *(cortical? trabecular?)* bone, increasing the risk of fractures in bones with large amounts of this type of bone. Name two such sites:_____ and _____

(e) Circle each of the following that is an effect of postmenopausal loss of estrogen that tends to lead to osteoporosis:

   (1) Cytokines such as 1L-6 (that stimulate osteoclast production) are increased.

   (2) Production of OPG (that normally inhibits osteoclast production: Question A1[h]) is decreased.

   (3) Osteoblast activity is decreased.

(f) OP that has a known cause is known as *(primary? secondary?)* osteoporosis. Identify factors that increase risk for OP in the following patients:

   (f1) Gina, age 17, 5'6" and 98 pounds, is a gymnast. She works out "40 to 50 hours a week to try to stop from getting any more fat on me." She is a nonpurging bulimic and much of her diet consists of diet cola.

   _____

   _____

   (f2) Mrs. McAllister, age 46, takes aluminum containing antacids for her peptic ulcer and corticosteroids for flare-ups of her Crohn disease; she had a panhysterectomy last year, in which her ovaries were removed, but she wears an "estrogen patch."

   _____

   _____

   (f3) Mr. Latimer, age 64, eats a 12-oz steak each night and then drinks two 6-packs of beer with cheese and crackers; he is a self-proclaimed "couch potato" and "two-pack-a-day man."

   _____

   _____

(g) Are osteoporotic bones likely to be painful? *(Yes? No?)* Describe the first clinical signs or symptoms likely for osteoporosis.

   _____

   _____

(h) How is a "dowager's hump" related to OP?

   _____

   _____

(i) With aging, height typically *(increases? decreases?)*. This change occurs primarily in length of the:

   (1) Leg bones

   (2) Vertebral column

(j) Write the meaning of the memory aid *ABONE* that describes risk factors for osteoporosis. _____

(k) List three diagnostic methods for detecting osteoporosis:

   _____

(l) Given the risk factors for OP, list four or more healthy behaviors that could help prevent this condition.

   _____

   _____

(m) Match the types of chemicals used in the treatment of OP with the descriptions that follow.

   Biphosphonates   Calcitonin   Estrogen

   (m1) Decreases osteoclast activity:

   _____

   (m2) Chemicals (such as Fosamax) that bind to bone tissue to prevent osteoclastic bone destruction:

   _____

   (m3) A powerful treatment to reduce incidence and progression of OP; includes plant forms and SERM:

   _____

A3. Answer the following questions about osteomalacia (OM).

(a) Osteomalacia is a condition in which bones are deficient in *(minerals? organic matrix?)*, specifically in _____ or _____. As a result bones are *(softer? more brittle?)* than normal. This condition is also known as adult _____.

(b) List several types of medications that can lead to osteomalacia.

   _____

(c) Circle the typical signs or symptoms of OM:

Bowlegs   Hip fractures
Muscle weakness   Pain
Severe hypocalcemia   Hyperparathyroidism

(d) List two effective and inexpensive treatments for OM.

_____

_____

A4. Answer the following questions about vitamin D.

(a) It is a *(fat? water?)*-soluble vitamin that is absorbed from foods with the help of bile or synthesized in _____. This vitamin is necessary for absorption of the mineral _____ from foods.

(b) Vitamin D deficiency in the United States results mainly from *(deficient dietary intake? impaired absorption?)*. List three countries in which vitamin D often is lacking in the diet.

_____

A5. Answer the following questions about how kidney disorders can lead to osteomalacia.

(a) Kidneys, along with the liver, normally are sites of _____ of vitamin D.

(b) In chronic renal failure (CRF), kidneys excrete *(more? less?)* than normal phosphate and *(more? less?)* than normal calcium ions. Resulting *(hyper? hypo?)*calcemia acts as a stimulus for *(increased? decreased?)* secretion of parathyroid hormone, which then stimulates bone *(formation? resorption?)*. This is known as _____ rickets.

(c) Vitamin D–resistant rickets involves excessive loss of _____ from kidneys. State one additional cause of phosphate deficiency.

_____

_____

A6. Answer the following questions about rickets in children.

(a) Rickets involves *(brittle? softened?)* and deformed bones caused by *(de? over?)*mineralization. Symptoms of this condition are most commonly identified in

children *(6 months to 3 years? 3 to 6 years? 6 to 10 years?)* old.

(b) What causes nutritional rickets?

_____

_____

(c) Use these key phrases to describe characteristics of rickets in children:

(c1) Buddha-like appearance

_____

(c2) Rachitic rosary

_____

(c3) Skull

_____

(c4) Hypocalcemia

_____

(d) List two effective and inexpensive treatments for rickets.

_____

A7. Alice, age 42, has been diagnosed with Paget disease. Write a one-sentence description of this condition.

_____

_____

(a) Paget disease typically begins in *(children? adults?)*.

(b) Explain Alice's manifestations of headache, vertigo, and hearing loss.

_____

_____

(c) Explain how Alice's waddling gait is related to Paget disease.

_____

_____

(d) Alice is at increased risk for pathologic fractures. Define this term.

_____

(e) What condition poses the greatest risk of death for Alice?

_____

_____

(f) Alice is experiencing severe pain. Is this typical of Paget disease?

_____

B. RHEUMATIC DISORDERS

B1. Circle the two true statements about arthritis. (Pay particular attention to whether the **bold-faced** word or phrase makes the statement true or false.)

(a) There are **more than** 100 different types of arthritis.

(b) Arthritis is a **rare** cause of disability in the United States.

(c) Arthritis **can** affect persons in any age group.

(d) **All** forms of arthritis are systemic.

B2. Answer the following questions about rheumatoid arthritis (RA).

(a) The incidence of RA is greater in *(women? men?)*, especially those in *(adolescence? middle age?)*.

(b) The exact cause of RA *(is? is not?)* known. The rheumatoid factor (RF) is present in body fluids of *(few? most? all?)* people who have RA.

(c) The RF *(is? reacts with?)* a fragment of the IgG autoantibody. The result is known as an immune _____. Explain why some people begin to develop antibodies (RF) that react with their own IgG.

_____

_____

_____

B3. Refer to Figures 43-4 and 43-5 in *Essentials of Pathophysiology* and select the key word or phrase that describes each major event in the progression of RA.

Ankylosis
Immune complex
Pannus formation
Phagocytosis

Extra articular changes
Granulation tissue formation

(a) RF combines with altered IgG in the synovial joint: _____

(b) Inflammation begins as neutrophils and macrophages are attracted and "eat up" immune complexes: _____

(c) Excessive numbers of blood vessels (granulation tissue) grow within the synovial membrane, leading to a red, warm, swollen, and spongy joint: _____

(d) Pannus exacerbates the synovitis and interferes with joint movement: _____

(e) Ligaments stretch and alter joint stability with possible dislocation; muscles associated with the joint atrophy from disuse; weakness and fatigue result: _____

B4. Circle correct answers about rheumatoid arthritis (RA).

(a) Pannus formation is found in *(RA only? many forms of arthritis?)*. This growth of blood vessels is *(helpful by nourishing? destructive to?)* joint tissues.

(b) Limitation of joint motion early in the course of RA is caused by *(fibrosis of? pain in?)* joints.

(c) Joints most affected by RA are *(large, such as hip and shoulder? small, such as hands and feet?)*, and the effects typically are *(unilateral? bilateral?)*.

(d) Which joints are least likely to be affected by RA?

Distal interphalangeal
Metacarpophalangeal
Proximal interphalangeal

(e) Swan-neck deformity affects *(great toes? neck? thumbs?)*. Subluxation also may occur; this is *(dislocation? spraining?)* of a joint. The bulge sign and genu vulgus are both possible signs of RA in the *(great toes? hand? knee?)*.

(f) If vertebrae are affected by RA, they are most likely to be *(cervical? lumbar? thoracic?)*, leading to *(lower back? neck?)* pain. The *(hip? knee? shoulder?)* is a commonly affected large joint, accompanied by severe atrophy of *(hamstrings? quadriceps?)* muscles.

(g) Which of the following are included in criteria for RA by the American Rheumatism Association (ARA)?

Anemia
Elevated ESR
Nodules
X-ray changes of hand joints

Cloudy synovial fluid
Evening stiffness
Swelling of at least three joints for at least 6 weeks

B5. List several treatment goals for persons with RA.

_____

_____

B6. Match the medications used to treat RA with the descriptions that follow.

Corticosteroids   Infliximab
Methotrexate   Nonsteroidal
                                 anti-inflammatory
                                 drugs (NSAIDs)

(a) Monoclonal antibody ("mAb") that blocks formation of the proinflammatory cytokine, tumor necrosis factor-α (TNF-α):_____

(b) Anti-inflammatories, including aspirin and ibuprofen: _____

(c) Reduce discomfort but do not prevent joint destruction; can be injected directly into inflamed joint; should not be repeated more than several times a year because of long-term side effects: _____

(d) A form of second-line drug therapy; potent, fast-acting drug that modifies the course of RA: _____

B7. Select the name of the surgery with the description that best fits.

Arthrodesis   Arthroplasty
Synovectomy   Tenosynovectomy

(a) Total joint replacement: _____

(b) Common surgery for RA that involves repair of damaged tendons: _____

B8. Answer the following questions about Ms. Wu's systemic lupus erythematosus (SLE).

(a) Because she is a woman, Ms. Wu's risk of SLE is considerably *(higher? lower?)* than that for men; *(androgens? estrogens?)* seem to protect against lupus. This condition also is more common in *(African Americans and Asians? whites?)*. List three other factors besides gender, race, and hormones that contribute to development of SLE:

_____, _____, _____

(b) Ms. Wu is likely to have *(deficient? excessive?)* production of _____ against her own tissues. These include ANAs that are antibodies against _____ of Ms. Wu's own cells. As a result, lupus is categorized as an _____ disease.

(c) Ms. Wu's autoantibodies combine with _____ to form immune complexes. How are consequences of this process similar to those in RA?

_____

(d) Explain why SLE is called "the great imitator."

_____

_____

List five or more of Ms. Wu's organs likely to be targeted by SLE.

_____

(e) Explain why arthropathies of SLE can be confused with those of rheumatoid arthritis.

_____

(f) Explain what is likely to cause these manifestations of SLE in Ms. Wu:

(f1) Fatigue

_____

_____

(f2) Increased tendency to bleed

_____

_____

(f3) Protein in her urine

_____

_____

(f4) Small strokes

_____

_____

(g) Ms. Wu exhibits the classic "butterfly rash" of SLE. Where is this located?

_____

(h) Diagnosis of SLE requires *(one single? many?)* test(s). The most common test for SLE is for high levels of *(antinuclear antibodies [ANA]? lactic dehydrogenase [LDH]? rheumatoid factor [RF]?)*.

B9. Circle the drugs that may be used to treat SLE and RA.

Corticosteroids   NSAIDs
Hydroxychloroquine
   (antimalarial)

B10. Match the systemic autoimmune rheumatic disorder with the best description below.

Discoid systemic lupus erythematosus (DSLE)
Systemic lupus erythematosus (SLE)
Scleroderma

(a) Mr. Isaac's rare disorder involves thickening of skin with fixation to tendons and muscles; Mr. Isaac has the CREST variant, which is limited to face and hands: _____

(b) The name of Ms. Wu's disorder (Question B8) indicates that many systems are affected, including skin with a red facial rash that was thought to resemble a wolf bite: _____

(c) A form of SLE that affects only the skin in 90% of persons with this disorder: _____

C. ARTHRITIS ASSOCIATED WITH SPONDYLITIS

C1. "Spondylo-" refers to _____, and "ankyl" means _____. Answer the following questions about these conditions.

(a) Spondyloarthropathies exert their main effects on the (axial? appendicular?) skeleton, primarily joints involving (ligaments that insert into bone? a synovial membrane?). These conditions (are? are not?) inflammatory.

(b) Rheumatoid factor (RF) (is? is not?) involved in spondyloarthropathies. Therefore, these conditions are known as sero(positive? negative?). Approximately 90% of people with ankylosing spondylitis (AS) have the HLA-_____ antigen genetic marker.

C2. Mr. Murray, age 68, has severe, debilitating AS. His thoracic spine has such a pronounced anterior curvature that he appears to look at the floor all of the time; seldom can he hold his head high enough to look ahead. Mr. Murray can barely maintain balance in walking. His weight is 105 lb, 35 lb less than his ideal weight. Answer the following questions related to his case.

(a) Describe the primary problem with AS.

_____

_____

_____

(b) Explain how this pathogenesis leads to the rigid "bamboo spine."

_____

_____

_____

(c) List reasons Mr. Murray may be at increased risk for:

(c1) Fractures

_____

(c2) Fatigue, shortness of breath, and recurrent infections

_____

_____

(c3) Lower back pain and hip pain

_____

(c4) Insomnia

_____

(d) Circle each of the following that is an intervention that may help Mr. Murray.

(1) Exercise for extensor muscles
(2) Getting flu shots
(3) Taking a cold shower before exercising
(4) Swimming
(5) Weight loss
(6) Taking NSAIDs

C3. Identify the spondyloarthropathy that best fits each description.

Ankylosing spondylitis   Enteropathic arthritis
Psoriatic arthritis   Reiter syndrome

(a) Most likely to involve inflammation of the uvea (middle layer of the wall of the eyeball) and the urethra: _____

(b) Almost all cases involve inflammation of the sacroiliac joint; seldom involves joints of hands or feet: _____

(c) A skin condition involving rapid turnover of epidermal cells; joints are involved in 5% to 7% of persons with this T cell–mediated immune disorder: _____

(d) Classic sign is bamboo-like spine seen on x-ray: _____

(e) Inflammatory bowel disease, such as Crohn disease or ulcerative colitis: _____

(f) Forms of reactive arthritis, for example, occurring considerably after an infection:

_____, _____

C4. Answer the following questions about reactive arthritis.

(a) The trigger for reactive arthritis is most likely to be *(rheumatoid factor? bacterial infection? high blood levels of uric acid in blood?)*. Such arthritis is sero*(negative? positive?)*.

(b) Identify the microorganism most likely to trigger reactive arthritis in each of the following patients.

Chlamydia   Salmonella or *Shigella Streptococcus*

(b1) Claudia, age 46, who contracted bacterial dysentery earlier this summer: _____

(b2) Bill, age 19, who presented at the university clinic 6 months ago with a sexually transmitted disease manifested by severe urethritis: _____

(c) List four extra-articular organs that may be affected by seronegative inflammatory arthropathies. _____, _____, _____, _____

D. OSTEOARTHRITIS SYNDROME

D1. Refer to Chart 43-3 in *Essentials of Pathophysiology* and identify which categories of disorders can lead to osteoarthritis (OA) in each of the following patients.

Anatomic   Idiopathic
Metabolic   Neuropathic
Post-traumatic

(a) Mr. Jeffrey, age 48, has frequent gout attacks related to his high serum urate levels: _____

(b) There is no known cause for Ms. Wright's OA: _____

(c) Junior, age 8, has a flattened head of the femur as a result of slipped capital femoral epiphysis: _____

(d) Mr. Plummer's type 2 diabetes has led to decreased proprioception in his feet and resultant injury known as Charcot foot: _____

(e) Torn menisci and other knee injuries have resulted from Joost's years of downhill skiing: _____

D2. Identify whether each of the following characteristics is indicative of osteoarthritis *(OA)* or rheumatoid arthritis *(RA)*.

(a) Primarily involves inflammation of the synovial membrane with subsequent damage to other joint structures: ____

(b) A disorder that starts with destruction of articular cartilage: ____

(c) Sometimes known as degenerative joint disease or wear and tear arthritis: ____

(d) An autoimmune disease that can manifest many extra-articular effects: ____

(e) Joints are warm and spongy, rather than hard: ____

(f) Involves pannus formation: ____

(g) Not a systemic disease: _____

D3. Circle the correct answers or fill in the blanks to answer the following questions about the pathogenesis of OA.

(a) The primary tissue injured in OA is:

Articular cartilage   Bone
Ligaments   Synovial membrane

(b) List two functions of cartilage in joints:_____ and _____

(c) Cartilage contains cells known as _____. Describe four chemical components of cartilage matrix surrounding these cells.

_____

_____

(d) Early in the course of OA, water content of cartilage *(increases? decreases?)* and proteoglycan content *(increases? decreases?)*. In addition, the protein collagen is *(increased? decreased?)*. As a result, cartilage becomes *(stronger? weaker?)*.

(e) As articular cartilage is injured, chondrocytes are thought to respond by releasing cytokines such as _____ and _____, which causes release of _____-digesting enzymes; these destroy cartilage components such as _____.

(f) As injured cartilage loses its smooth surface and cracks, underlying (subchondral) bone thickens (the process of _____) and appears polished and ivory-like (a process known as _____). Abnormal bone spurs known as _____ can lead to grating sounds (_____) as joints are moved.

(g) Describe how articular cartilage is injured in each case.

(g1) In Joost's knee joints (Question D1[e])

_____

_____

_____

(g2) Mrs. Shea, whose hip is immobilized after a fracture.

_____

_____

_____

D4. Osteoarthritis affects (only large? only small? both large and small?) joints. Circle the two most common sites for osteoarthritis (OA) out of the three sites listed in each case. (Identify these sites on yourself.)

(a) Hip joint   Knee joint   Sacroiliac joint

(b) Cervical   Lumbar   Thoracic
    vertebrae   vertebrae   vertebrae

(c) First carpo-   First metacar-   First metatarso-
    metacarpal   pophalangeal   phalangeal
    joint   joint   joint

D5. There (is? is not?) a cure for OA. Discuss nonpharmacologic treatments for osteoarthritis.

_____

_____

_____

_____

E. CRYSTAL-INDUCED ARTHROPATHIES

E1. Circle the two true statements about gout. (Pay particular attention to whether the **bold-faced** word or phrase makes the statement true or false.)

(a) Gout **is a systemic** disorder.

(b) Incidence of gout is highest in **middle-aged women.**

(c) Tophi are **deposits of crystals** in tissues.

(d) Gout is caused by deposits of **calcium carbonate** crystals in soft tissues.

(e) **All** people with hyperuricemia do eventually develop gout.

E2. Answer the following questions about the pathogenesis of gout.

(a) Primary gout (does have? has no?) known cause or is caused by inborn errors of metabolism and gout (is? is not?) the main disorder. About 90% of cases of gout are (primary? secondary?). Circle types of gout that are classified as secondary:

(1) Enzyme defects that cause overproduction of uric acid

(2) Increased breakdown of nucleic acids as in treatment that destroys malignant cells of leukemia

(3) Chronic renal failure

(4) Thiazide diuretics that interfere with excretion of uric acid

(b) Explain why joints become painful in people with gout.

_____

_____

_____

(c) Tophi are nodules that consist of _____ deposited in joint tissues. Tophi typically appear (immediately? about 10 weeks? about 10 years?) after the initial gout attack.

(d) Typically, the first gout attack involves (one? many?) joint(s). Subsequent attacks (almost always follow within days? may not occur for years?). Gout is most likely to affect (shoulder and hip joints? toes and other parts of feet and hands?). Explain.

_____

_____

_____

E3. Answer the following questions related to management of an acute gout attack in Mr. Jeffrey (Question D1[a]).

(a) Treatment of an acute attack is focused on reducing (serum urate levels? joint inflammation?). Which anti-inflammatory is likely to be the drug of choice to control Mr. Jeffrey's acute gout attack?

Colchicine   Corticosteroids   NSAIDs

(b) Explain how uricosuric medications help to control gout throughout life.

_____

(c) How can allopurinol help Mr. Jeffrey?

_____

(d) Uric acid can be produced by the breakdown of chemicals known as _____ such as adenine and guanine. List several foods that are high in purine content and thus should be avoided by Mr. Jeffrey.

_____

_____

F. RHEUMATIC DISEASES IN CHILDREN AND THE ELDERLY

F1. Explain why a team approach is important in managing rheumatic diseases in children.

_____

_____

F2. Identify the rheumatic disorder that fits each description.

Pauciarticular arthritis   Polyarticular arthritis
Systemic JRA

(a) The most common form of juvenile rheumatoid arthritis (JRA) in which no more than four joints are affected; onset younger in girls; ANA tests typically are positive: _____

(b) Form of JRA that closely resembles the adult form; more than four joints affected: _____

(c) A form of JRA characterized by episodic high fever, rash, high white blood cell count, and enlargement of liver, spleen, and lymph nodes; in most cases, joints are involved: _____

(d) A form of late-onset arthritis that occurs mostly in boys; in most cases HLA-B27 tests are positive: _____

F3. Circle the correct answer within each statement about rheumatic diseases in children.

(a) NSAIDs are *(first-line? seldom-used?)* drugs for treating JRA.

(b) The prognosis for most children with JRA is *(good? poor?)*.

(c) JRA *(always? sometimes? never?)* stunts growth.

(d) Ankylosing spondylitis, reactive arthritis, and psoriatic arthritis *(sometimes? never?)* occur in children.

(e) In children, spondyloarthropathies are likely to affect the *(sacroiliac joints? joints of extremities?)* earlier in the disease.

(f) *(Hepatic? Renal? Splenic?)* involvement is the best indicator of the prognosis of lupus (SLE) in children.

(g) Juvenile dermatomyositis (JDMS) affects *(brain and heart? muscles and skin?)*. The most debilitating symptom of JDMS involves *(calcifications? rash?)*.

F4. Arthritis is a *(common? rare?)* complaint among elderly persons. *(Osteoarthritis? Rheumatoid arthritis?)* is more common among the elderly. Explain how arthritis can affect quality of life in older adults.

_____

_____

_____

F5. The prevalence of rheumatoid arthritis, pseudogout, and polymyalgia rheumatica all *(increase? decrease?)* with aging. In which of these conditions are calcium pyrophosphate crystals deposited into articular cartilage that is deteriorating from osteoarthritis.

_____

F6. Mrs. Thielens, age 60, has received a diagnosis of polymyalgia rheumatica. Circle the correct answers within each statement about her condition.

(a) To meet criteria for this disorder, she must have experienced pain and stiffness for at least 1 *(week? month? year?)*, and her erythrocyte sedimentation rate (ESR) must be *(higher? lower?)* than normal.

(b) When a test dose of corticosteroid (prednisone) is administered to patients with polymyalgia rheumatica, pain relief is achieved in 1 to 2 *(days? weeks?)*.

(c) It is likely that Mrs. Thielens *(will? will not?)* need ongoing steroid therapy to control her condition.

F7. How is giant cell arteritis related to polymyalgia rheumatica?

_____

_____

Giant cell arteritis affects *(blood vessels? cartilage? synovial membranes?)*. Circle a serious potential consequence of giant cell arteritis.

Blindness   Deafness   Stroke

CHAPTER 44

Structure and Function of the Skin

■ Review Questions

A. STRUCTURE OF THE SKIN

A1. Skin may be one of the most underestimated organs in the body. What functions does your skin perform while it is "just lying there" covering your body?

_____

_____

_____

A2. Choose the two true statements. (Pay particular attention to whether the **bold-faced** word or phrase makes the statement true or false.)

(a) Skin is also known as the **integument.**

(b) The outermost layer of the skin is the **dermis.**

(c) Hair, nails, and glands are all formed from **dermis.**

(d) Epidermis is composed of **stratified squamous** epithelium.

A3. Epidermis contains four distinct cell types. Name the type of cell that fits each description. Choose from these answers:

Keratinocyte   Langerhans cell
Melanocyte   Merkel cell

(a) These cells contribute to the sensation of touch: _____

(b) Part of immune responses, these cells recognize, process, and present antigens in immune processes: _____

(c) These cells produce the pigment that gives skin brown or black color and protects skin from UV light: _____

(d) The most numerous cell type in skin, they produce the protective protein, keratin: _____

A4. Arrange epidermal layers from deepest to most superficial. Stratum:

Corneum   Germinativum   Granulosum
Lucidum   Spinosum

_____, _____, _____,
_____, _____

(a) Which is the thickest layer and composed of all flattened, dead cells? _____

(b) Which layer is present primarily in skin of palms of hands and soles of feet? _____

(c) Which of these layers is the site of formation of all new epidermal cells? _____

A5. Identify the chemical that fits each description.

Melanin   Sebum   Tyrosinase

(a) An enzyme missing in albinos: _____

(b) Oily substance produced by glands surrounding hair follicles; lubricates hair and skin: _____

A6. Choose the two true statements. (Pay particular attention to whether the **bold-faced** word or phrase makes the statement true or false.)

(a) As epidermal cells develop, they are pushed to more **superficial** layers.

(b) Melanocytes **do migrate** to more **superficial** layers.

(c) In psoriasis, turnover of epidermal cells takes place at a **slower** than normal rate.

(d) The basal lamina connects the **epidermis** to the **dermis.**

A7. Circle the correct answers within each statement.

(a) The dermis is _(thicker? thinner?)_ than the epidermis. The dermis is composed of _(connective? epithelial?)_ tissue and is _(vascular? avascular?)_.

(b) Dermal dendrocytes are thought to *(produce sebum? present antigens to immune cells?)*.

(c) Most sensory receptors of the skin are located in the *(epidermis? dermis?)*.

(d) Subcutaneous tissue *(does? does not?)* typically contain fat tissue.

(e) *(Arrector pili muscles? The eponychium?)* is/are responsible for "goose bumps."

(f) Most sweat glands and all blood vessels of skin are supplied with *(sympathetic? parasympathetic? sympathetic and parasympathetic?)* nerves.

(g) *(Apocrine? Eccrine?)* sweat glands are more numerous and empty directly *(onto the surface of the skin? into hair follicles?)* to cool skin. *(Apocrine? Eccrine?)* sweat glands, found in axillary and inguinal regions, produce secretions that combine with bacteria on the skin surface and produce the characteristic body odor of sweat.

(h) *(Sebaceous? Sweat?)* glands enlarge during adolescence, and they become inflamed in acne. The function of *(sweat? sebum?)* is to lubricate skin and hairs.

(i) Formation of new hair cells takes place in the *(bulb? shaft?)* of the hair follicle. Hair color is related to the size of *(melanosomes? rete ridges?)*.

(j) Nails are composed of keratin produced from the *(dermis? stratum corneum?)*. Hair grows *(continuously? cyclically?)*.

B. MANIFESTATIONS OF SKIN DISORDERS

B1. Match each type of primary lesion below with the correct category.

Flat with color change   Elevated and solid
Elevated and fluid-filled

(a) Acne pustule: _____

(b) Vesicle caused by herpes simplex or bulla as in second-degree burn: _____

(c) Papule such as a mole (nevus) or nodule: _____

(d) Macule such as a freckle: _____

B2. Circle the correct answer within each statement.

(a) *(Purpura? Petechiae?)* are smaller lesions.

(b) A callus involves *(a? hyper?)*plasia of dead cells in the stratum corneum.

(c) *(Blanched? Erythematous?)* lesions are reddened.

(d) A(n) *(excoriation? lichenification?)* is a raw line of broken epidermis.

(e) Telangiectasis refers to a condition involving *(excessive pigmentation? dilated blood vessels?)* in skin.

B3. Choose the two true statements about the sensation of itch. (Pay particular attention to whether the **bold-faced** word or phrase makes the statement true or false.)

(a) The sensation of itch is known as **pruritus.**

(b) Morphine **increases** the sense of itch.

(c) Histamine, bradykinin, and substance P **reduce** itching sensations.

(d) Scratching itchy areas of skin usually **helps** heal the area.

B4. Ms. Taylor, age 35, is African American. She is at *(higher? lower?)* risk for skin cancer because the increased _____ in her skin protects from UV rays. Areas of her face appear "ashy"—gray and *(dry? oily?)*. Explain what may be the cause.

_____

Ms. Taylor's skin is *(more? less?)* likely to wrinkle as she ages compared with white skin.

CHAPTER 45

Disorders of the Skin

■ Review Questions

A. PRIMARY DISORDERS OF THE SKIN

A1. Primary skin disorders are those that begin *(in? outside of?)* the skin.

A2. Complete this exercise about fungal skin infections by circling the correct answers or filling in the blanks.

(a) Ringworm is a *(superficial? deep?)* skin infection. Name three sources of the fungi that cause these infections.

_____

(b) Most of these microbes secrete enzymes that digest _____, causing skin scaling and nail disintegration.

(c) Treatments include:

(c1) Topical agents that are typically *(more? less?)* effective than oral agents.

(c2) Oral agents that are likely to be *(more? less?)* toxic than topical agents. Explain.

_____

(d) Fingernail infections are *(more? less?)* easily treated than toenail infections. Explain.

_____

A3. Tinea, also known as _____, is a(n) *(arthropod? bacterial? fungal?)* infection. Identify the location of the following fungal infections.

(a) *Tinea unguium;* an onychomycosis that involves digestion of keratin by fungi leading to thickening and yellowing of tissue: _____

(b) *Tinea capitis;* the noninflammatory type can present as hairless patches or black dots on the head; the inflammatory type may lead to a secondary bacterial infection and a lesion known as a kerion. _____

(c) *Tinea corporis,* often transmitted from pets to children; circular patches look like donuts or targets: _____

(d) *Tinea pedis,* also known as "athlete's foot"; may be itchy and foul-smelling: _____

(e) *Tinea manus,* usually occurs as a secondary infection from tinea pedis; typically unilateral: _____

A4. Match the chemicals used for diagnosis or treatment of skin disorders with the related descriptions.

Acyclovir   Corticosteroids
Griseofulvin   Potassium hydroxide
Tretinoin or isotretinoin

(a) Derived from *penicillium,* this oral systemic agent protects new skin cells from fungal infections: _____

(b) Agent used to prepare skin scrapings for microscopic examination for tinea or *Candida* infections: _____

(c) Agents that reduce itching and erythema of bacterial infections, but they increase risk for viral infections: _____

(d) Antiviral agent often used against herpesviruses: _____

(e) Vitamin A product that can be used to treat acne; has teratogenic effects: _____

A5. Explain why the following patients are likely to have developed candidiasis.

(a) Alecia had a severe *Streptococcus* respiratory infection for 2 months. For 6 weeks of that time, Alecia took a broad-spectrum antibiotic. Now she has a case of vaginal candidiasis.

_____

_____

_____

(b) Frank has AIDS. His CD4 T-cell count is currently 52 cells/L.

_____

A6. Complete this exercise about skin infections by circling the correct answers or filling in the blanks.

(a) Impetigo is most common among *(adults? children?)*. It is a *(superficial? ulcerative?)* infection, typically caused by *Staphylococci* or BHS, which stands for

_____

streptococci.

(b) Acne is a condition that affects the hair follicles and *(oil? sweat?)* glands of skin. The extra sebum provides a medium for growth of _____. Acne lesions may involve *(blackheads? whiteheads?)*, which are melanin-containing plugs that block pores of glands. Acne vulgaris is a *(common? rare?)* form of acne that occurs in adolescents. *(Androgens? Estrogens?)* have been implicated in acne. Besides treatment with topical vitamin A (isotretinoin, see Question A4[e]), what other agents help prevent further outbreaks of acne? _____ and _____

(c) Warts are *(benign? malignant?)* conditions in which the epidermis is stimulated to become *(thicker? thinner?)*. Warts are caused by the HPV (or human _____virus). This type of virus can also cause genital warts, which *(can? cannot?)* be sexually transmitted.

(d) Herpesviruses typically affect *(sensory? motor?)* neurons, where they may lie dormant for months or years. Herpes infections present with prodromal symptoms that include

_____. The acute phase involves *(fluid-filled vesicles? solid macules?)* that *(do? do not?)* dry up and crust.

(e) Herpes simplex-1 (or HSV-1) virus is most likely to cause _____, whereas HSV-2 typically causes _____:

(1) Fever blisters (cold sores)

(2) Genital herpes

(3) Chickenpox or shingles

(f) Currently there *(is? is not?)* a cure for HSV. _____ may be used to prevent recurrences. Sunscreens *(can? cannot?)* prevent HSV-1 on lips.

A7. Mrs. Yaskolski, age 86, has shingles. Answer the following questions about her condition by filling in the blanks or circling the correct answers.

(a) Shingles is caused by herpes _____ virus that can be reactivated decades after it caused _____. List two categories of persons at high risk for shingles: _____, _____

(b) Mrs. Yaskolski has lesions along the dermatome of her C8 spinal nerve. Vesicles are likely to appear *(bi? uni?)*laterally along this single dermatome. The lesions are likely to crust over and fall off within 2 to 3 *(days? weeks? months?)*.

(c) These lesions *(are not? can be?)* contagious. If the ophthalmic division of the trigeminal nerve is affected by shingles, Mrs. Yaskolski could experience _____. Postherpetic neuralgia can last for as long as several *(days? months?)* after the initial lesions.

(d) Describe treatments that may help manage shingles.

_____

_____

A8. Match the type of skin disorder with the correct description.

Acne conglobata	Atopic eczema
Nummular eczema	Plantar warts
Rosacea	

(a) Somewhat painful lesions on hands or feet, possibly transmitted in gym showers; likely to resolve spontaneously when immunity to the virus develops: _____

(b) Occurring later in life, this is a chronic form of acne with comedones, abscesses, cysts, and scars; often on back, chest, and buttocks: _____

(c) Called the "curse of the Celts," this facial erythema is often confused with acne; may involve bulbous thickening of the nose (rhinophyma): _____

(d) A type I hypersensitivity reaction that usually is hereditary; begins on the cheeks of children with oozing and crusting vesicles; treatments include moisturizers and antipruritics: _____

(e) Coin-shaped patches on the extremities, typically chronic with weeks to years between exacerbations; treatment is largely palliative, but frequent bathing should be avoided: _____

A9. Match the type of skin disorder with the correct description.

Lichen planus   Pityriasis rosea
Psoriasis   Toxic epidermal
Urticaria   necrolysis

(a) Also known as hives; involves reddened wheals that blanch with pressure; intense itching results from release of the vasodilator histamine, so antihistamine treatment helps; can be triggered by reactions to food, cold, pressure, or skin writing (dermographism): _____

(b) The most serious and possibly life-threatening drug reaction in which the epidermis can separate from the dermis in large areas of skin; trigger can be sulfonamide drugs: _____

(c) A hyperkeratosis due to rapid turnover of epidermal cells leading to thick red plaques covered by silvery-white scales; can accompany arthritis; has no cure but a variety of topical or systemic treatments exist: _____

(d) Rash with oval lesions; may form a "Christmas tree" pattern on the back; usually disappears within 6 to 8 weeks: _____

(e) Drug reaction (often to thiazide diuretics, beta blockers, or NSAIDs) that leads to pruritic, mossy skin lesions; usually self-limiting: _____

A10. Identify the type of psoriasis that fits each description.

Guttae   Plaque-type   Pustular

(a) When removed, lesions bleed from tiny points known as the Auspitz sign: _____

(b) Lesions are associated with streptococcal infections and are pink to salmon, teardrop-shaped: _____

A11. There *(is? is not?)* a cure for psoriasis. Circle the agents listed below that are topical rather than systemic. Then list a mechanism of action of each of these treatments of psoriasis.

(a) Topical emollients _____

(b) Keratolytic agents _____

(c) Coal tar _____
(d) Anthralin _____
(e) Calcipotriene _____
(f) Methotrexate _____
(g) Retinoids _____

A12. Classify each of the following skin infections according to the type of causative microbe.

Bacteria   Fungi   Virus

(a) Acne and rosacea: _____
(b) Candidiasis: _____
(c) Shingles: _____
(d) Verrucae: _____
(e) Cold sore: _____

B. ULTRAVIOLET RADIATION, THERMAL, AND PRESSURE INJURY

B1. Incidence of skin cancer has *(increased? decreased?)* over the past 2 decades. Answer the following questions about UV-induced skin damage.

(a) Which type of ultraviolet rays (UVR) are the "sunburn rays?"
  (1) UVA (long rays)
  (2) UVB (medium length rays)
  (3) UVC (short rays)

(b) Tanning salons deliver:
  (1) UVA (long rays)
  (2) UVB (medium length rays)
  (3) UVC (short rays)

(c) Exposure to UVR causes skin vessels to vaso*(constrict? dilate?)*, leading to reddening (or _____) of white skin. UVR also causes a(n) *(increase? decrease?)* in the pigment melanin in the epidermis.

(d) Carcinogenic effects of UVR result from direct damage to _____ of epidermal cells and also to a decrease in the number of _____cells.

(e) Drugs that cause an exaggerated response to UV light are known as:
  (1) Photosensitive drugs
  (2) Sunscreens

B2. Mary Beth is joining her friend Barbara for a run and a swim at the beach. Circle the correct answers related to reduction of risk of skin damage and possible skin cancer.

(a) Use of a sunscreen with an SPF of _____ is more advisable:

(1) 8

(2) 15

(b) A sunscreen containing the ingredient PABA can help protect Mary Beth's skin by:

(1) Absorbing sunlight

(2) Reflecting sunlight

(c) Skin products with a higher SPF will screen out _____ rays.

(1) UVA

(2) UVB

(d) Barbara is African American. Should she protect her skin from sunlight in order to avoid sunburn?

(1) Yes, black skin can burn

(2) No, black skin does not burn

B3. List five or more categories of causes of thermal injuries (or burns).

_____

_____

_____

B4. Complete this exercise about burns. Use these answers:

(1) First-degree

(2) Second-degree, full-thickness

(3) Second-degree, partial-thickness

(4) Third-degree

(a) Arrange in correct sequence the depth of burn from most to least extensive:

_____, _____, _____, _____

(b) A mild sunburn is an example; involves only the epidermis; healing usually occurs within 3 to 10 days:

_____

(c) Involves formation of blisters that actually protect underlying skin; white skin appears bright pink or red: _____

(d) Blister formation occurs and possibly some loss of sensation because all the dermis is involved; white skin appears mottled pink, red, or waxy white; some scar formation is typical: _____

(e) May extend into muscles and bone; skin is hard, dry and may vary in color from white to black; likely to require skin grafting and to leave permanent scars: _____

B5. Joel, age 19 years, has extensive third-degree burns covering all of his lower extremities and his buttocks from an incident in which his jeans caught on fire. Complete this exercise.

(a) Is Joel likely to experience pain from the burns? _____

(b) About what percentage of Joel's TBSA is burned? ___% The American Burn Association grading of Joel's burn severity would be (minor? moderate? major?).

(c) Circle the more likely manifestations of Joel's burns and then write a brief rationale.

(1) Cardiac output of (3? 5?) L/min

_____

_____

(2) (Increased? Decreased?) metabolic rate

_____

_____

(3) (Increased? Decreased?) risk of thromboses

_____

_____

(4) (Increased? Decreased?) risk of stomach ulcer _____

_____

(5) (Increased? Decreased?) urinary output

_____

_____

(6) Increase of fluid within (plasma? interstitial [between cells] areas?)

_____

(7) (Increased? Decreased?) levels of oxygen in blood _____

_____

(8) (Increased? Decreased?) risk for infection, including sepsis _____

_____

(d) Joel is likely to be receiving *(no? enormous amounts?)* of IV fluids and nutrients. Explain. _____

_____

_____

_____

B6. Describe treatments for Joel's burns by using the following key words in sentences or paragraphs.

(a) Water over burns

_____

_____

_____

(b) Cold (not ice)

_____

_____

_____

(c) IV fluids and antibiotics

_____

_____

_____

(d) "Nature's own blister" and protective isolation

_____

_____

_____

(e) Split-thickness autograft

_____

_____

_____

(f) Contractures prevention

_____

_____

_____

B7. Answer the following questions about pressure ulcers.

(a) Pressure ulcers are also known as _____. Describe the basic problem.

_____

_____

_____

(b) Identify the locations on the body where this skin condition is most likely to occur.

_____

_____

_____

(c) List several factors that increase risk for decubiti.

_____

_____

_____

(d) Define "shearing forces" that can lead to decubiti.

_____

_____

_____

B8. List specific interventions that nurses can take to help prevent decubiti in each of these patients.

(a) Mrs. Albertson, age 88, has Alzheimer disease and is in bed; she is dehydrated, anemic, and incontinent of bowel and bladder.

_____

_____

(b) Mr. Little, age 34, suffered a brain injury 5 years ago. He is in a wheelchair and requires assistance with all activities of daily living (ADL).

_____

_____

_____

B9. Select from this list to identify the stage of decubitus indicated in each case below:

Stage I   Stage II   Stage III   Stage IV

(a) Depth of necrosis extends into subcutaneous tissue; ulcer is a deep crater:

_____

(b) Black skin appears bluish-purple; no blistering or ulceration visible:

_____

C. NEVI AND SKIN CANCERS

C1. Choose the two true statements. (Pay particular attention to whether the **bold-faced** word or phrase makes the statement true or false.)

(a) Almost all adults **do** have nevi (moles).

(b) Nevi are **benign.**

(c) Nevi develop primarily from **keratinocytes.**

(d) Nevi typically have **poorly** defined borders.

(e) **Junctional** nevi have the ability to transform to malignant melanomas.

C2. Incidence of skin cancer has *(increased? decreased?)* significantly over the past several decades, especially among *(fair? dark?)*-skinned persons with _____ hair. List several reasons for the increased incidence.

_____

C3. Arrange these types of skin cancers from most serious and likely to metastasize to least serious:

Squamous cell carcinoma   Basal cell carcinoma
Malignant melanoma

_____ → _____ →
_____

(a) Which is the most common form of skin cancer and generally appears pink and pearly in white-skinned persons?

_____

(b) Which type appears red and scaly with a shallow ulcer and can develop from premalignant lesions such as actinic keratoses? _____

(c) Seventy percent of this category of cancer is of the "superficial, spreading" type.

_____

C4. Dixie, age 52, is seeing a dermatologist for a mole on her right leg that has changed over the past several months. Answer the following questions related to her case.

(a) Dixie has red hair with freckles on her face and upper back. She has visited tanning salons "to get a good base before summer" for about 10 summers. In her late teens, she worked as a lifeguard for 4 summers. Her mother died of metastatic malignant melanoma. Circle the factors in this history that are risk factors for malignant melanoma. Because of these risk factors, Dixie has a *(3.5? 20?)*-fold increased risk of malignant melanoma.

(b) Dixie's lesion has a diameter of 9 mm by 13 mm, is slightly raised, brown, with uneven borders. Which criteria of the ABCD(E) rule used to diagnose malignant melanoma does her lesion meet?

_____

(c) She is diagnosed with superficial spreading melanoma. This type of lesion is a *(common? rare?)* form of malignant melanoma that typically occurs on areas of skin that *(are? are not?)* sun exposed. With continued growth, it *(is? is not?)* likely to ulcerate and bleed.

(d) The fact that the lesion has a depth of 2.2 mm sets Dixie's likelihood of 8-year survival at about ___%. Treatment *(is? is not?)* likely to include surgical excision.

C5. List two preventive measures regarding skin cancers.

_____

_____

D. AGE-RELATED SKIN MANIFESTATIONS

D1. Choose the two true statements. (Pay particular attention to whether the **bold-faced** word or phrase makes the statement true or false.)

(a) Congenital melanocytic nevi are considered **harmless** lesions.

(b) Strawberry hemangiomas and port-wine stains are both disorders of **blood vessels.**

(c) **Port-wine stains** typically resolve by age 5 to 7 years.

(d) Port-wine stains **can** lead to neurologic problems.

D2. Answer the following questions about skin disorders of infants.

(a) Contrast the appearance of simple diaper rash with that of severe diaper rash.

_____

_____

(b) Prickly heat (heat rash) is more likely to occur when skin is *(moist? dry?)*.

(c) Cradle cap typically occurs when hair is washed *(too often? infrequently?)*.

D3. Circle helpful practices that can prevent or limit severity of episodes of diaper dermatitis.

Table 45-1.   Skin Disorders Associated With Infectious Diseases of Childhood

Disorder	Cause	Appearance	Location	Fever	Complications
Roseola	Herpesvirus-B			105° F	Usually none
Rubella (3-day or German)		Punctate	Starts on trunk; spreads to arms, legs		
Rubeola (7-day or hard)		Confluent; Koplik spots		100° F+	
Chickenpox (or shingles)	Varicella-zoster virus				Rarely

(a) Exposing irritated skin areas to the air

(b) Liberal use of corticosteroids, antifungal, and antibacterial agents

(c) Frequent diaper changes and cleansing of irritated areas

(d) Use of soap on baby's skin after each diaper change

(e) Application of creams or lotions with antiseptic properties

(f) Wearing plastic pants over diapers

D4. Complete Table 45-1 contrasting skin disorders related to infectious diseases of childhood.

D5. Arrange, in correct sequence, events in the typical course of chickenpox.

Scab formation
Vesicle formation
Macules on trunk, spreading to extremities and head

_____ → _____ →

_____

D6. Determine the probable diagnosis in each of the following cases and determine which condition has a greater potential for serious complications. Select from disorders listed in Table 45-1.

(a) Nicholas, age 13 months, is brought to the clinic on Monday. His mother reports that Nicholas "slept and cried a lot and pulled at his ears" last week, and she thought he had had a fever. His rash started on Saturday on his back and abdomen; it has now progressed to his arms and legs. Lymph nodes in his neck and behind his ears are normal. Probable diagnosis:

_____

(b) Anastasia is 4 years old. Her father reported that she had developed a "rash on her face, and then her arms and legs." Anastasia had been "whiny, complaining that she hurt." Her temperature had been "just under 101°." The probable diagnosis is:

_____

_____

_____

D7. Complete Table 45-2 relating observable changes in aging of the integument to their causes.

Table 45-2.   Skin Changes Related to Normal Aging

Changes	Causes
Decreased sensation of touch	
	Decreased in Langerhans cells
Dry, itchy, easily broken skin	
Less padding and insulation of skin	

Answers

Chapter 1

CELL STRUCTURE AND FUNCTION

A1. Most diseases begin at the cellular level.

A2. Water, proteins, lipids, carbohydrates

A3. (a) Lipids
(b) Carbohydrates
(c) Potassium
(d) Water

A4. Form structures of cells such as muscles, fibers in bones, hemoglobin, and antibodies; create enzymes that are required for synthesis of carbohydrates and lipids.

A5. (a) Transfer
(b) The nucleolus

A6. (a) Active (euchromatic) sections of cells stain more intensely (i.e., are heterochromatic).
(b) The nucleolus is large and prominent in active cells.

A7. (a) Rough ER
(b) Smooth ER
(c) Golgi
(d) Golgi
(e) Golgi
(f) Smooth ER
(g) Lysosomes
(h) Peroxisomes
(i) Mitochondria
(j) Mitochondria
(k) Smooth ER

A8. (a), (b), (d); but (c) mitochondria fit this description

A9. (a)

A10. (a) Flagella
(b) Cilia
(c) Actin and myosin
(d) Centrioles
(e) Basal bodies

A11. (a) Diabetic changes in microtubules alter ability of white blood cells to migrate to sites of infection.
(b) These structures indicate disruption of the cytoskeleton of brain neurons.

A12. (a), (c); but (b) hydrophobic and (d) integral

A13. (a) Cell coat
(b) Is

B1. (a) Anabolism
(b) Three; two; ATP
(c) Does not; begins; pyruvate; small; NAD
(d) Lactic; pyruvic
(e) Does; citric or tricarboxylic; mitochondria; pyruvic; oxaloacetic
(f) Transport; glycolysis; phosphorylation; cyanide

(g) Can; amino acids and portions of digested fat can enter the Krebs cycle
(h) 90; CO_2; H_2O

C1. The cell membrane normally forms a barrier that controls whatever enters and leaves the cell and determines chemical composition of fluids and electrical potential inside and outside cells. Errors in these functions provide the basis for many disorders.

C2. Active; "downhill" with
(a) Diffusion
(b) Osmosis
(c) Facilitated diffusion

C3. (a) Diffusion
(b) Facilitated diffusion
(c) Facilitated diffusion

C4. (a) Phospholipid bilayer (see question A12[a])
(b) Water molecules

C5. (a) Drinking
(b) Lysosome
(c) Leukocyte (white blood cell) or a macrophage
(d) Exo

C6. (a), (d); but (b) 14 times greater outside and (c) Primary

C7. (a) Integral proteins; gated
(b) Electrical changes
(c) Acetylcholine; high

C8. Any order:
(a–b) By movement of chemical messengers from cell to cell across gap junctions or through extracellular fluid to other cells.
(c) By chemicals (first messengers) that bind to receptors on or near the surface of a cell; this activates a G protein that acts upon an effector, which can lead to formation of a second messenger. Finally, this chemical causes a specific response within the cell.
(d) By lipid-soluble chemicals that can pass through the phospholipid bilayer of a plasma membrane.

C9. (c) Transduction; protein kinases

C10. (a) Down; decreasing
(b) Ion
(c) G; cAMP
(d) Protein; glucose
(e) Can; the nucleus

C11. (a) Are; negative; millivolts (-20 to -100 mV)
(b) Ions, permeability
(c) Na^+; positive

D1. (a) Epithelium
(b) Connective
(c) Muscle
(d) Nervous
Nervous

D2. (a), (d); but (b) avascular and
(c) single layer of flat cells

D3. (b), (c); but (a) simple columnar and
(d) lines urinary bladder

D4. (a) Exo
(b) Endo
(c) Endocrine

D5. (a) Gap (nexus) junctions
(b) Continuous tight junctions
(c) Adhering junctions
(d) Hemidesmosomes

D6. (a) Fibroblast
(b) Reticular
(c) Dense regular
(d) Dense irregular, bone
(e) Fat
(f) Matrix; polysaccharides, proteins
(g) Collagen; elastin

D7. (a), (d); but (b) vascular (does contain blood vessels)
and (c) smaller

D8. (b), (d), (e), (i); but (a) forms muscle cell membrane,
(c) from one Z line to another, (f) troponin,
(g) outside, and (h) slide

D9. (a) Involuntary
(b) One nucleus
(c) Does not
(d) Extracellular fluid
(e) Troponin

D10. (a) Brain, spinal cord
(b) Neurons
(c) Efferent

D11. (a) Cell body
(b) Ribosomes
(c) Axon; one; some

D12. (a) Ependymal cells
(b) Microglia
(c) Oligodendrocytes
(d) Schwann cells
(e) Satellite cells
(f) Astrocytes

Chapter 2

CELLULAR RESPONSES TO STRESS, INJURY, AND AGING

A1. Cells respond to changes in the internal
environment; (a)

A2. (a) Decrease in hormones
(b) Ischemia
(c) Disuse

A3. (a) Hyperplasia
(b) Hypertrophy
(c) Metaplasia
(d) Hypertrophy (because cells cannot undergo
mitosis)
(e) Hypertrophy (because cells cannot undergo
mitosis)
(f) Hyperplasia (because cells can undergo mitosis)
(g) Dysplasia
(h) Atrophy

A4. May. The liver's epithelial cells can increase in
number (hyperplasia) as in A3(a).

A5. The bladder's (detrusor) muscle works extra hard to
empty urine through the narrowed urethra. This
work causes smooth muscle cells of the bladder to
grow in number and size.

A6. (a) Alzheimer disease
(b) Fatty liver
(c) von Gierke disease
(d) Lead poisoning

A7. Excessive breakdown of RBCs (as by incompatible
blood transfusion); toxins that destroy RBCs
excessively; a "sick liver" (hepatitis or cirrhosis)
that is unable to remove bile pigments from RBCs;
blocked bile routes (from liver to intestine) caused
by gallstones or a tumor pressing on the bile duct
system, so that bile backs up into the liver; all of
these conditions cause retention of bilirubin.

A8. A brown chemical that builds up in aging cells; no

A9. Coal miners; coal dust (carbon particles) that
interfere with gas exchange in lungs

A10. (a) Metastatic
(b) Metastatic
(c) Dystrophic
(d) Dystrophic

B1. Reversible; liver and heart; Na^+/K^+ ATPase, into

B2. (a) Lactic; decrease
(b) Little, Na^+/K^+; Na^+; swell; increases; digestive

B3. (a) Temperature extremes
(b) Chemical injury
(c) Hypoxia (and chemical injury caused by carbon
monoxide)
(d) Electrical injury
(e) Temperature extremes
(f) Mechanical forces
(g) Biologic agents
(h) Chemical injury
(i) Ionizing radiation
(j) Nutritional imbalances

B4. (a) Vasoconstricting
(b) Increase
(c) Skin at entrance and exit sites
(d) Alternating current, or AC

B5. (a) Eating or inhaling lead paint or by playing in
lead-contaminated soil
(b) Can
(c) Blood cell formation; gastrointestinal tract;
kidneys
(d) Is

B6. Liver

B7. (c), (d); but (a) less, (b) localized irradiation for
cancer treatment

B8. (a) ATP; swell (as Na^+ and H_2O enter the cell), in
(b) Free radical
(c) Calcium

B9. An organ (could be heart, liver, brain, or muscle) is
damaged (possibly by hypoxia), causing cells to
open up and release contents (including these
enzymes) into blood. The higher the serum levels of
these enzymes, the more damage that tissue has
sustained.

B10. (a) Electron(s)
 (b) Oxygen in the air we breathe; the two outer electrons lead to reactive chemicals such as superoxide anion radical (O_2), and hydrogen peroxide (H_2O_2); also metals such as copper (Cu) and iron (Fe).
 (c) Smoking, excessive vadiation
 (d) Vitamins A (beta-carotene), C (ascorbic acid), and E

B11. (a) Protein
 (b) DNA
 (c) Lipid

B12. (a) Low; active (ATPase)
 (b) Increase; activate

B13. (a) Necrosis
 (b) Apoptosis

B14. Apoptosis accounts for death of some cells as other cells form to replace them. It functions to eliminate cells during embryologic development to make room for the next stage of development. Apoptosis decreases cell number as a normal part of aging. It accounts for death of endometrial cells (lining the uterus) that are sloughed off during menses when hormone levels fail to support the lining. Also, diminished breast size after cessation of breast-feeding is a result of apoptosis.

B15. Does. Inadequate apoptosis may be involved in cancer. Apoptosis may destroy neurons in Alzheimer disease, Parkinson disease, and amyotrophic lateral sclerosis (ALS or Lou Gehrig disease). Apoptosis may also be involved in some forms of hepatitis as well as thermal and radiation injury.

B16. (b), (c), (e); but (a) low oxygen level
 (d) irreversible

B17. Unlike; interferes with
 (a) Caseous
 (b) Liquefactive
 (c) Coagulative

B18. Large; (a), (d)

B19. (a) (5)
 (b) Clostridium
 (c) Fractured bones, skin, GI tract, vagina
 (d) Anaerobic; high

C1. (a) Decrease
 (b) Decrease
 (c) Decrease
 (d) Decrease

C2. (a) Genetically
 (b) Autosomal (Chromosome 8), faster
 (c) Changes resulting from an accumulation of environmental or other events; somatic mutation theory, free radical explanation, wear and tear theory
 (d) Sections of DNA; maintain their length; slowed down; accelerates

Chapter 3

GENETIC CONTROL OF CELL FUNCTION AND INHERITANCE

A1. (a) DNA; protein
 (b) Transcription
 (c) Messenger
 (d) The same as; only part

A2. Mitochondria; Leber's hereditary optic neuropathy

A3. (a) Phosphate; sugar (deoxyribose); nitrogenous base
 (b) Deoxyriboses; phosphates; deoxyriboses
 (c) Thymine; guanine
 (d) Helic; only one strand is
 (e) Proteins

A4. (a) Three; mRNA; amino acid
 (b) Lysine; synonyms
 (c) RNA; ribose; uracil; U A G
 (d) RNA polymerase; introns; may differ; many different
 (e) Smallest; 20; an mRNA codon
 (f) Most; nucleolus; nucleus; endoplasmic reticulum (ER); translation
 (g) 100–300

A5. (c); but (a) only a small number of (b) induction

A6. (a) DNA; base
 (b) Do not
 (c) Morphism; cannot; somatic

B1. (a), (d); but (b) similar, (c) males

B2. (a) Within a few days after conception, it is possible to determine which of a female embryo's X chromosomes (the one from the mother or the one from the father) will be active; the other will be the (inactive) Barr body.
 (b) None because the normal male's one X is active.
 (c1) 1
 (c2) 1
 (c3) 1

B3. (a) Meiosis and mitosis
 (b) Meiosis
 (c) Meiosis
 (d) Mitosis
 (e) Meiosis

B4. Bivalent formation with crossing over between homologous chromosomes. (Also independent assortment [the way in which homologous chromosomes align] during Metaphase I.)

B5. (a) Cytogenetics
 (b) Venous blood (lymphocytes)
 (c) The picture that shows all pairs of chromosomes from one cell
 (d) One with the centromere near the end of an arm
 (e) By a "p" (for petite); centromere outward
 (f) They allow the DNA in the end of the chromosome to be completely replicated.

C1. (a) Phenotype; genotype
 (b) Penetrance
 (c) Locus; allele
 (d) Multiple-gene; single-gene; multifactorial

C2. 19th; peas, round; Punnett

C3. (a) a
   (b) Katie's (AA); John's (Aa)
   (c) Heterozygous; does not
   (d) Pedigree

D1. The project that identified and localized the more than 30,000 genes present in cells of humans. Carried out between 1990 and 2003, the project provides critical information about genetic diseases and related screening and treatment.

D2. (a) In 1911, the first human gene to be mapped was found to be on the X chromosome of the mother.
   (b) In 1968, the location of the Duffy blood group was identified on the long arm of chromosome 1.

D3. mRNA; polypeptide (or protein)

D4. (a) The same; close together; are
   (b) X; only one; more (because they have no other X chromosome to override the harmful gene); hemizygous

D5. Both parents or only one

D6. (a) Another species, such as a mouse; gene
   (b) Radioactive DNA or RNA; gene (or DNA sequence)

D7. (a) Insulin; growth hormone
   (b) Bacteria; DNA; human gene
   (c) Bacteria

D8. A gene that is defective (in the patient with cystic fibrosis) can be replaced by normal DNA that is introduced into the patient within the genome of an adenovirus. The virus does not become part of the human genome but does deliver the normal gene product so that patients with cystic fibrosis produce normal mucus.

D9. DNA from the suspect is cleaved with restrictive enzymes, separated, and characterized by probes to reveal banding patterns.

Chapter 4

GENETIC AND CONGENITAL DISORDERS

A1. See Study Guide Chapter 3, Questions C1 and C3.

A2. (b), (c); but (a) some do not appear for decades after birth and (d) may affect many different parts

A3. (a)

A4. (a) 4; 2; 2
   (b) 2; 4
   (c) Circles; squares
   (d) Grandmother; mother
   (e) Yes; the partnered daughter on the left and one single son
   (f) Yes; grandmother to her son as shown here and also from woman in the second generation to a son and a daughter; this is not a sex-linked disorder

A5. See the text.

A6. (a) Only one parent
   (b) 50%
   (c) Can (in cases of reduced penetrance)
   (d) Expressivity

A7. (a) Connective; skeletal, cardiovascular, special senses [eyes]; cardiovascular; tall, thin; fibrillin-1 (FBN1), 15
   (b) Two; different; NF-1; café-au-lait spots; eyes; hearing; more

A8. (a), (c), and (d); but (b) usually do not,
   (e) PKU but not Tay-Sachs, and (f) lysosomal

A9. (a) Recessive
   (b) X, recessive; males
   (c) Cannot (because this disorder is transmitted on the X chromosome and males give only a Y to their sons)

A10. (a) 50% of children are likely to have the autosomal dominant disorder (short limbs); 50% would be normal.
   (b) Besides the 25% normal (CC: shown), 50% are likely to be carriers (heterozygous = Cc), and 25% (cc) to have the autosomal recessive disorder, CF.
   (c) Because hemophilia A is sex-linked, probabilities are described for children of each gender: 50% of females are normal, and 50% are carriers ($X^H X^h$); 50% of males are normal, and 50% have hemophilia ($X^h Y$). Note: no males are carriers.

A11. (a) Cannot
   (b) 100%
   (c) Mentally retarded
   (d) See text.

A12. Pyloric stenosis, clubfoot, diabetes mellitus, congenital heart disease, congenital hip dislocation, and coronary artery disease

A13. See text.

A14. (a), (c); but (b) boys, girls; (d) and/or;
   (e) single surgery

A15. (a) And also
   (b) 37; mother; ATP; apoptosis
   (c) More; (see Table 4–1 in *Essentials of Pathophysiology*)

A16. (a) Robertsonian translocation
   (b) Translocation of part of chromosome 21 with part of 14 or 22
   (c) Deletion

A17. (b), (c); but (a) 47, XX, +21 and (d) different numbers of chromosomes in different body cells

A18. (a) 47; 21
   (b) (The most) common; increases
   (c) Smaller; larger
   (d) Weaker; hypotonia
   (e) Leukemia; Alzheimer

A19. (a) (Maternal blood levels of) alpha-fetoprotein (AFP), human chorionic gonadotropin (HCG), unconjugated estriol
   (b) Amniocentesis, chorionic villi sampling (CVS), percutaneous umbilical blood sampling

A20. (a) Turner syndrome
   (b) Klinefelter syndrome
   (c) Fragile X syndrome

B1. (b), (d); but (a) first trimester, specifically during weeks 3 to 8 of gestation and (c) embryonic or fetal abnormality

B2. (a) Is not
(b) Few
(c) Lipid; small
(d) X
(e) 10,000
(f) At any time during

B3. (Any order)
(a) Facial abnormalities: flattened philtrum, thin upper lip, and short palpebral fissures
(b) Prenatal or postnatal height or weight less than the 10th percentile
(c) Central nervous system abnormalities such as cognitive defects or delays in motor functioning

B4. (c) No

B5. (a) Neural tube; spina bifida, myelomeningocele, and anencephaly
(b) Cereals, grains, orange juice, dark leafy vegetables
(c) Tooth

B6. (a) Microorganisms
(b) Protozoan, cats
(c) Viral, German measles
(d) Herpes

Chapter 5

NEOPLASIA: A DISORDER OF CELL PROLIFERATION AND DIFFERENTIATION

A1. (c), (d); but (a) cardiovascular disease, (b) differentiation

A2. Numbers; specialization
(a1) Labile
(a2) Permanent
(b) Lose

A3. (c), (b), (a)

A4. G_1, S, G_2

A5. (c)

A6. (a) Cyclin-dependent kinases (CDKs)
(b) Cyclins and CDKs
(c) Inhibitors

A7. These "checkpoints" allow for any defects in DNA to be repaired. Defective checkpoints may lead to cancer cell formation.

B1. (a) Parenchymal
(b) Stroma

B2. (c), (d); but (a) some, (b) connective or muscle

B3. (a) B
(b) B
(c) M
(d) M
(e) M
(f) B
(g) B

B4. (a) More
(b) Each other; IV
(c) Lesser; decreased; infiltrate other regions; enzymes
(d) Markers; less
(e) Hormones (in paraneoplastic syndromes) and coagulation factors

B5. Kidney carcinomas often metastasize to the lungs, where they are discovered. Examination of the lung tissue reveals that the cancer cells have characteristics of kidney cells, which points to kidneys as the site of the primary tumor.

B6. (a) By infiltration of the endometrial (uterine lining) cancer through all layers of the uterine wall, through the peritoneum, and then by seeding into the abdominopelvic cavity to peritoneum of GI organs, and then infiltration into walls of those organs
(b) Veins; because lymph empties into venous blood

B7. When radioactive tracer and blue dye is injected into the tumor, the "sentinel node" is the first node that the tracer and dye reaches. Biopsy of this node will indicate whether cancer cells have metastasized to this point. If not, then the malignancy is unlikely to have spread any further.

B8. (a) Testicular veins carry cancer cells from the testes, empty directly into the inferior vena cava to the right side of the heart, to the pulmonary artery, and then to the lungs.
(b) Veins from the intestine (including the colon) empty into the portal vein and directly into the liver.

B9. See text

B10. (a) (2)
(b) One billion

C1. Cancer; the transformation of normal cells into cancer cells

C2. Proto-oncogenes, tumor suppressor genes (or antioncogenes), genes that control apoptosis, and genes that repair DNA

C3. See text.

C4. (b), (d); but (a) multifactorial, (c) viruses are implicated in some cancers

C5. (b), (c), (f); but (a) irreversible, (d) is, (e) different from

C6. Breast (as well as other cancers, including ovarian adenocarcinomas); 10% to 20%

C7. $CD4^+$ helper T cells, $CD8^+$ cytotoxic T cells, natural killer (NK) cells, B lymphocytes

C8. (a) Emily
(b) Julia
(c) Robert

C9. (c)

C10. (a) Dominant
(b) Are (osteosarcoma)
(c) Only on tumor cells
(d) Coal soot and scrotal cancer
(e) Do not
(f) Many
(g) Plant

C11. Smoked meats (especially those with nitrates), foods fried in reused fat, high-fat diet, lack of dietary fiber, smoking and exposure to secondhand smoke (especially when combined with alcohol). (See Chart 5-1.)

C12. (a) Vaginal
    (b) Skin
    (c) Leukemia

C13. (a) Hepatitis B virus
    (b) Human T-cell leukemia virus-1
    (c) Human papillomavirus
    (d) Epstein-Barr virus

D1. (a) Blockage of the bowel by the tumor, breakage of vessels by straining, and pressure of the tumor against blood vessels
    (b) Growth of the tumor may exert pressure on ureters, bladder, or urethra.
    (c) Pressure of the tumor against nerves, ischemia, or metastasis of the tumor into pelvic bones
    (d) Cachexia accompanies most solid tumors and is related to effects of factors from tumor cells or host cells (including tumor necrosis factor [TNF]-α, interferons, or interleukin-6) that act on the satiety center (in hypothalamus) or injure tissues that then release anorexigenic chemicals. Side effects of treatments can lead to anorexia. Fluid in abdomen (ascites) may be due to blockage of venous flow or inflammation with increased permeability of the cancerous organs.

D2. (a) Mr. Feinstein's multiple myeloma may have caused bone breakdown (osteolysis), which moves calcium into blood (hypercalcemia). Some cancers also lead to paraneoplastic syndrome via production of PTH-related protein, which leaches Ca^{2+} out of bones.
    (b) Some tumors produce procoagulation factors that increase risk for thrombus formation, which is exacerbated by Mr. Feinstein's immobility related to his fracture.

D3. Lambert-Eaton myasthenic syndrome can accompany this type of lung cancer, causing weakness in his proximal muscles.

E1. (a) As cells become more abnormal, their cell surfaces change so they lose cohesiveness and are more likely to shed (exfoliate).
    (b) Breast and testicular self-examinations and colorectal screening; also biopsy and tumor markers

E2. PSA is a tumor marker, an antigen found on certain cancer cells, such as those of the prostate. An increase in PSA in circulating blood points to increase in the number of cancer cells from Mr. Rhodenberger's prostate cancer.

E3. (a) Carcinoembryonic antigen
    (b) Alpha-fetoprotein
    (c) Human chorionic gonadotropin

E4. (a) S (*Hint:* remember "S" for staging and "S" for spread of the tumor); lymph nodes; yes
    (b) G (grading studies the pathology of cancer cells to indicate degree of malignancy); grade IV.
    (c) Postsurgical staging

E5. Radiation and surgery debulk the tumor. Chemotherapy is then more likely to destroy remaining tumor cells because a smaller number of cells are rapidly dividing and more vulnerable to chemotherapy.

E6. (a) Rapidly; radiosensitive
    (b) Multiple fractionated; cancer cells die, but normal tissue is more likely to recover between treatments.
    (c) Rapidly dividing gastrointestinal tract, hair follicle cells, and bone marrow cells are vulnerable to radiation.

E7. (a) Only a specific proportion (percentage) of the cancer cells are killed with each course of treatment.
    (b) Combination
    (c) Specific; S; CMF

E8. Methods that alter the person's response to cancer; involves biologic response modifiers (BRMs)
    (a) A
    (b) A
    (c) P
    (d) P

E9. (a) Hematopoietic growth factors
    (b) Monoclonal antibodies
    (c) Interferons
    (d) Interleukins

F1. (c), (d); but (a) secondary to injuries/accidents, (b) blood, neuroglia, or connective tissue

F2. Prolonged fever and unexplained weight loss, especially if the latter occurs with a growing mass

F3. (a) Less; difficulty in
    (b) Of preschool age
    (c) Are known to

Chapter 6

DISORDERS OF FLUID, ELECTROLYTE AND ACID-BASE BALANCE

A1. (a) Intracellular fluid
    (b) Intracellular fluid
    (c) Plasma or serum
    (d) Interstitial fluid and plasma or serum

A2. (a) Bicarbonate, chloride, protein
    (b) Glucose
    (c) Osmosis
    (d) (1)
    (e) Iso
    (f) Swell
    (g) Pleural, pericardial, peritoneal, or synovial cavities or the lumen of the GI tract; third

A3. 60; 40; 20; interstitial fluid

A4. (a) Capillary (or BP); pushes out of; hypertension, CHF, high steroid level
    (b) Capillary; pulls into; decreased production of plasma proteins (starvation or liver failure) or loss of protein (burns or renal failure)
    (c) Increase; inflammation or burns
    (d) Lymphatic; removal of lymph nodes in cancer surgery

A5. (a) (2)

(b) (1), which is a relatively small protein and also the most common plasma protein

(c) (1)

(d) (1)

(e) (2)

(f) (2)

(g) (3)

B1. Creates osmotic pressure; takes part in buffer systems for maintaining acid-base balance; involved in nerve impulses

B2. GI tract (food); medication including sodium bicarbonate, IV solutions; kidneys

B3. (a) Save Na^+

(b) Save Na^+

(c) Lose Na^+

(d) Save Na^+

B4. 60; 40; 20-year-old woman, lean person, person with body temperature of 99.0°F, 2-month-old infant; see text

B5. (a) Food and drink; metabolism (burning up)

(b) 1500; 1 (1500 mL per day/1440 minutes per day)

(c) GI tract; skin and exhalations

B6. Early

(a) Hypothalamus; superior; de; walls of major arteries and veins, mouth

(b) ADH; pos

B7. (a) Hypo

(b) Psychogenic

(c) (3)

B8 (a) More; increases; decreased; opposite of

(b) Pressin; constrict

B9. Decreases

B10. (a1) Little; 15 (normal is 1.5 L); increase; concentrated

(a2) Nonsugary; large; sugary; insulin

(a3) Central; adequate; do not

(b1) Over; retention; edema; hypo; anemia

(b2) Stress and pain, head injuries, certain drugs, certain cancer cells, and HIV

B11. Na^+

(a) ADH; increases (hypernatremia); 135–145

(b) Aldosterone

B12. (a) (1)

(b) (2)

(c) (3)

(d) (2)

B13. (a) Hypernatremia

(b) FVE

(c) Hyponatremia

(d) FVE

(e) Hypernatremia

(f) FVD or hypernatremia

(g) Hyponatremia or FVE

B14. (a) FVE

(b) FVD

(c) Hypernatremia or FVD

(d) Hypernatremia

(e) Hyponatremia

(f) FVD

(g) FVD or hypernatremia

(h) Hyponatremia

C1. (a) ICF; 3.5 to 5.0 mEq/L

(b) Cantaloupe, dried fruits such as prunes or figs, avocado, orange juice, and bananas

(c) Into; into

(d) Kidneys; increases; H^+ also enters urine, and Na^+ and H_2O are reabsorbed from urine into blood

(e) H^+; 0.7, such as 4.2 to 4.9 (mEq/L)

(f) Non–potassium-sparing diuretics; H_2O and Mg^{2+}.

C2. (a) Deficient; hyper

(b) Hypo

(c) Hyper; hypo

C3. (a) Hypo; cardiovascular; 3.0

(b) Exacerbate = make worse; brady

(c) Decreases (such as from −70 to −90 mV); decrease; muscle weakness, fatigue, tingling of nerves (paresthesia)

(d) Increase dietary potassium (see Question C1[b]) or take K^+ supplements

(e) Ensure that urine output is adequate to avoid hyperkalemia and possible cardiac arrest

C4. (a) Hyper; common; rare

(b) Is, because her level is greater than 6 mEq/L

(c) K^+ level > 5.0 mEq/L and risk of cardiac arrest with extremely high K^+ levels (such as 8.0 mEq/L)

(d) Exacerbate, because acidosis tends to cause hyperkalemia (See Study Guide Fig. 6-1E.)

(e) Should not if they have their major ingredient as K^+ (which most do)

D1. Bones

(a) D; PTH (parathyroid hormone)

(b) Skin, liver, kidneys; PTH

(c) Posterior of thyroid gland (in the neck); hypo; Mg^{2+}

D2. (a) Increase; bones, food in intestine, and urine in kidneys

(b) Increases; decreases; renal; decrease

(c) Mg^{2+}

D3. Abnormal losses of calcium from kidneys, as in renal failure; dietary deficiency; low plasma protein levels

D4. (a) Failing kidneys do not secrete PO_4^{3-}, but they secrete excessive amounts of Ca^{2+}, which leads to hypocalcemia, which is the major stimulus for PTH growth and secretion.

(b) PTH pulls minerals Ca^{2+}, PO_4^{3-}, and Mg^{2+} from bones, weakening them.

D5. See text.

D6. (a) High; normal is 8.5 to 10.5 mg/dL = 4.5 to 5.3 mEq/L

(b) Cheese, milk, turnip or collard greens, almonds, peanuts

(c) Bone; rare

(d) Urine

(e) Ionized

(f) Hypo

D7. (a) Hypo

(b) Hyper: lack of stimulation of osteoblasts by movements causes bones to give up Ca^{2+}

(c) Hyper: these chemicals break down and demineralize bone

(d) Hypo

(e) Hyper

D8. Rapid. Transfused blood has calcium chelated (tied up) to citrate to prevent clotting in the blood bank. The recipient's liver requires some time to remove the citrate and free ionized Ca^{2+}.

D9. (a) Less; more; 7.0; hypo
   (b) Low serum Ca^{2+} triggers PTH production, which demineralizes bones.
   (c) Tapping on the face (over facial nerve), which causes muscle spasms of nearby muscles (a positive sign of hypocalcemia)
   (d) These are signs of hypocalcemia and also related to buildup of other toxic substances in the brain caused by ESRD.
   (e) Paresthesia; carpopedal; larynx (blocking her airway)
   (f) If acute, administration of IV calcium compounds; for chronic hypocalcemia, attempts at improvement of the underlying cause (renal function), and provision of calcium and activated vitamin D

D10. (a) Hyper
   (b) Hyper
   (c) Both hyper and hypo

D11. (a) Hypo
   (b) Hypo
   (c) Hyper

D12. 1.8–2.7. Magnesium is a cofactor to many aspects of metabolism that are dependent on ATP, including protein synthesis, and nerve conduction.

D13. Hypo; positive; weakness; hypo

E1. (b), (d); but (a) release, (c) less, (e) as bicarbonate or dissolved CO_2

E2. $CO_2 + H_2O \rightarrow H_2CO_3 \rightarrow H^+ + HCO_3^-$. Write CA above the first arrow.

E3. (a) Lactic, ketoacids, citrate, acetate
   (b) Sulfuric, hydrochloric, phosphoric

E4. (a) 7.4; 7.35 to 7.45
   (b) 20:1; Henderson-Hasselbach
   (c) 24; 31; 27
   (d) 1.35; 40 ($\times$ 0.03) – 1.2; less
   (e1) About 27 to 1.35 = 20 to 1
   (e2) About 24 to 1.2 = 20 to 1 (See textbook Fig. 6-16.)
   (f) 2.4; increase (double); 48 mEq/L; increase also; 48/2.4 = 20/1
   (g) $NaHCO_3$; H_2CO_3 = dissolved CO_2; respiratory

E5. Buffers attempting to maintain the 20:1 ratio just described; lungs altering amounts of CO_2 exhaled; and kidneys altering amounts of H^+ or HCO_3^- excreted; buffers, lungs, kidneys

E6. (a) HCO_3^-; 20; 1
   (b) Carbonic acid (H_2CO_3); Cl^-; $H_2CO_3 + NaCl$

E7. (a) Protein
   (b) Bicarbonate–carbonic acid
   (c) Transcellular H^+/K^+ exchange
   (d) Ammonia
   (e) Transcellular H^+/K^+ exchange

E8. (a) H^+; HCO_3^-
   (a1) Na^+; HCO_3^-
   (a2) Phosphate; Na^+; HCO_3^-
   (a3) Ammonia; NH_3; NH_4; Na^+; HCO_3^-
   (a4) These prevent urine from being so acid that it will injure renal tubules
   (b) Raise; carbonic

E9. (a) K^+; H^+; alkal
   (b) Na^+; H_2O; K^+; H^+; alkal; acid
   (c) HCl; HCO_3^-; alkal

E10. (a) Yes (80 to 100 mm Hg is normal)
   (b) No, moderately high, related to her COPD (38 to 42 mm Hg is normal)
   (c) No, somewhat acidotic, which fits with her elevated PCO_2 (7.35 to 7.45 is normal)
   (d) No, high to compensate for her acidosis (24 to 31 mEq/L is normal) (See text Table 6-1.)
   (e) No, high, related to her high HCO_3^- (± 3.0 is normal)

E11. His anion gap is calculated as 136 – 120 = 16 (normal range: 8–12). This is slightly high, probably related to high lactic acid levels in his blood. His HCO_3^- level is raised as it buffers the increased PCO_2 from the run. His Na^+ and Cl^- levels have dropped somewhat from sweat production.

F1. (a) Correction of metabolic acidosis
   (b) Renal compensation for her respiratory alkalosis

F2. (a) Increases; decreases; decreases; weakness, fatigue, confusion, lethargy, and stupor that can lead to coma; malaise, headache, anorexia, nausea, vomiting, abdominal pain
   (b) Decreases; increases; increases; muscle spasms or tetany

F3. (a) Mr. Hershey's high serum levels of BUN, creatinine, K^+, and H^+ relate to his renal failure, and his ECG changes, abdominal cramping, and diarrhea relate to high K^+.
   (b) Mrs. Litzinger's carpopedal spasms from alkalosis
   (c) Mrs. Litzinger's renal secretion of HCO_3^-

F4. (a) Metabolic acidosis
   (b) Respiratory acidosis
   (c) Metabolic acidosis related to lactic acid production
   (d) Metabolic acidosis
   (e) Metabolic acidosis
   (f) Metabolic alkalosis
   (g) Metabolic alkalosis
   (h) Metabolic alkalosis

F5. (a) Kussmaul; metabolic; 5.0 as kidneys excrete H^+; can
   (b) Repeated vomiting causes metabolic alkalosis with loss of both K^+ and Cl^-; to replace lost K^+ and Cl^- acidosis
   (c) Increased; slowly so the acid pH (with its effects) continues for hours or days
   (d) 7.5 (respiratory alkalosis); hyper; breathing into a paper bag so she rebreathes air high in CO_2

F6. The key is to determine which is the "problem" value because it "matches" the pH. Mr. Feinberg's high PCO$_2$ "fits" his low (acidic) pH. Therefore, this is respiratory acidosis. His high HCO$_3^-$ must be due to a compensatory mechanism because a high (alkalotic) HCO$_3^-$ value does not "match" a pH of 7.33 (when PCO$_2$ goes up, so will HCO$_3^-$; see Questions E4[b] and [f]). Emily's high pH (7.54) is related to her loss of Cl$^-$ (through emesis) that causes plasma HCO$_3^-$ to increase (metabolic alkalosis). To compensate for her high HCO$_3^-$, she automatically increases PCO$_2$ by hypoventilating.

Chapter 7

STRESS AND ADAPTATION

A1. (a) Claude Bernard
(b) Walter Cannon
(c) Hans Selye
A2. (a) Increase; dilate; negative; opposite
(b) Negative; stability; elevated; lower
A3. (a) Processes that oppose change; change
(b) Does; cognitive
B1. See text.
B2. Adrenal enlargement, atrophy of the thymus, and gastric ulcer
B3. General adaptation syndrome
(a) Alarm, resistance, exhaustion
(b) Alarm
(c) Resistance; exhaustion
B4. Mild headaches, insomnia, upset stomach, GI ulcer, joint and muscle problems, cardiovascular and renal diseases
B5. (a) Exo
(b) External; decrease (although they may have strengthened her coping skills)
B6. Nervous (releasing neurotransmitters), endocrine (releasing hormones), and immune (releasing chemical mediators)
B7. (a) Thalamus
(b) Reticular activating system, cerebral cortex
(c) Limbic system
(d) Hypothalamus, locus ceruleus–norepinephrine pathway
(e) Locus ceruleus–norepinephrine pathway
(f) Hypothalamus
B8. (a) Catecholamines, such as NE and epinephrine, and glucocorticoids, such as cortisol; receptors
(b) Lymphocytes and monocytes; pituitary; adrenal
B9. For discussion
B10. (a) (2); timing of onset
(b) (2); age
(c) (2); health status
(d) (1); psychological factors
B11. Insomnia: inability to fall asleep or stay asleep
Increased somnolence: tendency to sleep excessively
C1. (a) Chronic intermittent
(b) Chronic sustained
(c) Acute time-limited

C2. The compensatory sympathetic response of vasoconstriction of vessels in kidneys (as well as GI organs and skin) can further injure Mr. Clement's already compromised kidneys. Because patients with diabetes are at increased risk for heart disease, the high blood pressure may cause cardiac overload.
C3. Higher levels of salivary cortisol, possibly increased risk of herpes simplex type 1 infections, more severe symptoms of a common cold or flu, decreased immune response to influenza vaccine, and delayed wound healing.
C4. Post-traumatic stress disorder
C5. (a) Avoidance, depression, alcohol or drug abuse, survival guilt
(b) Sleep disturbances, intrusions
C6. (a) War, bombings, or other violence (including rape and child abuse); airplane or automobile crashes; fires; natural disasters such as tornados, floods, hurricanes, or earthquakes
(b) Fear; amygdala; hippocampus; hippocampus
(c) Sympathetic; increased; norepinephrine
(d) Decreased; increased; differ from
(e) Decrease
(f) Relaxation; guided imagery; music, art, or massage therapy; biofeedback; and psychotherapy
C7. Decreases; constriction; electrothermal

Chapter 8

ALTERATIONS IN BODY NUTRITION

A1. See text.
A2. Fats, alcohol, carbohydrates, or proteins; kcal (if the slice weighs about 25 g)
A3. (a) 90; metabolism
(b) Cushions, protects, and insulates the body; site of fat storage and source of chemicals that can provide energy or be used for synthesis of important lipids in the body, such as cholesterol, estrogen, progesterone, testosterone, and aldosterone; also secretes leptin, adiponectin, some cytokines, and growth factors
(c) Do
(d) Stimulate; decrease
(e) Decrease, lipodystrophy
(f) White; brown fat releases more heat than white fat
A4. (a) (1)
(b) (2)
(c) (2)
(d) (1)
(e) (2)
(f) (1)
(g) (2)
(h) (2)
(i) (2)
(j) (1)
(k) (1)
(l) (2)

A5. (a) Carbohydrates
(b) Fats
(c) Proteins
(d) Proteins
(e) Fats
(f) Carbohydrates
(g) Fats
(h) Carbohydrates (specifically, glucose)
(i) Proteins

A6. No. Health consequences would occur, so at least 50–100 grams per day are recommended. Because protein is an expensive source of calories and no more than 30% of the calories in the diet should be derived from fat, most of the diet must consist of carbohydrates.

A7. (a) Appetite; satiety
(b) Hypothalamus; signals from the gastrointestinal tract about presence or absence of food there, signals indicating blood levels of chemicals such as glucose, and messages from the cerebral cortex about sight, smell, or taste of food
(c1) IL
(c2) IL
(c3) S
(c4) S
(c5) S

A8. Breakdown of sizable amounts of body fats leads to the formation of ketoacids (ketones) and these depress appetite.

A9. (a) Biologic impedance
(b) Relative weight
(c) Laboratory studies
(d) Biologic impedance, BMI, relative weight, waist-to-hip circumference

A10. (a–c) Compare your answers with those of a colleague. (Watch decimal points when squaring meters.)
(d) See Table 8-2 in *Essentials of Pathophysiology*.

A11. (a) 14%
(b) 14% and 21%
(c) Increase

B1. (a) 25
(b) 30; 30
(c) Live below the poverty level
(d) Both genetic and environmental
(e) Certain antidiabetic agents (insulin, sulfonylureas, and TZDs), steroids, and some antipsychotic, antidepressant, and antiepileptic agents

B2. See text.

B3. Fat distribution
(a) 0.933 (42"/45"); upper; upper; upper body or abdominal
(b) Visceral. Hypertension, heart disease, stroke, type 2 diabetes, some forms of cancer, arthritis, sleep apnea, social and psychological effects, and others

B4. See text.

B5. (a) (1) Because older than 45 years; (2) because his waist is over 40"; (3) because HDL is less than 35 mg/dL and LDL is more than 160 mg/dL; not (4) because BP is less than 140/90 mm Hg; not (5), (6), or (7) because his BMI is just over 30. (Calculation of his BMI: 220 pounds = 100 kg; 6 feet = 72 inches × 2.54 cm/inch = 182 cm = 1.82 m. 1.82 m² = 3.31 m². BMI = 100 kg/3.31 = 30.2 kg/m².)
(b) 300–500 (based on a BMI between 27 and 35); 30%
(c) One-half; most days each week
(d) See text.
(e) Is not

B6. Common; 15; 120; that obese children grow up to be obese adults, and psychosocial concerns for children, such as low self-esteem and discrimination

B7. Highly educated parents, obese parents

C1. (a) Physical health problem
(b) Willful eating behaviors
(c) Lack of food availability

C2. 200 million
(a) Marasmus
(b) Marasmus
(c) Kwashiorkor
(d) Kwashiorkor

C3. Respiratory, cardiac, and other muscle weakness, problems with digestion and absorption, diminished immunity and healing.

C4. (a) Fat
(b) Fat
(c) Protein
(d) Protein
(e) Protein

C5. Slowly; is; should not

C6. (a) Females; 56
(b) Reproductive (amenorrhea) and skeletal (osteoporosis)

C7. (b), (c), (d); but (a) not quite low enough to meet DSM-IV-TR criterion of 85%, (e) and (f) are a part of the anorectic profile but are not listed as part of the DSM-IV-TR criteria

C8. Decreased fat intake reduces estrogen production, which stops the monthly thickening (then sloughing) of the uterine lining. Because estrogen protects against bone loss, estrogen deficiency in the anorectic can mimic osteoporosis of the elderly, complete with kyphosis and fractures.

C9. (a) Binge eating two or more times a week, self-induced vomiting
(b) Purging
(c) Action of gastric acid on teeth and on the esophageal lining
(d) Repeated bouts of emesis are likely to result in aspiration of vomitus into lungs with resulting infection.
(e) Bulimia, since not as dramatically low as that of an anorectic

C10. See text.

Chapter 9

DISORDERS OF WHITE BLOOD CELLS AND LYMPHOID TISSUES

A1. Blood formation
   (a) Pluripotent; (either order) lymphoid, myeloid
   (b) Bone marrow; myeloid; platelets
   (c) Specific; colony-forming units
   (d) Granulocytes (see Question A4[e]) and monocytes; lymphocytes; erythrocytes

A2. (a) Central; all
   (b) The thymus
   (c) Lymph nodes, the spleen, mucosa-associated lymphoid tissues (MALT), and the immune cells in the skin

A3. (a) Leukocytes; infection control
   (b) Neutrophil; unlike "mononuclear" leukocytes such as monocytes or lymphocytes, polymorphonuclear cells have nuclei divided into many (three to five) lobes.
   (c) Marginating
   (d) They function as lysosomes to release enzymes that destroy such invaders.
   (e) Hours; days

A4. (a) Lymphocytes
   (b) Monocytes
   (c) Basophils
   (d) Eosinophils
   (e) Neutrophils, eosinophils, and basophils
   (f) Basophils and eosinophils

A5. (a) B
   (b) Clusters of differentiation; CD4

B1. (a) 6,000; leukopenia
   (b) Neutrophils; common, neutropenia
   (c) Agranulocytosis; respiratory; recombinant human granulocyte colony-stimulating factor

B2. (a) Felty syndrome
   (b) Congenital neutropenia
   (c) Drugs that interfere with normal marrow function
   (d) Drugs that interfere with normal marrow function
   (e) Aplastic anemia
   (f) Bacterial or viral infection
   (g) Metastatic solid tumor cancer
   (h) Hemopoietic cancer

B3. A reaction to a drug that differs from reactions of most persons taking that drug and that is not due to an allergic reaction

B4. These manifestations indicate pancytopenia. Chemotherapy not only destroys rapidly dividing cancer cells, but it also kills normal body cells that rapidly divide, such as those lining the mouth, stomach, intestine; hair-forming cells; and bone marrow. Destruction of blood-forming cells in marrow decreases RBCs, increasing fatigue; destruction of WBCs leads to infections that may exacerbate her mouth sores (ulcerations); the drop in platelet count causes bleeding that exacerbates anemia.

B5. (a) Epstein-Barr virus
   (b) B, genome; heterophil; they can react with cells from other species, such as sheep cells; IM
   (c) T; eliminate or destroy

B6. Incubation period (4 to 8 weeks) → Prodromal phase (several days) → Acute phase (2 to 3 weeks) → Recovery phase (up 3 months)

B7. (b), (c), (d)

B8. 20 to 30

B9. The excessive number of immature WBCs are very mobile and tend to infiltrate (and enlarge) those organs that are ordinarily sites that remove old blood cells.

B10. (b), (c), (f); but (a) middle to upper socioeconomic levels, (d) do not, and (e) mostly by asymptomatic persons who shed the virus even when healthy

C1. (a) Lymphomas
   (b) Multiple myeloma
   (c) Leukemias

C2. (a) HL
   (b) NHL
   (c) HL, NHL
   (d) NHL
   (e) NHL
   (f) NHL

C3. Common; see text
   (a) Epstein-Barr virus (EBV)
   (b) Persons with AIDS or who are immunosuppressed congenitally; individuals who have had bone marrow transplantation.

C4. Reed-Sternberg; lymph tissue and bone marrow biopsy, blood studies, abdominal CT, and PET imaging

C5. (a) The stage determines the treatment and points to the prognosis, for example, greater severity if infected lymph nodes are found both superior and inferior to the diaphragm.
   (b) Fever, night sweats, and significant weight loss

C6. A combination of chemotherapy and radiation for NHL; monoclonal antibodies (MOAs); possibly bone marrow and peripheral stem cell transplantation

C7. For discussion

C8. Lymph tissue; bone marrow

C9. Huge numbers of immature WBCs ("-blasts") form and circulate in blood and in the lymphatic system; proliferation of these cells prevents normal blood cells from forming (see Question B2[h]). In persons of all ages; common

C10. (a) Acute; gradual; chronic
   (b) Lymphocyte; spleen, lymph nodes, and central nervous system; myelogenous; bone marrow
   (c) Are not; exposure to high levels of radiation and chemotherapy (for example for Hodgkin lymphoma); and chromosomal abnormalities as in Down syndrome and the Philadelphia chromosome
   (d) Are; deficiency of all types of blood cells occurs as leukemic cell lines crowd the marrow
   (e1) R
   (e2) W
   (e3) P

C11. (a) ALL
(b) AML
(c) CLL
(d) CML

C12. (a) Rapid formation of immature WBCs (blasts)
(b) Because of the presence of huge numbers of immature WBCs, blood becomes so sluggish that it comes to a standstill.
(c) Immature WBCs have crossed the blood-brain barrier into the brain, affecting the N/V center, and producing extra intracranial fluid that exerts pressure on the cranial nerves; one effect is papilledema of the optic nerve.
(d) Chemotherapy destroys WBCs and leads to excessive breakdown of purines to uric acid.
(e) Necrosis of huge numbers of WBCs leads to life-threatening imbalances in blood electrolytes.
(f) By organ infiltration of leukemic cells

C13. Induction→ Intensification→ Maintenance

C14. (a) Chemotherapeutic agents do not cross the blood-brain barrier to destroy WBCs that have entered the central nervous system (CNS).
(b) Antibiotics treat infections caused by neutropenia.
(c) Allopurinol is used to treat renal complications by inhibiting excessive production of uric acid.

C15. (a) Plasma; 71; immune disorders such as autoimmunity and HIV; exposure to ionizing radiation, exposure to pesticides, herbicides, or Agent Orange; genetic factors (for example, on chromosomes 4 and 14).
(b) Immunoglobulins (Igs); G, A; M; increased.
(c) Bence Jones, kidneys.
(d) Enhanced; interleukins, interferon, CSF
(e) Osteoclasts; destruction; early; common; hyper
(f) Heart and nerves; kidneys

C16. Multiple myeloma and treatments both injure bone tissue leading to signs and symptoms of pancytopenia: fatigue, infections, and bleeding problems. As osteoclasts destroy bone tissue, calcium is released into the blood (causing hypercalcemia) and deposited in the kidneys, destroying them and leading to chronic renal failure (CRF). Bone tissue is rigid and rich with sensory nerves. Any invasion of cancer into bone (possibly also effects of treatment) damages bone tissue, stimulating pain nerves there.

C17. Do, but do not; 20%

Chapter 10

ALTERATIONS IN HEMOSTASIS

A1. Stoppage (or standing) (either order)
(a) Excessive clotting (thrombosis)
(b) Bleeding

A2. (a) Platelets
(b) Clotting factors in plasma
(c) Anticoagulants produced by body cells
(d) Properties (such as smoothness) of blood vessel lining

A3. (a) Megakaryocytes; thrombo; liver, kidneys, smooth muscle, and bone marrow
(b1) Glycoproteins that serve as receptors, some of which bind fibrinogen and form bridges between platelets
(b2) Clotting factors (fibrinogen), fibrinolytic factors (plasminogen), and platelet-derived growth factors (PDGF) that function in platelet aggregation, coagulation, and vessel repair
(b3) Contain ADP, ATP, serotonin, and histamine that function in platelet adhesion and local vasoconstriction
(b4) Actin and myosin filaments that facilitate clot retraction
(c) Does not, does

A4. (a) The fact that each of the many steps is designed to activate the next step normally prevents massive episodes of clotting.
(b) Inactive factors in blood can be quickly activated.

A5. Vasospasm → Platelet plug formation → Coagulation → Clot retraction → Fibrinolysis

A6. (a) Constrict, less than a minute; thromboxane A_2 (TXA$_2$), platelets
(b) Aggregation; are not; spiny; collagen; vWF; endothelial cells lining blood vessels, VIII
(c) vWF; platelets; ADP and the prostaglandin thromboxane A_2 (TXA$_2$)
(d) Increases; fibrin
(e) Bleeding

A7. Fibrin
(a) Within; collagen of an injured vessel wall factor XII
(b) By trauma to the blood vessel or surrounding tissues; rapidly; less
(c) K
(d) Calcium (Ca^{2+})

A8. (a) IV (Ca^{2+})
(b) X
(c) VIII

A9. (a) Fibrinogen (made in the liver) is the inactive form of fibrin, which is insoluble and constitutes the meshwork of clots (thrombi).
(b) Thrombin is the active enzyme that converts fibrinogen to fibrin to form clots (coagulation); plasmin is the active enzyme that breaks down fibrin clots (fibrinolysis).
(c) An anticoagulant (heparin or Coumadin) prevents (or limits) clot formation, whereas fibrinolytic agents (e.g., TPA or urokinase) break down clots that have already formed.
(d) Both are anticoagulants: antithrombin III inactivates coagulation factors such as factor Xa and thrombin, whereas protein C inactivates factors V and VIII.

A10. (a) Warfarin (or Coumadin)
(b) Heparin
(c) Plasminogen
(d) Plasminogen activator

A11. (a) Calcium ions (factor IV), coagulation factors VII–XII, fibrinogen, thrombin
  (b) Antithrombin III, heparin, protein C, warfarin
  (c) Tissue-plasminogen activator
B1. Blood clots can stop unwanted bleeding. However, formation of inappropriate clots (thrombi) can be harmful, even lethal (e.g., in cerebral or coronary arteries).
B2. Veins. (For a–b, see text Chart 10-1.)
B3. (a) Damaged blood vessel lining, platelet adhesiveness and aggregation
  (b) Damaged blood vessel lining, platelet adhesiveness and aggregation
  (c) Damaged blood vessel lining, platelet adhesiveness and aggregation
  (d) Platelet adhesiveness and aggregation (related to high platelet count)
  (e) Stasis of blood flow (leading to increased clotting factors)
  (f) Stasis of blood flow (leading to increased clotting factors)
  (g) Increased clotting factors and deficiency of anticoagulant production
  (h) Deficiency of anticoagulant production.
B4. Long-term sitting (e.g., in a car, plane, or bus) increases risk of pulmonary embolism (PE) because venous return from legs into iliac veins is impeded (at flexed hips)—especially in obese persons. Taking frequent walks and drinking adequate fluids keeps circulation moving and helps prevent PE formation. Mr. Longstreth's age also puts him at risk for slower circulation so clotting factors have a greater chance of grouping together.
B5. (a) A
  (b) G
  (c) A
B6. Persons with a history of deep venous thrombosis; arterial thrombosis (including stroke, myocardial infarction, or gangrene); thrombocytopenia; fetal loss at 10 weeks or more gestation; or those with premature delivery due to pregnancy-induced hypertension or uteroplacental insufficiency.
C1. (a) (3) A normal platelet count is 150,000–400,000.
  (b) (2)
  (c) (3)
C2. (a) Blood backs up from the liver into abdominal organs, enlarging the spleen so that it sequesters more platelets than normal.
  (b) Sulfa-containing antibiotics destroy platelets.
  (c) Chemotherapy leads to bone marrow suppression with decreased production of megakaryocytes.
  (d) He has developed heparin-dependent antiplatelet antibodies; these lead to platelet aggregation, which removes platelets from circulation.
  (e) Thrombotic thrombocytopenic purpura (TTP)
C3. Newborns lack the normal flora in the colon required to synthesize vitamin K. After ingesting food in the digestive tract, Kareenya will begin to establish an intestinal flora that will produce vitamin K.

C4. (a) The liver is the source of many clotting factors, including prothrombin, fibrinogen, and factors V, VII, and IX to XII.
  (b) Aspirin and nonsteroidal anti-inflammatory drugs (NSAIDs) often taken as analgesics are platelet inhibitors.
  (c) Antibiotics can destroy the normal intestinal flora that produce vitamin K.
  (d) Hemophilia A, an X-linked recessive disorder that occurs almost entirely in males.
  (e) Von Willebrand disease, the most common hereditary bleeding disorder, which may not manifest until dental extraction leads to prolonged bleeding due to reduced platelet adhesion.
  (f) Blood stored more than 24 hours has no viable platelets, so transfusions can lead to a dilutional thrombocytopenia.
C5. Splenomegaly; lack of vitamin K; lack of factor VIII (as in the most common form of hemophilia); taking a baby aspirin each day; heparin or Coumadin. Factors that lead to hypercoagulability are aneurysm (stasis); smoking; smoking and taking oral contraceptives; dehydration (stasis of thickened blood); and diabetes mellitus.
C6. Disseminated intravascular coagulation
  (a) See text.
  (b) Massive clotting occurs in "unneeded" areas (leading to organ ischemia and failure), using up clotting factors so they are not available for needed clots (leading to extreme bleeding and bruising).
  (c) Bleeding; see text.
  (d) Kidneys, heart, lungs, and brain
C7. (a) Thin-walled, dilated capillaries and arterioles
  (b) Bruising in the elderly

Chapter 11

THE RED BLOOD CELL AND ALTERATIONS IN OXYGEN TRANSPORT

A1. Transport oxygen; transport carbon dioxide; the biconcave disk shape provides much cell membrane surface area for diffusion and deformability allows RBCs to squeeze through narrow capillaries. Spectrin increases flexibility of the RBC membrane.
A2. (a) Four; heme; four
  (b) HbF; gamma; higher; it allows fetal blood to transport more oxygen through the relatively inefficient fetal circulatory system.
A3. (a) Meats (or green, leafy vegetables); transferrin; ferritin; ferritin
  (b) (3)
A4. (a) Pluripotent stem cells → Erythroblasts → Reticulocytes → Erythrocytes
  (b) Reticulocytes; lacks; 1
  (c) 120; 1; nucleus
  (d) Kidneys
  (e) Hypoxia

A5. Failing kidneys do not produce erythropoietin, so RBC production is limited. LaVerne's Hb level is well below a normal range of 12 to 15g/dL. Fatigue is a classic sign of anemia and it becomes more intense as anemia worsens. Erythropoietin therapy can help bring red blood cell count back to its maximum level within 5 days.

A6. Bilirubin; observe his sclera ("whites of the eyes") and note if they appear yellow. Significant RBC destruction (as by transfusion reactions or HDN [see Question D2]) or obstructions of bile pathways.

A7. Maturing RBCs lose their mitochondria, which are the site of aerobic metabolism in other body cells. Anaerobic; red blood cells die prematurely due to denaturation of hemoglobin

A8. (a) 4
(b) 14 (not 42, which would be hematocrit)
(c) 4
(d) 120
(e) (close to) 98

A9. (a) 37% to 47% (for women)
(b) (3) because reticulocyte count focuses on the newly formed ("adolescent") RBCs, which will rise more dramatically than the entire RBC count or hematocrit
(c) 15; 1 is a normal count, but the goal of therapy is an increased reticulocyte count. Values for reticulocytes are in "% of total RBCs," so can never exceed 100%. A number greater than 100 would indicate an error in documentation.

A10. (a), (d); but (b) jaundice may accompany anemia if the cause of anemia is breakdown of RBCs, but jaundice is a sign of hyperbilirubinemia and (c) because males have the effect of testosterone stimulating blood cell formation, and the female population as a whole has a lower RBC count related to regular menstrual flow among much of the female population

B1. (a) Hemorrhage (bleeding); RBC destruction
(b) Nutritional (iron, folic acid, or vitamin B_{12}); bone marrow

B2. (a) Fatigue, weakness, faintness, angina, or dyspnea; increased; pallor; increased
(b) Size
(c) Fracture or brain injury

B3. (a) Acute; diluted; normal
(b) Chronic; is; reduced; hypochromic
(c1) E
(c2) I
(c3) E

B4. (a), (d); but (b) 1 in 10, or 10%; and (c) less; (e) 40%

B5. (a) Hypoxia-triggered events in which RBCs sickle because of defective hemoglobin; sickled cells occlude vessels and cause painful ischemia and organ damage
(b) Cold exposure, stress, physical exertion, dehydration, acidosis, or infection
(c) (3)
(d) (4) because HbF is typically replaced by HbS by then

(e) The spleen (also brain and lungs); the spleen normally destroys encapsulated microorganisms when a child's ability to produce antibodies is still undeveloped; microbes may enter bloodstream (septicemia)
(f) Is not; are
(g) Hydroxyurea; it allows synthesis of more HbF and less HbS, thereby decreasing sickling
(h) Avoidance of situations that lead to sickling crises (see Question B5[b]), including prophylactic administration of pneumococcal vaccine and antibiotics (penicillin); pain control and hydration

B6. (a) B_{12} deficiency
(b) Folic acid deficiency
(c) Hemorrhagic
(d) Chronic disease
(e) Iron-deficiency
(f) Hemolytic
(g) Aplastic
(h) Sickle cell (also a form of hemolytic)
(i) Thalassemia (also a form of hemolytic because RBC membrane is fragile)
(j) Spherocytosis

B7. Women
(a) Because of blood lost in menstruation
(b) People with gastric irritation and bleeding, hemorrhoids or polyps, and those having blood drawn frequently; persons requiring more iron for increased growth, such as pregnant women or growing children; those with decreased dietary intake of iron, such as individuals who cannot chew meat and lack other dietary sources of iron

B8. (a) Red blood; myelin; stomach (or gastric); small
(b) Cancer cells compete with normal cells for folic acid, and methotrexate, often used in chemotherapy, blocks activation of folic acid
(c) Neural tube

B9. (a), (b); but (c) it is not likely that a newborn baby will have been exposed to factors such as radiation, chemotherapy, or toxins that typically cause bone marrow destruction and (d) splenomegaly is more likely to "snag" RBCs and cause hemolytic anemia.

C1. (d)

C2. (a) All except (6)
(b) All
(c) (2)
(d) All except (1)

C3. (a) Relative
(b) Absolute secondary
(c) Absolute primary

D1. (a) Declined; HbA
(b) Less; are; common

D2. (a) Second or third; negative
(b) Higher; kernicterus; brain; mild: lethargy and poor feeding; severe: rigidity, tremors, seizures, and death
(c) Photo; fluorescent lights; urinary and digestive
(d) Negative
(e) Antibodies (that will destroy fetal Rh-positive cells that have entered the mother's circulation)

D3. Decrease; iron-deficiency anemia; see text.

Chapter 12

MECHANISMS OF INFECTIOUS DISEASE

A1. (a) Normal microflora
(b) Host, virulent, colonized
(c) Pathogenic; opportunistic infection

B1. (a) Viruses
(b) Prions
(c) Viruses
(d) Bacteria
(e) Bacteria
(f) Mycoplasma
(g) Fungi
(h) Rickettsiae
(i) Chlamydiae
(j) Parasites
(k) Bacteria
(l) Bacteria

B2. (a) Cocci; spirochetes
(b) Clusters; pairs; species
(c) Increase; acid-fast
(d) (2)
(e) (2)

B3. (a) Superficial; cool
(b) Antibiotic therapy kills the normal microflora but does not touch fungi (see Question B1[g]). As a result, yeast overgrowth causes a "yeast infection."

B4. (a) Protozoa; by direct contact between humans, through infected fecal contamination of food or water, or through arthropod vectors
(b) Roundworms, tapeworms, and flukes; developing nations
(c) Ecto; lice

C1. Study all the factors that contribute to the spread of disease with the goal of interrupting the spread of the infectious agent, as well as predicting and preventing future outbreaks.

C2. (a) Incidence
(b) Epidemic
(c) Endemic

C3. (a) Inhalation
(b) Ingestion
(c) Ingestion
(d) Penetration
(e) Direct contact
(f) Penetration

C4. Direct contact: passage of HIV, rubella, or other viruses across the placenta during pregnancy; infection leading to blindness caused by *Neisseria gonorrhoeae* or trachoma as the baby passes through the mother's infected vagina during birth. Ingestion: HIV infection through breast milk.

C5. (a) Mucus and cilia, coughing, antibodies, and phagocytic cells of alveoli
(b) Low pH (acidity) of the stomach
(c) Intact skin provides a mechanical barrier with its tightly packed epithelial cells.

C6. (a) Fomites
(b) Zoonoses
(c) Nosocomial

C7. Incubation → Prodromal → Acute → Convalescence and recovery (See also Chapter 16, Question B6 about stages of infectious mononucleosis)
(a) Incubation
(b) Prodromal
(c) Convalescence and recovery
(d) Prodromal

C8. (a) Blood
(b) Diverticulitis
(c) Fulminant
(d) Gastric ulcers

C9. (a) Evasive factors
(b) Evasive factors
(c) Invasive factors
(d) Adhesive factors
(e) Toxins

D1. (a) Pathogenic microbe (or pathogen)
(b) Signs and symptoms (or manifestations)

D2. (a) Serology
(b) Culture
(c) Genome sequences
(d) Antigen detection (antigens on the pathogen bind to specific antibodies)

D3. Antimicrobial agents, immunologic approaches, and surgery

D4. Destroy or interfere with some key component of the anatomy or metabolism of the harmful microbe without destroying or interfering with host (human) cells, which would cause side effects

D5. (a) Cephalosporins
(b) Aminoglycosides
(c) Sulfonamides

D6. See the text.

D7. (a) Antibiotic
(b) Antiviral
(c) Antiparasitic
(d) Antifungal
(e) Antifungal

D8. (a) Immunizations (against measles, mumps, rubella and diphtheria, pertussis and tetanus)
(b) White; phagocytosis, antibody production, leukocytosis, and fever
(c) Cytokines
(d) Intravenous immunoglobulin; bodies

D9. (a) Debridement
(b) Gas gangrene
(c) Infected heart valve
(d) Appendectomy

E1. Use of microorganisms as weapons
(a) *Bacillus anthracis;* plant-eating animals; rare
(b) Integumentary (by cutaneous exposure), respiratory (by inhalation), and digestive (by ingestion); intentionally contaminated envelopes delivered via the U.S. Postal Service
(c) The laboratory response network (LRN) in which the CDC collaborates with federal, state, and local agencies

E2. A
  (a) C
  (b) C
  (c) B
  (d) B
  (e) A
  (f) A
E3. Emergency room personnel, infectious disease doctors, laboratory personnel, and public health workers
E4. (a) MV
  (b) WNV
  (c) SARS

Chapter 13

THE IMMUNE RESPONSE

A1. See text.
A2. (a) Innate
  (b) Innate
  (c) Innate
  (d) Adaptive
  (e) Adaptive
A3. Phagocytic; a variety of pathogens, walls; eyes
A4. (a) Antigens; stimulate; immunogens
  (b) Bacteria, bee venom, fungi, pollen, protozoans, transplanted organs, viruses (Note that penicillin is a hapten that must complex with body proteins to form an antigen.)
  (c) Epitope
  (d) Hundreds of
  (e) Hapten. The molecular weight of penicillin is too low for this antibiotic to serve as an antigen. Christopher must have body proteins that can combine with penicillin to form an antigen that leads to an allergic response.
A5. (a) Antigen-presenting cells (APCs)
  (b) Lymphocytes
  (c) Effector cells
A6. (c), (d); but (a) 25% to 35%; (b) 60% to 70%
A7. (a) Gen
    (a1) Immunoglobulins [antibodies]
    (a2) MHCs
  (b) Antigen-presenting cells (see Question A5[a])
  (c) Kines; divide (or clone)
  (d) Plasma; humoral
  (e) Cell; cytotoxic
A8. (a) Membrane molecules known as "clusters of differentiation" that distinguish different subsets of T cells
  (b) CD8$^+$, CD4$^+$
  (c) CD4$^+$
A9. (a) Major histocompatibility; tissues; 6; nonself; gens
  (b) Autoimmune; destroy
  (c) MHCs ensure that Kate's own healthy cells will not be destroyed by her immune system.
A10. (a) Nearly every cell of the body; cytotoxic
  (b) APCs such as macrophages, dendritic cells, and B cells; CD4$^+$ helper

A11. (a) Human leukocyte; white; HLA-B; HLA-C; also
  (b) Haplotype; is (except for identical twins); very similar
A12. (a) Monocytes; white; liver; brain and spinal cord (CNS)
  (b) Both innate and adaptive; innate
  (c) Cytokines, stimulate
  (d) APCs; CD4$^+$
A13. They are both APCs, so present antigens to T-lymphocytes; lymphoid; Langerhans
A14. (a) Viral; direct killing action; cell-mediated or CMI; T, B
  (b) Bone marrow, thymus; CD8$^+$
  (c) 4; II; cytokines; macrophage or white blood
  (d) 8; I; see text
A15. (a) Bone marrow; antibodies (or immunoglobulins such as IgM or IgD); does not
  (b) Antigen receptors, class II MHC proteins, complement receptors, and specific CD molecules
  (c) Migrate to peripheral lymphoid tissue; plasma, memory
  (d) Bacteria and their toxins; causing production of antibodies; humoral
A16. (a) Proteins; 4; 2
  (b) D, E, and G
  (c) Antigen; forked; antigen; variable; constant
A17. (a) IgM
  (b) IgG
  (c) IgA
  (d) IgE
  (e) IgD
A18. (a) Natural killer; are; directly; do not; they recognize MHC self-molecules on normal human cells
  (b) T; perforins, enzymes, and toxic cytokines
A19. (a) Bone marrow and thymus; the remainder are peripheral organs
  (b) Thorax, anterior to his heart; smaller
  (c) Cytokines; thymic; do not
  (d) Foreign from self; thymic; peripheral lymphoid tissues
  (e) Trunk and proximal ends of his extremities; both B and T; removal and phagocytosis of antigens from lymph
  (f) Stomach; left; red; B; T
  (g) Tonsils (including adenoids) and mucosa-associated lymphoid tissue (MALT) lining airways
A20. (a) Are made by and act on; T; nearby; receptors; more than one
  (b) IL-1, IL-6, and TNF
  (c) IL-1 to IL-7, IL-11, and CSFs
  (d) IL-2
  (e) They stimulate cells near cells infected with viruses (or other microbes such as parasites or rickettsiae) to produce antiviral proteins; IFNs are not pathogen specific, so they are effective against different types of microbes.
  (f) TNF

A21. (a) A
     (b) A
     (c) P
     (d) P
     (e) P
A22. B (see Question A7[d]); see text.
A23. The second—the secondary or memory response. (See text Fig. 13-11.)
A24. (a) Viruses, cancer cells, and intracellular bacteria (because antibodies cannot penetrate living cells)
     (b) T; helper; cytotoxic
A25. (a) Proteins; cascade of reaction; humoral
     (b) Classic; alternate; lectin; on pathogen surfaces so pathogens are better recognized by phagocytes or released into fluids to enhance inflammation
     (c) Classic; C9
     (d) Dilate; increased; anaphylaxis
     (e) Opsonization; chemotaxis
     (f) Attack; red blood cells, platelets, and lymphocytes.
A26. Antigens, as well as antibodies and cytokines are short-lived; tolerance to self-antigens, which normally prevents autoimmune diseases
B1. (b) (c) (a)
B2. (a) IgGs
     (b) Deficient, because most IgGs cross the placenta from mother to fetus during final weeks of pregnancy.
     (c) Will; because IgG antibodies in mother's blood can cross the placenta into fetal blood; although Celia's blood tests positive for HIV (because she does have the antibodies), Celia may not have received sufficient HIV viruses from mother to be infected. Further testing can determine her HIV status.
     (d) Cannot; Jill has been exposed to antigens and is producing antibodies against them.
     (e) Through breast milk; reduce diarrheal infections in Miji
B3. Cell-mediated immunity, antibody-mediated immunity, T-cell count, IL-2 cytokine production

Chapter 14

INFLAMMATION, TISSUE REPAIR, AND FEVER

A1. Inflammation is designed to mobilize defenses against infection, but does cause some discomfort and sometimes serious side effects.
A2. -itis
A3. Infection, trauma, surgery, caustic chemicals, extremes of heat or cold, and ischemia.
A4. (a) Dilation of blood vessels that bring more (warm) blood into the area
     (b) Increased permeability of vessels to allow more white blood cells and defensive chemicals to reach tissues
     (c) Edema and chemical stimulation of nerves by release of prostaglandins and bradykinin

A5. Vascular; (3)
A6. (a) Neutrophils; adhesion; margination; 1.5
     (b) Emigration; enzymes; chemotaxis
     (c) Increases; cytosis; bands
     (d) Baso; eosino; basophils; dilates
     (e) Mono; longer; macrophages; lymph nodes
A7. Cytokines, bacterial and cellular debris, complement fragments
A8. Adherence/opsonization→ engulfment→ intracellular killing
A9. (a) Prostaglandin
     (b) Bradykinin
     (c) Platelet-activating factor
     (d) Leukotrienes; platelet-activating factor
     (e) Histamine
     (f) Serotonin
     (g) Complement
     (h) Arachidonic acid
     (i) Cytokines
A10. Dilators; cell; bradykin and complement
A11. Watery; red blood cells; leukocytes, proteins, and tissue debris
A12. See text.
A13. (a) Increases
     (b) Increases
     (c) Increases
     (d) Increases
     (e) Decreases (lethargy sets in)
A14. (a) Increase; 15,000 to 20,000
     (b) Hours; left
     (c) Bacterial infection
     (d) Viral infection and cancer
     (e) Allergic reaction, parasitic infection
     (f) Inflammation; cancer
A15. (a) Monocytes; macrophages; fibroblast
     (b) Granulomatous; granulomatous; cheesy (like cottage cheese)
B1. Labile, stable, permanent
     (a) Permanent
     (b) Labile
     (c) Stable
B2. (b), (d); but (a) stroma, (c) slower, worse
B3. (a) Inflammatory, proliferative, remodeling
     (b) (3), (4), (1), (2)
B4. (a) Macrophages are critical to wound healing; their roles include cleaning up debris, releasing growth factors such as TAF, and attracting fibroblasts.
     (b) Stimulate growth of new blood vessels (angio)
     (c) These WBCs (mainly neutrophils) ingest bacteria and cell debris.
     (d) The key cells during the proliferative phase, fibroblasts secrete the collagen used to form collagen fibers.
     (e) With fibroblasts, endothelial cells form soft, pink granulation tissue that serves as the foundation for a scar.
B5. (a) G and B, because granulation tissue is a sign of the beginning of healing but excessive amounts are "proud flesh" and may need to be removed.
     (b) B, because a keloid is excessive scar tissue.
B6. (a), (b); but (c) 10%, (d) 70%–80%

B7. (a) Vitamin B
(b) Vitamin A
(c) Vitamin C (also vitamin A)
(d) Vitamin K

B8. (a), (b); but (c) decreases, (d) decrease, delay; (e) pulling apart

B9. Activates killing of bacteria by neutrophils; decreases growth of anaerobic microbes; promotes growth of blood vessels and fibroblasts

B10. Overall, this is true because sutures approximate (bring together) the two sides of the wound, prohibiting entrance of most microbes. However, sutures themselves are foreign bodies that can serve as routes for infection. So sutures are removed (unless they are the type that dissolve) a number of days after suturing.

C1. (c), (d); but (a) 36.0°C to 37.5°C, (b) late afternoon or evening, (e) good (insulator)

C2. (a) P
(b) P
(c) P
(d) L
(e) L
(f) P
(g) P (because less blood volume is available to reach skin surface)

C3. (a) Convection
(b) Conduction
(c) Evaporation
(d) Radiation

C4. (a) Resetting the temperature set point in the hypothalamus
(b) 41 (105.8); convulsions or higher ambient temperature
(c) Pyrexia; decrease; resetting the temperature set point
(d) Exo; endo; interleukin; prostaglandin
(e) Shivering and vasoconstriction (so less blood is cooled at skin surface)
(f) Interleukin-1

C5. (a) Injured heart cells or macrophages can release pyrogens.
(b) Cytokines can be released by the lymphocytes present in excessive numbers in Hodgkin disease.
(c) Neurogenic fever

C6. Slight fever does activate the immune system (leukocytes and interferon) and retards growth of some microbes.

C7. (a) Relapsing
(b) Remittent

C8. Increase; increased

C9. Prodrome→ Chill→ Flush → Defervescence
(a) Chill
(b) Flush, defervescence

C10. Increased body temperature activates the dormant virus.

C11. Fever of unknown origin with a temperature of 101°F or higher for at least 3 weeks. See text.

C12. More poorly; 38°C (100.4°F)

C13. Elderly persons typically maintain a lower baseline temperature, which may mean that a temperature of 100.2°F is considerably elevated. Oral temperature may not be accurate due to tongue tremors and mouth breathing associated with PD. Mr. Baker's diuretic medication reduces the volume of blood that can cool his body.

Chapter 15

ALTERATIONS IN THE IMMUNE RESPONSE

A1. Protect against microorganisms, protect against cancer, and facilitate healing

A2. Immunodeficiency disorders; allergies or hypersensitivity reactions; transplantation rejection; autoimmune disorders

A3. Induce an immune response. Inhalation, ingestion, injection, or skin contact

A4. (a) I, II, and III; B; I; II and III
(b) IV; cytokines; delayed; days
(c) II and III
(d) III; joints by rheumatoid arthritis; joints and kidneys in SLE (lupus); kidneys by damage to glomerular vessels

A5. (a) Mast; IgE; ragweed pollen
(b) Inflammatory; histamine, kinins, leukotrienes, prostaglandins, and acetylcholine
(c) I; immediate, minutes
(d) Rhinoconjunctivitis; seasonal; dilation and increased permeability of mucosal vessels
(e) See Question A6(c2)
(f) (Any order)
(f1) Produce cytokines that stimulate B cells to form plasma cells that secrete IgEs
(f2) Act as growth factors for mast cells
(f3) Activate eosinophils
(g) Atopic (hereditary); high

A6. (a) Proteins; E; I
(b) Children; rash or hives, dilation of blood vessels with drop in blood pressure (anaphylaxis); difficulty breathing (dyspnea) as airways constrict
(c1) Widespread dilatation of blood vessels
(c2) Contraction of smooth muscle in airways (causing bronchoconstriction) as well as increased permeability of blood vessels in airway mucosa, leading to swelling and airway obstruction
(d) Epinephrine mimics sympathetic nerves as it vasoconstricts (which helps raise blood pressure) and relaxes smooth muscle of airways (bronchodilates).
(e) Being tested for allergies and avoiding those foods that cause allergic reactions; being prepared with treatments such as epinephrine and antihistamines
(f) Reactions to (and destruction of) intestinal parasites

A7. Hemolytic (disease of the) newborn; II; Rh antibodies; G (because IgMs are too large to cross the placenta); anemia and hyperbilirubinemia (if severe, can lead to kernicterus)

A8. Purified protein derivative; subcutaneously; has enough sensitized T cells to cause a hypersensitivity reaction; IV

A9. IV
(a) Cosmetics or medications applied to skin; metals (e.g., in jewelry such as rings or necklaces); poison ivy
(b) Check the location(s) of the affected area and get a good history.
(c) Swollen, red, and warm. Avoid contact with the allergen; use topical creams to treat symptoms.

B1. (a) Ability of the immune disease to distinguish its own antigens from non-self antigens and to not mount an immune response against one's own tissues.
(b) CD4$^+$ helper T-cell receptors recognize MHC (major histocompatibility) molecules that identify "self" and are presented along with "non-self" antigens.
(c) T cells that would react with self are eliminated centrally in the thymus; self-reactive B cells are eliminated centrally (in bone marrow); self-reactive T or B cells that escape thymus or bone marrow may be removed or inactivated peripherally (from blood or lymphoid tissue).

B2. See Chart 15-1 in the textbook.

B3. (a) Specific antigens are highly associated with autoimmune conditions including joint disorders such as ankylosing spondylitis, Reiter syndrome, rheumatoid arthritis, and lupus.
(b) Because not all persons with a genetic predisposition do develop an autoimmune disorder; also a virus or chemical attached to the antigen-MHC complex may alter it and cause CD4 cells to fail to recognize MHC as self.
(c) The autoimmune disease lupus (SLE) occurs more commonly in women, thus suggesting a role of estrogen in development of lupus.
(d) Results in failure to delete T cells that react to self.

B4. (a) Strepto; heart
(b) Streptococcal; mimicry; HLA; increased; failure

B5. Antibodies; enzyme-linked immunosorbent

C1. (a) (1)
(b) 95%; match closely
(c) (2)
(d) T; B; blood vessels; humoral

C2. Hyperacute→ acute→ chronic; hyperacute

C3. (b), (c); but (a) most commonly, (d) commonly

C4. (a) Nausea, bloody diarrhea, and abdominal pain
(b) Bleeding and coma
(c) Rash and itching beginning on palms and soles, but often spreading and leading to skin peeling (desquamation)

C5. Removal or destruction of T cells from the transplanted tissue; T-cell-blocking drugs (e.g., cyclosporine)

D1. (a) S
(b) S
(c) P
(d) S
(e) P

D2. (a) Combined B-cell and T-cell deficiencies
(b) T-cell (cellular) deficiency
(c) T-cell (cellular) deficiency
(d) Combined B-cell and T-cell deficiencies
(e) B-cell (humoral) deficiency

D3. (c), (d); but (a) many such genes are on X-chromosomes, (b) IgGs, (e) less

D4. (a) IgA; 50%; does not
(b) IgG; polysaccharide; polysaccharide
(c) IgMs are too large to pass across kidney membranes.

D5. Secondary; few persons survive primary T-cell deficiencies very long; autosomal (chromosome 22). Failure of thymus and parathyroid gland to develop (with hypocalcemia); heart defects; increased risk of infections

D6. (a) Viruses; cancers; opportunistic; negative skin test reaction to antigens
(b) Severe combined immunodeficiency syndrome; both B and T; 2; bone marrow or stem cell transplantation; ADA enzyme replacement

E1. (b), (c); but (a) in Sub-Saharan Africa (d) under age 25

E2. Blood, semen, and vaginal fluids; breast milk. HIV has not been shown to be transmitted by any of the other fluids listed.

E3. Their use alters perceptions of risk and reduces inhibitions to risk-taking behaviors.

E4. (b), (c); but (a) acquired—meaning not hereditary and (d) uncommon

E5. (b)

E6. (a), (c), but (b) can and (d) can

F1. (b)

F2. CD4$^+$ T helper cells and macrophages

F3. (b), (e), (f); but (a) HIV-1, (c) RNA, (d) RNA

F4. (b) → (h) → (e) → (d) → (g) → (f) → (c) → (a)

F5. (a) gp 120 and gp 41
(b) p24

F6. (b)

F7. Carl: category 2C; Terry: category 1B; Kelsey: category 3C
Carl and Kelsey because both are in clinical category C and Kelsey is category 3.

F8. (a) Primary (acute) infection phase
(b) Primary (acute) infection phase
(c) Latent period
(d) Overt AIDS (or sympathetic)

F9. Slow

F10.

Name of Microbe	Class of Microbe	Commonly Infected Systems
Candida albicans	Fungus	D-E, N-S, and R
Cryptosporidium parvum	Protozoan	D-I
Cytomegalovirus (CMV)	Virus	D-E, D-I, N-S, R
Herpes simplex (HSV)	Virus	D-E, D-I, N-S
Mycobacterium avian complex (MAC)	Bacterium	D-I, R
Mycobacterium tuberculosis	Bacterium	R
Pneumocystis carinii (PCP)	—	R
Toxoplasma gondii	Parasite	N-S, R

F11. (a) *Cryptosporidium*; also CMV, MAC
 (b) *Candida*
 (c) PCP
 (d) *Mycobacterium tuberculosis*
 (e) *Candida*, CMV, HSV
 (f) *T. gondii*
F12. AIDS dementia complex, progressive multifocal leukoencephalopathy (PML) caused by the JC virus, and *T. gondii* infection
F13. Kaposi sarcoma (KS); non-Hodgkin lymphoma, cervical carcinoma (in women)
F14. (a) HIV-wasting syndrome
 (b) Lipodystrophy
F15. (b), (c); but (a) not the first test because it is more expensive and slower than the ELISA test and (d) the reverse is true
 (e) the antibody to the virus.
F16. Highly active anti-retroviral
 (a) Cleavage, which requires protease (F4[c])
 (b) Reverse transcription (F4[e])
F17. For prevention of infections
 G1. (b), (d); but (a) perinatally, (c) will not necessarily, and (e) for all pregnant women
 G2. (a), (c), (e)
 G3. Different from; early; less; do

Chapter 16

CONTROL OF CARDIOVASCULAR FUNCTION

A1. The heart, blood vessels, and blood
A2. (a), (b); but (c) pulmonary artery and (d) about one-eighth
A3. (a) Venules and veins → Arteries and arterioles → Heart (See Figure 16-2 in *Essentials of Pathophysiology.*)
 (b) Arteries → Capillaries → Veins
 (c) Superior vena cava → Right side of the heart → Pulmonary artery
A4. The same amount of; high to low; seven times

B1. (a) 16; vasoconstriction as a result of sympathetic nerve impulses or epinephrine, atherosclerosis, or stenosis
 (b) Blood pressure (P): resistance (R); P/R
 (c) Higher (see Chapter 11); high; increases
 (d) Aorta; capillaries; blood flows swiftly through the aorta to reach organs, but maximum time is permitted within capillaries for exchange of gases and nutrients
 (e) Within the center; laminar; in curving or branching
 (f) More; increases; Laplace
 (g) Veins
C1. (a) Right
 (b) Ventricles; pumps; reservoirs
 (c) Myo
C2. Fibrous pericardium → Parietal pericardium → Pericardial cavity → Visceral pericardium → Myocardium → Endocardium
C3. (a) S
 (b) C
 (c) C
 (d) C
 (e) C (myocardial function)
C4. Connective tissue that separates atria from ventricles. Serves as an attachment point for valves and helps produce orderly contractions by "forcing" electrical impulses to pass through the AV node.
C5. (a) Aortic
 (b) Bicuspid
 (c) Bicuspid, tricuspid
 (d) Aortic, pulmonary
 (e) Bicuspid, tricuspid
C6. (a) Can; faster
 (b) SA node → AV node → Bundle and bundle branches → Purkinje fibers
 (c) SA node; right
 (d) Slow; ventricles can completely fill before their contraction is initiated
 (e) AV node; because atria and ventricles are otherwise completely separated, ventricles are protected from excessively high rates that arise in the atria
 (f) Within the interventricular septum
 (g) Rapid; this increases the likelihood that all parts of the ventricles will contract virtually simultaneously to swiftly eject blood
C7. (a) Sudden change in voltage involving depolarization and repolarization
 (b) −90; K^+; Na^+
 (c) Na^+; depolarization threshold; +20; 0; de
 (d) Downward; negative
 (e) Plateau; slow influx of Ca^{2+} into the cell so cardiac muscle can sustain a contraction 3 to 15 times longer than skeletal muscle
 (f) Dramatically; out of; ceases
 (g) Out of; into
C8. (a) SA node and AV node; SA; AV
 (b) Atria, ventricles
 (c) De
 (d) Increase; parasympathetic; increases; de

C9. (a) (1); cannot
(b) Supernormal excitatory; ectopic
C10. (a) Complete heart block
(b) Ventricular dysrhythmia
(c) Supraventricular dysrhythmia
(d) Bradyarrhythmias
(e) PVCs
C11. (a) 12; see Figure 16-14 in *Essentials of Pathophysiology*
(b1) T wave
(b2) QRS complex
(b3) PR interval
(b4) RR interval
C12. (a) Electrical; atria; QRS complex
(b) (C)→(A)→(B)→(E)→(G)→(F)→(D)→(H)
(c) (c1) A
(c2) F
(c3) Rapid ventricular filling occurring between D and H
(c4) H
(d) F (specifically, aortic semilunar valve closure)
(e) AV; semilunar
(f) Ventricular; early; stroke
(g) Great arteries; 120
(h) Elastic recoil; 80
(i) (1) B; 120 mL − 50 mL = 70 mL
(2) A; 70/120 = close to 60%
(j) Decrease; increase
C13. (a) Normal
(b) Weak; bulging (as right atrial blood backs up in jugular veins)
C14. (a) 70 mL/beat × 72 beats/minute = about 5,000 mL/minute = 5 L/minute
(b) 300%
(c) More; increasing; more
(d) Greater; actin (and) myosin; Frank
(e) Dehydration, hypovolemic shock, lack of exercise
(f) Increase; decrease; inversely
C15. (a) Her cardiac muscle is "overstretched" (beyond the optimum for the Frank-Starling law), so her stroke volume decreases whereas EDV and preload increase.
(b) Contractility
(c) 0.5 (120 cycles/60 seconds); 0.33 (180 cycles/60 seconds); diastole; fill; low
D1. Externa → Media → Intima; media
D2. (a) Help to prevent clot formation along the inside of the vessel; secrete chemicals that alter the diameter of blood vessels by contracting or relaxing smooth muscle in the tunica media
(b) See text.
D3. (a) Waves of pressure that are generated by the alternate contraction and relaxation of the left ventricle that eject blood into the aorta and on into smaller vessels
(b) Pressure pulse is felt when a pulse is taken and pressure pulses produce Korotkoff sounds heard during measurement of blood pressure.
(c) Dissipates; cannot

D4. (a) Capillaries
(b) Arterioles
(c) Arteries
(d) Venules
(e) Veins
(f) Veins
(g) Lymphatic vessels
(h) Arterioles, capillaries, and venules
D5. Just superior to medial aspects of clavicles at the junctions of subclavian veins with internal jugular veins
D6. Removal of lymph nodes lowers her defenses against infection; interference with lymph pathways by node surgery leads to stasis of fluid in her arm.
D7. (a) Precapillary sphincters
(b) Nutrient flow
(c) Metarterioles
(d) Lymphatic vessels
D8. Increase; reactive
D9. (a) Vasodilator
(b) Vasoconstrictor
(c) Vasodilator
(d) Vasoconstrictor
(e) Vasoconstrictor
D10. Collateral arteries parallel the femoral artery much like side streets that maintain traffic flow when a major highway is blocked.
E1. (a) Medulla (oblongata); baroreceptors (sense changes in blood pressure) and chemoreceptors (sense changes in blood chemistry such as low oxygen level)
(b) Parasympathetic; 2
(c) Spinal cord segments T1-L2; 1, 3, and 4
E2. (a) Acetylcholine
(b) Norepinephrine
(c) Epinephrine

Chapter 17

DISORDERS OF BLOOD FLOW AND BLOOD PRESSURE

A1. (a) Externa → media → intima
(b) Intima; media
A2. (a) Regulate the following: movement of chemicals across the tunica intima; platelet adhesion and blood clotting; blood flow and resistance to flow; hormone metabolism; immunity and inflammation; and growth of smooth muscle in the tunica media
(b) Inflammatory agents such as hypoxia; cytokines and bacterial products; viruses; complement products; lipids; and stresses of blood flow on walls of vessels
A3. (a) Sympathetic; norepinephrine, constriction
(b) Atherosclerosis; growth promoters (some derived from endothelium) including platelet-derived growth factor (PDGF), thrombin, fibroblast growth factor, and cytokines (such as interferon-gamma and interleukin-1)

B1. (a) LDL; bad; high; low density lipoprotein
     (b) HDL; good; high; decrease
     (c) VLDLs
     (d) Can
     (e) Apo; some play roles in metabolism (getting rid) of cholesterol

B2. (b), (c); but (a) secondary and (d) LDLs

B3. (a) Dominant; can; 50; 2
     (b) High (over 240 and 160, respectively, which are considered normal); low. Yet most (70%) removal of LDLs from blood requires LDL receptors on cells. As a result, Amy's body must call on the limited number of non–receptor-dependent mechanisms, so her blood levels of LDLs are likely to rise.
     (c) Cholesterol deposits (xanthomas) along tendons are a sign of this disorder.
     (d1) Increased; increase
     (d2) Fruits, vegetables, and fish
     (d3) Cholesterol and fats; saturated
     (e1) Statins
     (e2) Ezetimibe

B4. (a) High cholesterol, smoking, diet high in saturated fats and calories, and inactivity; his blood pressure is in the prehypertensive range.
     (b) Male gender, probable family history of heart disease
     (c) His high lipid levels (hyperlipidemia)
     (d) Studies have indicated that fatty streaks may be present even in infancy.

B5. (a) Increased; blood vessels; meats; folic acid, and vitamins B_6 and B_{12}
     (b) C-reactive
     (c) *Chlamydia pneumoniae,* herpesvirus hominis, cytomegalovirus

B6. D → E → A → B → C → F

B7. (a) Thrombosis (or thrombus formation)
     (b) Occlusion
     (c) Ischemia
     (d) Infarction

B8. Vasculitis
     (a) Secondary to other disease
     (b) Immune process
     (c) Physical agent

B9. (a) Raynaud phenomenon
     (b) Acute arterial occlusion
     (c) Polyarteritis nodosa
     (d) Thromboangiitis obliterans
     (e) Giant cell temporal arteritis
     (f) Atherosclerotic occlusive disease

B10. Acute arterial occlusion, atherosclerotic occlusive disease, Raynaud phenomenon, and thromboangiitis obliterans

B11. Both Mr. Whitehead (Question B9[d]) and Mr. Vonnahme (Question B9[f]) have pain on exercise that subsides with rest.

B12. Chemicals in cigarette smoke act as vasoconstrictors and can trigger an immune reaction that affects clot formation. Inflammation of the vessel can then result.

B13. (b), (c), (e) where clots form due to stasis of blood in abnormally dilated vessels; but (a) dilatation, (d) brain, and (f) more

B14. An abdominal aorta dissection. Clues: the ripping pain, and syncope (from hypovolemic shock as blood accumulates within the wall of the aorta).

C1. (a), (c); but (b) lower and (d) 40 to 50

C2. Cardiac output and vascular resistance; factors through *n* through *r* in Study Guide Figure 17-1

C3. (a) ↑CO
     (b) ↑Stroke volume
     (c) ↑Venous return
     (d) ↑Exercise
     (e) ↑Blood volume
     (f) ↑Heart rate
     (g) ↑Sympathetic impulses
     (h) ↑Norepinephrine and epinephrine
     (i) ↓Vagal impulses
     (j) ↑ADH
     (k) ↑Aldosterone
     (l) ↑NaCl in diet
     (m) ↑Peripheral vascular resistance (PVR)
     (n) ↑Vasoconstriction
     (o) ↑Angiotensin II
     (p) ↑Viscosity of blood
     (q) ↑Erythrocyte count
     (r) ↑Plasma protein

C4. (a) (1), (2)
     (b) (1)
     (c) (1), (2)

C5. (a) L
     (b) S
     (c) S
     (d) L

C6. Increases; (d) → (b) → (a) →(c)

C7. (a) Constrictor
     (b) Constrictor
     (c) Constrictor

C8. Both are located in carotids and the aorta and both signal a need for altering BP. However, chemoreceptors respond to changes in chemical (O_2, CO_2, H^+) levels in blood, and baroreceptors respond to changes in BP.

C9. (a) Medulla, vasomotor, sympathetic, elevate; stimulating vasoconstriction that increases PVR and increasing heart rate
     (b) Orthostatic ("standing up straight")

D1. (a) Man
     (b) *55*
     (c) Lower
     (d) African

D2. (a) (4)
     (b) (4)

D3. No; increase; increase; sympathetic; increase; retention

D4. (b), (e), (f), (i); but (a) "apple" shape, (c) high salt and high fat foods, (d) beginning use of oral contraceptives, (g) high stress level, and (h) abuse of alcohol

D5. (a) No

   (b) Kidneys, heart, brain (stroke), eyes, extremities—any part of the body because hypertension increases risk for arteriosclerosis

   (c) Systolic

   (d) Increase. Left ventricular hypertrophy develops, increasing oxygen demands, but diastolic BP (needed for coronary perfusion) does not increase.

   (e) LVH does regress with therapies that reduce systolic BP.

   (f) Nephropathy can decrease urinary output; resulting fluid retention increases blood volume, venous return, and workload of the heart.

D6. (a) (2) (40% of circumference); over

   (b) (3)

D7. (a) 20% (1,200/6,000 g of sodium)

   (b) Saturated

   (c) Does

   (d) Brisk walking

D8. (a) Central adrenergic blockers

   (b) Calcium channel blockers and α_1-receptor antagonists

   (c) β-blockers

   (d) Diuretics

   (e) Angiotensin-converting enzyme inhibitors (ACE-I)

D9. (a) (3)

   (b) 56 (148/92); greater; see text

   (c) Low; step-wise; one

E1. (b), (d); but (a) only 5% to 10% with the rest being primary (essential) (c) most often, such as hypertension secondary to renal artery stenosis and coarctation of the aorta

E2. (a) Hypertension caused by any condition that reduces renal perfusion and activates the RAA mechanism

   (b) Renin; constrictor; aldosterone; retain; hypo

   (c) (2), (3)

   (d) Medulla; catecholamines; pheochromocyt(oma); sympathetic; headache; (2), (3)

   (e) Narrowing; arms

E3. (c), (d); but (a) no, it is a fast and fatal form of secondary hypertension, (b) 120, and (e) immediately in intensive care

E4. (a), (c), (e); but (b) less and (d) increased, indicating liver damage

E5. Sometimes. Women with PIH lose protein in urine; this lowers plasma protein, which leads to edema; decreased glomerular filtration rate (GFR) leads to decreased urinary output.

E6. (b), (c), (d), (e); but (a) multiple fetuses

E7. Hemolysis, elevated liver function tests, and low platelet count

E8. Eclampsia superimposes convulsions with no other explanation onto signs and symptoms of preeclampsia.

E9. (a) Preeclampsia/eclampsia

   (b) Gestational hypertension

   (c) Chronic hypertension

E10. (a), (b), (c); but (d) can injure the baby and (e) not unless on a salt-restricted diet before the pregnancy

F1. (a) Higher

   (b) Secondary; kidney disorders

   (c) 95th; stage 1 hypertensive; should

F2. Alcohol, oral contraceptives, and medications such as steroids or immunosuppressants

F3. (c), (d), but (a) 50, 75, and (b) systolic, but not diastolic

F4. See text.

F5. See text.

G1. (a) Lower; decreases

   (b) Thorax (aorta) and neck (carotids); increase; constriction; increase

G2. A drop in BP when the person stands (or sits) up often manifested by dizziness and syncope

   (a) Excessive sweating, vomiting, or diarrhea or production of large volumes of urine (diuresis), and loss of fluid volume with prolonged bed rest

   (b) Antihypertensives, antipsychotics, or diuretics

   (c) Neuropathy slows autonomic (sympathetic) nerve reflexes

G3. (a) Low blood pressure decreases cerebral perfusion. Her BP is low because of fluid loss from bed rest, increased respiratory work, possible fever with infection, and leg muscle weakness that decreases venous return. Elderly people are at greater risk for orthostatic hypotension.

   (b) See text.

H1. Contraction of the gastrocnemius and other skeletal muscles of the legs; inspiration that increases size of lungs and decreases intrathoracic pressure, "inviting" blood to move through the inferior vena cava back to the heart; and valves in veins that prevent backflow of blood.

H2. (a) Superficial, perforating or communicating, and deep

   (b) Valves in perforating veins prevent such flow

   (c) Deep; secondary; deep venous thrombosis

H3. All except male gender

H4. Superficial; they lack the support of muscle and connective tissues possessed by deep veins.

H5. Avoid prolonged standing; elevate feet when sitting; apply support hose before standing.

H6. (a) Superficial; lower

   (b) Venous; arterial

   (c) Lung (because blood from legs cannot enter the portal vein to directly reach the liver)

H7. (a) Varicose veins

   (b) Peripheral arterial disease

   (c) Deep venous thrombosis

   (d) Chronic venous insufficiency

H8. (a) Venous stasis

   (b) Hypercoagulability and some venous stasis related to pressure of the fetus or reduced mobility

   (c) Vessel injury with some venous stasis during recovery period

   (d) Vessel injury

   (e) Hypercoagulability

   (f) Venous stasis (and some hypercoagulability related to dehydration)

H9. Often, pulmonary embolism, which can be fatal

H10. Prevention is best. Early ambulation after childbirth or surgery; avoiding severe flexion at hips or knees or prolonged standing; antiembolism stockings or sequential pneumatic compression devices; anticoagulants, thrombolytic agents; insertion of devices into the inferior vena cava to filter emboli before they become pulmonary emboli.

Chapter 18

DISORDERS OF CARDIAC FUNCTION

A1. (a) Parietal pericardium; visceral pericardium
  (b) That accumulation of excessive fluid will compress the heart and prevent filling of the heart, and that this will lower stroke volume and cardiac output.

A2. (a) Increases; decreases; decreases; decreases; 2 to 4
  (b) Less; is; extra compression of the heart decreases stroke volume and systolic blood pressure to even lower values than normal during inspiration

A3. (a) Constrictive pericarditis
  (b) Cardiac tamponade
  (c) Acute pericarditis
  (d) Pericardial effusions
  (e) Acute pericarditis

A4. (b), (c); but (a) sharp pain, (d) expands the pericardial cavity, compressing the heart, (e) withdrawal of fluid from this cavity

B1. (a) Left
  (b) Right
  (c) Small

B2. (a) Neural
  (b) Physical
  (c) Metabolic
  (d) Endothelial chemicals

B3. (a) Is
  (b) Proximal
  (c) Stable; stable
  (d) Grayish-white, unstable

B4. Lower. Coronary arteries normally perfuse during diastole; perfusion can be inadequate when diastolic pressure is low and in association with tachycardia, which especially reduces the time spent in diastole.

B5. (a) Limitation of blood flow
  (b) Atherosclerotic plaque and vasospasm
  (c) Stress, exercise, exposure to cold, excessive production of thyroid hormone that increases metabolic demands, or aortic valve stenosis

B6. (a) Chronic ischemic heart disease; chronic ischemic heart disease
  (b) Stable; choking (angina) of the chest (pectoral region); squeezing or suffocating; sometimes
  (c) Sit; lying down would increase venous return, preload (and therefore workload of the heart)
  (d) Stop smoking, lose weight, reduce cholesterol and saturated fats in his diet, exercise regularly
  (e) Place the pill under his tongue but not swallow it
  (f1) Antiplatelet drugs such as aspirin, β-blockers, calcium channel blockers, long-acting nitrates
  (f2) Angioplasty or coronary artery bypass surgery
  (g) Variant angina; spasms; calcium channel blockers and long-acting nitrates

B7. (a) Unstable
  (b) She might have had "silent myocardial ischemia" (without pain) related to her lack of sufficient exercise to cause angina at that point; her perception of pain may have been diminished as a result of diabetic neuropathy.
  (c) Disruption
  (d) Some; (2)
  (e) (3), (2), (1)
  (f) (3)
  (g) Present; dip

B8. Intact myocardial cells; directly; days
  (a) Myoglobin
  (b) Troponin
  (c) Total creatine kinase; CK-MB levels specifically indicate injury to cardiac muscle cells

B9. (b), (d); but (a) vasospasms, rest or minimal exercise, and during the night (c) is not

B10. (b)

B11. (a) 30% to 50%; transmural, ST-AMIs; transmural
  (b) 20; stunned; may

B12. (a) Some; vasodilates; decrease
  (b) Oxygen
  (c) Intravenously
  (d) Should
  (e1) Percutaneous transluminal coronary angioplasty, balloon percutaneous coronary interventions; skin (to reach the lumen of a femoral or brachial artery)
  (e2) Radiation
  (e3) Coronary artery bypass graft; saphenous; internal mammary

B13. (a) Necrotic
  (b) Soft; week; rupture; fever; increase
  (c) Months; is not; ECG; aneurysm
  (d) Peri

C1. MI is caused by coronary artery disease (CAD) leading to ischemia; the other disorders are not.

C2. (a), (b); but (c) not fatal, (d) bed rest

C3. Idiopathic (cause unknown)
  (a) Hypertrophic
  (b) Dilated
  (c) Restrictive
  (d) Hypertrophic
  (e) Peripartum
  (f) All

C4. (a) Bacteria; do; acute
  (b) Endocardium; portal of entry
  (c) Microbes, cellular debris, and fibrin
  (d) (2) → (3) → (1)
  (e) Is; see text
  (f) Blood culture during a chill (that precedes a fever) to determine choice of antibiotic; transesophageal echocardiography

C5. (a) Group A (β-hemolytic) streptococcal; can; poor
  (b) Is systemic; central nervous system, joints, skin
  (c1) Skin
  (c2) Central nervous system

(c3) Joints

(c4) Skin and joints

(d) Temporary (for about a month)

(e) Permanent; decades; mitral

(f) Penicillin; dental

D1. (a) Rheumatic fever or bacterial endocarditis; congenital defects

(b) Workload of the heart is increased and may lead to heart failure; if mitral or aortic valves are involved, blood accumulates in lungs causing pulmonary edema and dyspnea.

(c) Opening; closing; regurgitation

(d) They result from turbulent blood flow over diseased valves

D2. (a) Mitral valve stenosis

(b) Mitral valve stenosis

(c) Mitral valve regurgitation

(d) Mitral valve prolapse

(e) Aortic valve stenosis

(f) Aortic valve regurgitation

(g) Aortic valve regurgitation

D3. Auscultation for heart murmurs with a permanent record by phonocardiography; ECG changes; echocardiography (ultrasound) to detect changes in heart function; and client history of fatigue, dyspnea, palpitations

E1. (a) 40,000; does

(b) Weeks; during

(c) AV; septa

(d) Atrial; ovale

E2. (a) Umbilical arteries

(b) Ductus venosus

(c) Ductus arteriosus and foramen ovale

E3. Umbilical arteries → Placenta → Umbilical vein → Ductus venosus → Foramen ovale

E4. (a) Lower

(b) Fluid; hypoxic; constrict; high; ductus arteriosus

(c) Increase; decrease; lowers; increases; foramen ovale; remain open

(d) Thinning of smooth muscle in the walls of pulmonary vessels during the first two months postnatally

E5. (a) (1)

(b) (2), because blood enters systemic circulation without having passed through lungs

(c) By observing for duskiness in mucous membranes, tongue, lips, fingernails and toenails

E6. Poor perfusion deprives tissue of oxygen and nutrients necessary for growth; fatigue may reduce ability to feed and also limit muscle development because children are inactive.

E7. (a) Tetralogy of Fallot, and ventricular transposition of the great vessels septal defects; possibly endocardial cushion defects

(b) Atrial septal defect

(c) Tetralogy of Fallot

(d) Coarctation of the aorta

(e) Transposition of the great vessels

(f) Patent ductus arteriosus

(g) Ventricular septal defect

(h) Endocardial cushion defects

(i) Pulmonary stenosis, transposition of the great vessels

E8. Hypercyanotic periods with deep breathing (hyperpnea), irritability, diaphoresis, possibly limpness and unconsciousness; children may assume a squatting position that increases blood flow to the upper body so they feel better

E9. (a) (The most) common

(b) Blood vessels; is

(c) Many systems; coronary arteries, which leads to myocardial ischemia

E10. (a), (d), and (e); but (b) not itchy, (c) no discharge, and (f) in subacute or convalescent phase

Chapter 19

HEART FAILURE AND CIRCULATORY SHOCK

A1. See study guide

A2. (a) Heart

(a1) Myocardial infarction related to atherosclerosis and vasoconstriction (as in chronic hypertension); valve disorders, congenital heart disorders; cardiac myopathies; cardiac tamponade

(a2) Excess blood volume (secondary to renal failure or IV overload); extreme exercise; thyrotoxicosis; and effects of adaptive mechanisms (see Question A2b).

(b) Adaptive

(b1) Aldosterone (from the renin-angiotensin-aldosterone mechanism) or ADH

(b2) High preload and also high peripheral vascular resistance caused by excess vasoconstriction (resulting from sympathetic nerve stimulation, catecholamines such as epinephrine, angiotensin II, endothelins, and other vasoactive chemicals)

(b3) The Frank-Starling mechanism; increased myocardial wall tension; myocardial hypertrophy and remodeling (as the heart responds to high preload and afterload)

A3. The Frank-Starling mechanism; sympathetic nerve stimulation, the renin-angiotensin-aldosterone mechanism, and local vasoactive chemicals

A4. (a1) Increase

(a2) Increase

(a3) Increase

(b) Constrict; hyper; stenosis

(c) Contractility; digitalis, epinephrine, sympathetic nerve impulses

A5. (a) Overstretched; increases; decreases; inadequately

(b) Cardiac output, ejection fraction, stroke volume, cardiac reserve

(c) (2), (3), (4), (5)

(d1) Pros: increased heart rate, heart contractility, and vasoconstriction are attempts to improve cardiac output and perfusion of vital organs

(d2) Cons: vasoconstriction increases afterload; this factor as well as stimulation of the heart will increase workload of the heart

(e1) Constrictor; decrease; decreases; increases; exacerbates

(e2) Aldosterone; cortex; Na^+ and H_2O

(e3) Constrictor; retain

(e4) Increase

(e5) Natriuretic peptides; opposes; ANP (atria), BNP (brain), and CNP (blood vessels)

(e6) Angiotensin II, atrial natriuretic peptide (ANP), and endothelin-1 (AT-1)

A6. (a) EWD
(b) EWD
(c) EWD
(d) ICF
(e) ICF
(f) ICF

A7. Low. Anemia in which even a normal cardiac output does not provide enough oxygen to tissues. Hyperthyroidism (or thyrotoxicosis—sudden increase in thyroid hormone) increases metabolism; tissues then require unusually large amounts of oxygen.

A8. (a) Forward; ejection; increases; increases; ischemia
(b) Backward; filling; edema
(c1) D
(c2) S
(c3) S (as blood backs up in left ventricle, overstretching it)
(c4) D (because filling time is reduced)

A9. (a) Left: APE, DN, F, ICP-P, PSOB
(b) Right: AA, Asc, F, HS, ICP-S, JVD

A10. (a) Shortness of breath while lying flat because blood backs up into the heart, overloading it (increasing preload)
(b) Sweating: a sympathetic response
(c) Skin is cool related to vasoconstriction and clammy because it is both cool and sweaty (sympathetic responses).
(d) Increased need to urinate at night as fluid from edematous legs returns to the heart and increases perfusion of kidneys
(e) Deep breathing when PCO_2 is high, and slight breathing when PCO_2 is low
(f) Limited exercise tolerance related to dyspnea

A11. (a) L
(b) L
(c) R
(d) R
(e) L

A12. (a) IV
(b) Her cachexia may be caused by fatigue, depression, ascites and congestion of blood in GI organs that have led to anorexia and malnutrition.
(c) Edema may be manifested by a weight gain of 2.2 lb for 1 liter of fluid; she also may be gaining some weight from her tube feeding.

(d) Persistent left-sided failure with pulmonary congestion increases pulmonary resistance and workload of the right ventricle, leading to its failure.
(e) 67%

A13. (a) Chest x-ray
(b) Echocardiography
(c) BNP
(d) History and physical examination

A14. (a) Dietary modifications
(b) ACE inhibitors
(c) Digitalis
(d) Diuretics; also dietary modifications, digitalis (by increasing effectiveness of heart contractions), and ACE inhibitors (by increasing renal flow and urinary output)

A15. (a), (d), (f), (g), (h); but (b) tachycardia as a compensatory mechanism, (c) agitation, and (e) moist (diaphoretic) skin

A16. (a) Left
(b) Prevent total assessment of bluish tinge (cyanosis) of lips and nail beds
(c) Assist her in sitting up so that blood will move out of her lungs and to lower (i.e., dependent) body parts by gravity
(d) Remove excess fluid from lungs; but the decrease in circulating blood volume can lower diastolic blood pressure so that inadequate coronary perfusion occurs
(e) Reduces anxiety and pulmonary vasoconstriction

A17. Heart. (b), (c) and (d); but (a) myocardial infarction (heart attack)

A18. (a) Dilators; decrease; decrease; decrease
(b) Increase; constrictors; increase
(c) An intra-aortic balloon pump; increases
(d) Heart failure that does not respond to medication or surgery; ventricular assist devices (VADs) or heart transplantation

B1. Inadequate blood supply to body tissues
(a) Functional heart, effective vessels, adequate blood, and tissues that can make use of the oxygen
(b) Hypovolemic, obstructive, distributive
(c1) Hypovolemic
(c2) Hypovolemic
(c3) Hypovolemic
(c4) Obstructive
(c5) Distributive
(c6) Distributive

B2. (a) Increases; tachy; increased
(b) Constriction; much; increases; Frank; increase
(c) (3)
(d) Increased; cool, clammy
(e1) Thirst; ADH
(e2) Sympathetic; endothelins and ADH (vasopressin); aldosterone and ADH
(f) Increase; increase

B3. (a) Hemorrhage; 25 to 30 (3 pints lost of 10 to 12 pints total)

(b) Cardiac output, because vasoconstriction maintains his mean arterial pressure (MAP) temporarily

(c) (1), (2), (4); not (3) because his circulating blood volume is already decreased. If his shock is severe and prolonged, then dopamine may be given to restore blood to kidneys and GI organs.

(d) Progressive

(e) Vasoconstriction deprives the brain and kidneys of oxygen. The Na^+/K^+ pumps fail, cells swell, and mitochondrial function decreases, leading to ATP deficit. Release of lysosomal enzymes further destroys cells of these organs.

B4. Normal (normovolemic shock); decreases; dilate; decreased; dilators; anaphylactic, neurogenic, septic

B5. (a) Histamine; increases; decreases; urticaria or hives

(b) Histamine constricts smooth muscle of airways.

(c) Epinephrine constricts blood vessels but dilates airways.

B6. (a) Neurogenic

(b) Septic

(c) Cardiogenic

(d) Obstructive

(e) Neurogenic

B7. TNF and interleukins; (d through g); but (a) fever and (b and c) warm, flushed skin

B8. (a) (2); vasoconstriction of renal blood vessels is a compensatory mechanism for shock, and endotoxins released in septic shock are vasoconstrictors; by measuring her urinary output and checking her blood levels of BUN and creatinine

(b) Vasoconstriction of vessels to the stomach and duodenum increases risk for ulcers.

(c) Acute respiratory distress syndrome; days; stiffer

(d) 30% to 50%

B9. Multiple organ dysfunction syndrome; decompensated; is. Hypoxia, lactic acid buildup, compensatory vasoconstriction (which causes more hypoxia), and complications such as ARDS, DIC, renal failure, and malnutrition (partly related to peptic ulcer)

C1. (a) (4 to 8) and (12 to 14); but (2) tachycardia, (10) grunt on expiration, and (11) cool hands and feet

(b) Weight assesses fluid retention associated with heart failure: 1 lb means 1 pint.

(c) All except supine positioning; upright position will decrease preload and heart workload.

C2. (a), (c); but (b) common, (d) carefully prescribed exercise, and (e) early

Chapter 20

CONTROL OF RESPIRATORY FUNCTION

A1. Nose or mouth → Pharynx → Larynx → Trachea → Bronchi → Bronchioles → Alveolar ducts → Alveolar sacs

A2. Slows down or paralyzes cilia, which allows particles to accumulate in lungs

A3. Pharynx; food there (specifically in the oropharynx) must be kept out of the larynx to prevent airway obstruction and risk of aspiration pneumonia.

A4. Larynx; glottis; epiglottis

A5. Warming, humidifying, and filtering air

A6. Do not; bronchospasms can collapse airways

A7. (b), (c), (d); but (a) larynx, (e) I, stay open or not collapse, and (f) 300 million

A8. Bronchial

A9. Pleural cavity (which normally contains only a few drops of serous fluid); Parietal pleura → Pleural cavity → Visceral pleura

B1. (a) 760

(b) Oxygen; 152; partial pressure

(c) 3; 456 (152 × 3)

(d) Water vapor; alveoli in Jillian's lungs—which should have 100% humidity unless she is dehydrated

B2. (a) Intrapulmonary (or alveolar)

(b) Intrapleural; negative; elastic recoil tends to cause lungs to collapse, yet the chest wall (because of flexibility of ribs and "give" of other tissues) tends to pull away from lungs.

(c) Intrapulmonary (or alveolar)

(d) Both pressures

B3. (a) Closed; sternum, thoracic vertebrae, ribs, intercostal muscles, and diaphragm; trachea

(b) Diaphragm; phrenic; cervical; inferiorly

(c) Increases; decreases; sucked into; in

(d) Passive; relaxes; up; increase; pushed out of; recoil

(e) External; ins; lift; in; ex

B4. Internal intercostals and abdominal muscles. (Note that scalenes and sternocleidomastoids would aid with forced inspiration.)

B5. (a) Ease of; (2)

(b1) Surfactant-producing cells do not usually mature until weeks 26 to 28 of gestation; infant respiratory distress syndrome (IRDS)

(b2) Interstitial lung disease causes lungs to stiffen (lose compliance).

B6. (a), (e); but (b) lipoproteins, (c) outside, and (d) dry

B7. (a) Small; Poiseuille

(b) Ex; ex

(c) Compressing

B8. (a) Tidal volume

(b) Vital capacity

(c) Functional residual capacity

(d) Minute volume

B9. (a) 500

(b) 4,600

(c) 2,300

(d) 6,000

B10. (c), (d); but (a) lung volumes (b) volume exhaled in 1 second

C1. Ventilation (movement of air into and out of alveoli), pulmonary perfusion (movement of blood into and out of pulmonary capillaries), and exchange of gases (O_2 and CO_2) across the alveolar-capillary membrane

(a) Base. Because of gravity, alveoli in the base are more collapsed (much like balloons that are almost empty), so they can accommodate more air (i.e., are farther from being fully inflated).

(b) Posterior or dependent, for the same reason as in C1(a)

(c) Blood; base

(d) Veins

C2. Constrict

(a) Blood is shunted away from hypoxic areas of the lungs to regions that are well ventilated.

(b) If all lung areas are hypoxic (as in chronic bronchitis), pulmonary vasoconstriction will force blood back into the right ventricle and overload it, possibly leading to right-sided failure (cor pulmonale—see Chapter 22)

C3. (a) Surface area for gas exchange (because emphysema involves destruction of alveolar walls)

(b) Diffusion distance (related to extra fluid between alveoli and pulmonary capillaries)

(c) Partial pressure of gases (because PO_2 is lower at high altitudes)

(d) Diffusion distance, which is increased in pulmonary edema. Also solubility and molecular weight of gases: CO_2 is considerably more soluble than O_2 so readily diffuses out of blood and into alveoli.

C4. Tidal; 350; 150; anatomic

C5. (a) Pulmonary embolism

(b) Atelectasis

C6. Ventilation without perfusion; anatomic

C7. (a) About the same as

(b) No, ABGs should be the same as aortic or alveolar values with $PO_2 = 80–100$ mm Hg and $PCO_2 = 35–45$ mm Hg. Jeremy's values indicate inadequate gas exchange.

(c) 98; 75; venous; about 98 to 99

(d) Blood plasma; hyperbaric; carbon monoxide

(e) Increase in temperature and CO_2, decreased pH (as in lactic acidosis), and also increased blood level of 2,3-DPG, which is an intermediate chemical in metabolism

(f) Right; more

(g) PO_2; SO_2; only PO_2 because SO_2 is a percentage (% of Hb that is saturated with SO_2) that cannot exceed 100

C8. (a) (2)

(b1) H_2CO_3

(b2) HCO_3^-

(c) See Figure 20-1A.

(d) It is the enzyme that catalyzes the first reaction shown in Figure 20-1A.

(e) Increase

(f) 30

D1. (b) (Pons and medulla)

D2. (c), (d); but (a) apneustic and (b) hypercapnia, or elevated blood level of PCO_2

D3. Hypoxia (with PO_2 less than 60 mm Hg) serves as his major stimulus for ventilation.

D4. (a) Stretch; ins; ex; stretch

(b) Trachea and bronchi; vagus; medulla

D5. Weak abdominal and respiratory muscles as in persons who have multiple sclerosis, are post-surgery, have brain disorders, or are taking drugs that depress the cough center

Chapter 21

RESPIRATORY TRACT INFECTIONS, NEOPLASIA, AND CHILDHOOD DISORDERS

A1. (a) Viruses

(b) The common cold; 2 to 4

(c) More than 100 types of viruses; rhino

(d) Can; infected fingers

(e) Have not; related to the large number of types of viruses that cause the common cold

A2. Fingers are the greatest source of spread. Your fingers can pick up viruses by contact with infected surfaces and then spread the viruses to mucous membranes of your nose or eyes.

A3. (e)

A4. (a) Frontal, ethmoid and sphenoid, maxillary

(b) Paranasal; nose; polyps can block the openings (ostia) into nose

(c) Mucous; do

(d) Acute; is not

(e) (1), (2), (4)

(f) (1), (3)

A5. (a) 3; rapidly; 2; 7

(b) Fever, chills, malaise, muscle ache, headache, "runny nose" (rhinitis), sore throat, and nonproductive cough

(c) 4–6; 8–11

(d) (2)

(e) (2), (4); but (1) antivirals (3) warmth discourages viral growth, which is optimal at cooler temperatures of about 35°C (95°F)

(f) Is (she is in a high-risk group because of her age); each fall

(g) A; more

A6. (a) Alveoli, bronchioles

(b) Is (sixth most common); leading

(c) Bacteria; atypical

(d) Aspiration of gastric contents; inhalation of fumes

Carbonic anhydrase

$$CO_2 + H_2O \xrightarrow[\text{Enzyme}]{} H_2CO_3 \longrightarrow H^+ + HCO_3^-$$

Binds to Hb — Shifts to plasma in exchange for Cl^- — **FIGURE 20-1A**

A7. (a) Community

(b) *Streptococcus;* pneumo; positive; capsule

(c) Decreased; increased (as a compensatory mechanism)

(d) To identify the causative microbe and to determine appropriate antibiotic therapy

(e) Antigens from 23 types of pneumococcal capsular polysaccharides; yes, she is over 65

A8. (a) Hospital; nosocomial; bacterial; 48

(b) Persons with inadequate cough reflex or damaged ciliated epithelium; compromised immune function (possibly following chemotherapy for cancer) affecting T cells, antibody function, and phagocytes; chronic lung disease; airway instrumentation or mechanical ventilation; infection with a highly virulent strain of bacteria

A9. (a) SACG

(b) B

(c) VFMP

A10. Sickle cell is likely to cause destruction of the spleen (see Chapter 11, Question B5[e]). The spleen's macrophages and antibody production normally combat pneumococci.

A11. (a) Common

(b) Negative; in warm, standing water, as air-conditioning systems

(c) Respiratory, digestive, nervous, articulations, and skin (temperature elevation)

A12. *Mycoplasma pneumoniae,* viruses (such as herpes simplex or varicella), and *Chlamydia pneumoniae*

A13. (a) Common; crowded; is

(b) Capsules; acid-fast

(c) Lungs; miliary

(d) (2)

A14. (c) → (b) → (a) → (d) → (e) → (f)

A15. (a) Immunosuppressed patients lack the normal T-cell–mediated responses that prevent further spread of TB bacilli by encapsulating the bacilli within Ghon foci or complexes.

(b) Calcified scar tissue is evident on x-rays.

(c) Primary TB typically has no symptoms; symptoms of secondary TB include low grade fever, night sweats, fatigue, weight loss, cough, and dyspnea.

(d) Previous exposure to TB bacilli, but not necessarily that the person has active TB

(e) Negative because they cannot mount a cell-mediated response to TB antigens

(f) Check for reactions to common microbes to which most people have been exposed such as mumps virus or *Candida;* negative responses to these indicate that the negative TB test came from immunosuppression and that the person may actually have been exposed to TB.

(g) The most widely used drug for TB treatment; long (months or years); TB bacilli become resistant to one drug

A16. Are; productive cough, fever, night sweats, weight loss

(a) Blastomycosis

(b) Histoplasmosis

(c) Coccidioidomycosis

(d) Candidiasis

B1. (a) Leading

(b) Greater than

(c) Is not; chronic cough, dyspnea, and wheezing

(d1) Blood in sputum

(d2) Related to pressure of the tumor on the recurrent laryngeal nerve (a branch of cranial nerve X that supplies vocal cords)

(e) Lung cancer may have spread to distant sites, and cytologic studies will indicate that the primary tumor was in a lung.

(f) These are signs of paraneoplastic syndromes: Many bronchogenic carcinomas are so poorly differentiated that they become sites of ectopic production of hormones ADH or ACTH or parathyroid-like peptide (causing hypercalcemia).

(g) 13% to 15%

B2. (a) Squamous cell carcinoma

(b) Large cell carcinoma

(c) Adenocarcinoma

(d) Small cell carcinoma

(e) Adenocarcinoma, squamous cell carcinoma

(f) Adenocarcinoma, large-cell carcinoma, and squamous cell carcinoma

C1. (b), (c); but (a) more slowly and (d) age 5 to 6 years

C2. (a) Compliant because tissues are soft; easier

(b) Abnormal; inspiration

(c) Nose

(d) Smaller; more; less; increases

(e) 80–100; 25–30; 50–70

C3. (a) Restrictive; helps to increase her lung volume at the end of expiration (FRC), which can increase gas exchange

(b) Intra; wheezing or whistling; ex

(c) Obstructive; extra; slower; ins; inspiratory stridor

C4. (a) Male infant born prematurely by cesarean section of an insulin-dependent mother

(b) Increases; decreasing; higher

(c) A clear membrane forms inside alveoli, decreasing gas exchange

(d) Do; tachy; restrictive

(e) Surfactant and oxygen administration, continuous positive airway pressure (CPAP)

C5. Premature infants who were on mechanical ventilators; lung damage increases pulmonary vascular resistance, and blood flows retrograde into the right ventricle leading to hypertrophy and ischemia.

C6. Common; young children have not yet built immunity to common pathogens, and airways are of small diameter

C7. (a) Younger; viral

(b) (3), (4), (6)

C8. (a) Croup (spasmodic or viral)
  (b) Epiglottitis
  (c) Epiglottitis
  (d) Viral croup
  (e) Spasmodic croup
  (f) Viral croup
  (g) Epiglottitis
  (h) Bronchiolitis
  (i) Bronchiolitis

C9. (a–c) Conditions in all answers are possible.

Chapter 22

DISORDERS OF VENTILATION AND GAS EXCHANGE

A1. See Chapter 20, Questions A9 and B2 (b).

A2. (d)

A3. 2 to 4 (Note: 4 to 5 mL = 1 tsp); serous; effusions; atelectasis. (1–2) Increased capillary pressure or permeability (as occurs in inflammation), (3) decreased blood colloidal osmotic pressure (due to deficient plasma protein), and (4) blocked lymphatic pathways

A4. (a) Hemothorax
  (b) Empyema
  (c) Chylothorax
  (d) Hydrothorax
  (e) Pneumothorax

A5. (a) Dyspnea; dullness or flatness; diminished
  (b) Removal of fluid from the pleural cavity as a diagnostic procedure or to allow lung re-expansion

A6. (a) Traumatic
  (b) Tension
  (c) Primary spontaneous
  (d) Secondary spontaneous

A7. (c), (d), (e); but (a and b) increase as compensatory mechanisms

A8. (a) O
  (b) O
  (c) C

A9. Similar to: (c), (d), (e), as in Question A7

A10. Reinflating the collapsed lung (or portion of it)

B1. (a), (c); but (b) dilate and (d) increasing

B2. (a) Inflammatory; during the night and early morning
  (b1) E
  (b2) I
  (b3) E
  (b4) E
  (c) 10 to 20; mast; E
    (c1) Constriction
    (c2) Permeability
    (c3) Increased; decrease
  (d) Macrophages, several types of white blood cells; may not be
  (e) T_H2; T_H1, decrease

B3. (a) Younger; do; house dust mite allergens, cockroach allergens, animal dander, and the fungus *Alternaria*
  (b) Common; cold
  (c) Viruses
  (d) Tobacco smoke (including secondhand smoke), smog, occupational fumes, gases, dusts
  (e) Appear to
  (f) Aspirin and NSAIDs (nonsteroidal anti-inflammatory drugs)

B4. (c–d, f–h); but (a, b, and e) the reverse is true because the patient with asthma has difficulty with expiration

B5. Lung hypoxia causes vasoconstriction and increased resistance of pulmonary vessels, retrograde flow into the right ventricle, and overload and hypertrophy of the right ventricle (see Chapter 20, Question C2[b]).

B6. (a) (2)
  (b) Peak expiratory flow rate

B7. (a) Education regarding avoidance of exposure, relaxation and breathing techniques
  (b) Prophylactic
    (b1) Dilators; sympathetic or adrenergic; parasympathetic or cholinergic or vagal; relax
    (b2) Inflammatories
    (b3) Leukotriene
  (c) Quick-relief

B8. Four visits to ER in 1 year, one in the past month; has been intubated for asthma

B9. (a), (c); but (b) common, and (d) is

B10. A cold with runny nose, nonproductive cough, irritability, rapid heart rate and rapid, difficult breathing with prolonged expiration

B11. (a) Chronic obstructive pulmonary disease; emphysema and chronic obstructive bronchitis
  (b) Common (the fourth leading cause of death); smoking
  (c) Are not
  (d) (1), (3), (5); but (2) true of asthma but not COPD and (4) true of the COPD emphysema but not asthma

B12. (a) Breakdown; decreased
  (b) Smoking; inflammatory cells (such as neutrophils or macrophages); elastase, protein; hyper

B13. (a) CB
  (b) CB
  (c) CB
  (d) CB
  (e) Emph
  (f) Emph (Chronic bronchitis causes excessive fluid in ankles [edema] and abdomen [ascites] so less weight loss.)
  (g) Emph

B14. (a) History and physical examination, pulmonary function tests (PFT), chest x-rays (CXR), and lab tests
  (b1) Ex
  (b2) 7 to 8
  (b3) Less
  (b4) Greater (exhalation is compromised)

B15. (a), (b), (d)

B16. (a), (b), (c); but (d) to maintain PO_2 at 60 to 65 mm Hg, or SO_2 at about 90%

B17. (a) Dilatation; infection; decreasing
(b) Tumors, foreign bodies, or mucus plugs in airways
(c) Cystic fibrosis, immunodeficiency states, lung infection, or exposure to toxic gases
(d) Permanent
(e) Infection and inflammation lead to dilatation of airway walls, pooling of secretions, and new infection
(f) Fever; large; blood (hemoptysis), microbes, and leukocytes (purulent); is; loss; clubbing

B18. (a) Common; autosomal recessive; no
(b) 7; CFTR; Cl^-; exocrine; high; thick
(c) Lungs and pancreas; infections; *Pseudomonas Burkholderia cepacia*; bronchiectasis
(d) Pancreas; steat; lower
(e) Vas deferens

B19. So that early treatment can delay onset and limit severity of CF
(a) Trypsinogen; pancreas; elevate (as the trypsinogen accumulates in the pancreas)
(b) Sodium levels of sweat; CFTR

B20. 35; pancreatic; airways; chest percussion and postural drainage, as well as use of bronchodilators and mucolytic agents

C1. (a), (c), (f); but (b) alveoli and interstitium—located between airways or alveoli and blood vessels, (d) may be, and (e) commonly

C2. (a), (d), and eventually (f), (g); note that interstitial lung disease differs significantly from COPD, although both involve dyspnea, tachypnea, and eventually cyanosis and hypoxemia

C3. (a) Asbestos, silica, chemicals in coal mines
(b) Chemotherapy agents such as methotrexate, and ionizing radiation
(c) SLE (lupus), rheumatoid arthritis, scleroderma

C4. History (especially occupational) and physical examination, chest radiographs and gallium lung scans, lung biopsy

C5. Similar; see text

D1. (a) Air, fat, or amniotic fluid (in maternal blood)
(b) Deep venous thromboses; lower
(c1) Immobilization after surgery, childbirth, fracture, or spinal cord injury; heart attack or heart failure
(c2) Surgical injury or inflammation of veins (phlebitis)
(c3) Pregnancy, use of oral contraceptives, hormone replacement therapy, smoking, or cancers that release clotting factors
(d) Direct obstruction to flow through pulmonary vessels and reflex vasoconstriction related to pulmonary hypoxemia
(e) Chest pain, dyspnea, and tachypnea; hypoxemia; large

D2. (a) III
(b) I
(c) I

D3. 28/8, 15 (8 + [1/3 of 20]); low; thin and compliant

D4. Secondary
(a) PHPV
(b) EPPV
(c) PHPV
(d) IPBF
(e) OPV

D5. Signs or symptoms of the underlying cause; also dyspnea, fatigue (because blood is not getting oxygenated), and signs of cor pulmonale (right-sided heart failure related to a lung problem)

D6. (a) 26; higher (15 would be normal)
(b) Rare; million; 20
(c) Same as in Question D5 except no signs of an underlying cause
(d) Oxygen, anticoagulants, and calcium channel blockers that both dilate and decrease heart workload; also dilators (such as epoprostenol)

D7. Lung; (c) → (b) → (f) → (a) → (d) → (e) → (g)

D8. Hypoxemia stimulates kidneys to produce erythropoietin, which stimulates erythrocyte production that causes skin redness.

D9. (a) Acute respiratory distress; chest trauma, burns and related infections, fat emboli (from fractures), and reactions to smoke and other inhaled gases
(b) Increase; inactivation; hyaline; decrease; increase
(c) Oxygen

E1. Hypoxemia; hypercapnia (or hypercarbia)

E2. (a) Ventilation
(b) Perfusion
(c) Exchange of gases

E3. (a) 88 and 102 are considered in the normal range; 72 is somewhat low
(b) 60; hypoxemia
(c) 38 and 42 are normal; 30 is too low; 52 and 64 are values congruent with respiratory failure
(d) 50; hypercapnia

E4. (a) Hypoxemia because CO_2 is more permeable
(b) Both but hypoxemia is more severe
(c) Hypercapnia
(d) Hypoxemia

E5. (b), (c), (e); but (a) fresh air (20% oxygen) and (d) commonly

E6. (a) Shunt (also cyanosis, hypercapnia, and hypoxemia)
(b) Impaired diffusion
(c) Cyanosis
(d) Hypercapnia
(e) Hypoxemia

E7. Pulse oximeter with sensors placed on ear, finger, toe, or forehead

E8. (a) Central; H^+; high blood levels of CO_2
(b) Decreases; peripheral; common carotid
(c) Increase. Because a low level (less than 60 mm) of PaO_2 serves as the major "drive" for ventilation in persons with COPD, she would be likely to hypoventilate and build up her $PaCO_2$ levels.

E9. (a) When lungs are hyperinflated or airway resistance is increased, as in COPD

(b) In malnutrition, anemia, hypoxia, heart failure, electrolyte imbalances, or degenerative neuromuscular diseases

E10. (a) Acidosis; 7.25

(b) Markedly; 38 to 42 (or 35 to 45); decrease; dilatation

(c) Decreasing the work of breathing, strengthening respiratory muscles, oxygen therapy to keep PaO$_2$ about 60 mm Hg, and possibly mechanical ventilation

Chapter 23

CONTROL OF KIDNEY FUNCTION

A1. (a) At waist level; retroperitoneally; renal surgery does not require operative entry into the peritoneal cavity

(b) Capsule → Cortex → Medulla

(c) Pelvis; ureters

(d) Renal artery → Intralobular artery → Afferent arteriole → Glomerular capillary → Efferent arteriole → Peritubular capillary → Intralobular vein → Renal vein

A2. (a1) Glomerulus; Bowman; corpuscle

(a2) Tubule; peritubular

(b) Basement membrane; prevents

(c) Mesangial; phagocytosis and contraction to control blood flow through glomeruli

(d) PCT → DLLH → ALLH → DCT → CD

(e) Short; juxtaglomerular; concentrated

A3. (a) Glomerular filtration

(b) Tubular reabsorption

(c) Tubular secretion

A4. (a) 125; glomerular filtration; blood cells and plasma proteins

(b) 124; 1; 60; 1440 (60 mL/hour × 24 hours/day)

(c) 60; higher; vasoconstriction; decreased; decreased; increased

A5. (a) Interstitial fluid and blood; Na$^+$; reabsorption; co; secondary

(b) Opposite; counter; secretion; bicarbonate, phosphate, and ammonia

(c) Passive; PCT

(d) Higher; more; transport; does

A6. More

(a) Smaller; concentrated

(b) Countercurrent; opposite; vasa recta; hyper

A7. (a) Increase; on Figure 23-2: H$_2$O in circle, blood volume and BP ↑ and UO↓

(b) DCT, Na$^+$; K$^+$; H$^+$; on Figure 23-3: Na$^+$ and H$_2$O in circles on left, K$^+$ and H$^+$ in circles on right; blood volume and BP ↑ and UO↓

(c) Decrease; raise; right atrium; opposes

(d) DCT; Ca^{2+}; mimics; increase; on Figure 23-4: Ca^{2+} in circle on left, PO$_4^{-3}$ in circle on right; ↑ Ca^{2+} and ↓ PO$_4^{-3}$

(e) DCT; thick

A8. 25%

(a1) Antidiuretic hormone (vasopressin), angiotensin II, sympathetic nerve activity

(a2) Dopamine, nitric oxide

(b) Autoregulation; decreasing

(c1) Macula densa

(c2) Afferent; angiotensin; aldosterone

(d) Increases; inhibits; inhibits

A9. Well; poorly; inulin; not at all

A10. Uric; aspirin, sulfinpyrazone, probenecid, and certain diuretics

A11. (a) Urea; 8 to 20; high

(b) Proteins; decreased; de

(c) Intestine; liver; kidneys

(d) Degradation of proteins in blood released by GI bleeding (related to long-term use of analgesics for arthritis); tissue wasting (caused by muscle inactivity) or anorexia related to the pain of arthritis; dehydration (which increases blood concentration of urea) associated with high blood glucose; and increased risk for renal damage (indicated by a GFR that is 20% of normal [see Question A4]) related to diabetes

(e) Increase; she may need lower dosages of her medications because her kidneys do not eliminate these drugs

(f) A low red blood cell (RBC) count may result from reduced erythropoietin production by failing kidneys and from iron deficiency anemia (related to anorexia); epoetin-alfa will stimulate RBC production.

(g) Failing kidneys do not activate vitamin D (1,25-dihydroxycholecalciferol) needed to maintain calcium levels, and they excrete excessive calcium because they excrete little phosphate (see Chapters 6 and 25).

B1. Casts, glucose, pink color (red blood cells or hemoglobin), and 400 mL total volume in a 24 hour urine sample

B2. (a) 1.025 (concentrated urine); colorless; higher; SIADH

(b) Such kidneys lose the ability to concentrate urine

(c) High, acidic

B3. Normal

(a) Is not; 120; good

(b) Less; increase; poor

(c) 1.0; one third; higher because GFR and creatinine clearance decrease with age

(d) 10:1, 1.2; 1

B4. Creatinine. The other chemicals may increase because of many other factors besides renal function: BUN by high protein intake, GI bleeding, and dehydration; levels of K$^+$ and H$^+$ by fluctuations of aldosterone; serum K$^+$ increases with tissue damage; and H$^+$ increases with respiratory disorders and ketoacidosis.

Chapter 24

DISORDERS OF RENAL FUNCTION

A1. (a), (d), (f); but (b) bilateral, (c) less, and (e) less—a condition known as oligohydramnios

A2. Ureters are likely to kink, thus obstructing urine flow and causing urinary tract infections and possibly backflow that leads to kidney damage.

A3. (a) Fluid-filled; 2 inches; they cause damage by compressing blood vessels or kidney tissue
    (b) Common; commonly
        (b1) ADPKD
        (b2) ARPKD
    (c) PDK 1; protein, polycystin 1; renal tubules

A4. (a) Compression of renal vessels activates the renin-angiotensin-aldosterone mechanism
    (b) From bleeding into a cyst
    (c) Caused by pressure within kidneys or against adjacent structures
    (d) Ascending urinary tract infections move into cysts

B1. See text.

B2. (a) Stasis; infections; stones
    (b) Hydronephrosis

B3. (a) Acute; rate; flank area
    (b) Unilateral; increased
    (c) Renal calculi (or kidney stones); nidus
        (c1) Saturation
        (c2) Matrix
        (c3) Inhibitor

B4. (a) Uric acid
    (b) Struvite
    (c) Calcium oxalate or calcium phosphate

B5. (a) Colicky; left; uni
    (b) Drinking fluids can help prevent formation of kidney stones; but after they have formed, large amounts of fluid can cause them to move into a ureter.
    (c) Are (unless formed of uric acid); is not; (1) (extracorporeal shock-wave lithotripsy)
    (d) Urinary outflow from the bladder is impeded so urine concentrates.
    (e) Immobilization causes calcium depletion from bones and leads to hypercalcemia.
    (f) Unilateral; irreversible

C1. (b), (c), (e); but (a) second most and (d) lower to upper urinary tract

C2. (a) (2) has less estrogen and less protective mucin
    (b) (1) has a shorter urethra, which limits the washout phenomenon; also potential trauma to the urethra by sexual activity
    (c) (1) obstruction leads to urinary stasis
    (d) (2) has urinary stasis from neurogenic bladder (result of her MS), urethral irritation by catheter insertion, and possible growth of a biofilm on the catheter

C3. (a) C. These filaments allow bacteria to adhere to receptors on cells of the urinary tract.

    (b) C. In some persons, ureters attach to the bladder at such an angle that urine is forced back into ureters during micturition.
    (c) P. The mucin layer may bind water to form a protective barrier between bacteria and the bladder.
    (d) P. These antibodies protect against bacteria.

C4. (a) (1) (indicated by lack of flank pain and only mild fever)
    (b) 15 and 24
    (c) Increased; drinking large volumes of fluid increases the washout phenomenon

C5. Can. Scarring can obstruct urine flow and lead to stasis and more infection; a vicious cycle of chronic UTIs can occur.

C6. UTIs during pregnancy typically are asymptomatic, so diagnosis of UTIs existing prepregnancy is important.

C7. (a) Children in this age group are at increased risk for pyelonephritis that can lead to renal scarring with permanent kidney damage.
    (b) UTIs are common among elderly in nursing homes or extended care facilities. UTIs are related to such factors as immobility, bladder ischemia, prostatic enlargement, senile vaginitis, or constipation. Virtually all persons with indwelling catheters develop UTIs. In some persons, no symptoms are noted until the UTI is advanced, possibly leading to kidney damage.

D1. Endothelial layer of the capillary, basement membrane, epithelial layer forming the outer layer of the capillary and the lining of Bowman's capsule; lack

D2. (a) Nephritic; common; is
        (a1) Azotemia
        (a2) Oliguria; hypertension; edema
        (a3) Hematuria; pyuria
    (b) Nephrotic
        (b1) Proteinuria; hypoalbuminemia
        (b2) Edema
        (b3) Infections; coagulation disorders

D3. Her GFR is likely to decrease, which does decrease urinary output (see Question D2[a2]). However, this may be offset by the damaged kidneys' loss of ability to concentrate urine. Large amounts of dilute urine may then result.

D4. (a) Are; bodies; gens; DNA in a person with lupus or chemicals in infective streptococci
    (b) Diffuse; segmental
    (c1) Sclerotic
    (c2) Proliferative
    (c3) Membranous

D5. (a) Nephrotic syndrome (Note: Normal protein in urine is less than 150 mg/day = 0.15 g/day.)
    (b) Focal segmental glomerulosclerosis
    (c) Acute proliferative glomerulonephritis
    (d) Rapidly progressive glomerulonephritis
    (e) Chronic glomerulonephrosis
    (f) Minimal change disease
    (g) IgA nephropathy

D6. (a) 3; glomerulus
  (b) Thicker; glucose
  (c) High; slightly; are
  (d) Is
D7. Both. See Chapter 17.
E1. (a) DCT, interstitium, PCT
  (b) Acute hypersensitivity reaction to drugs, acute pyelonephritis
  (c1) Chronic pyelonephritis
  (c2) Acute pyelonephritis
  (c3) Acute hypersensitivity reaction to drugs
E2. Aspirin (salicylate), NSAIDs (ibuprofen), acetaminophen, furosemide (Lasix), methicillin
E3. (a) Increased urinary output especially at night when the person lies flat; cause: damaged kidneys lose the ability to concentrate urine.
  (b) Inflammation of tubules increases their permeability.
E4. Renal perfusion is high (25% of cardiac output) and kidneys metabolize (destroy) many toxic chemicals in the body.
E5. Older adults are likely to have somewhat reduced renal function and may take multiple medications (polypharmacy), such as analgesics and diuretics.
F1. Young children; higher; uni; hyper; 90
F2. 60; hematuria; late; nephr; I

Chapter 25

RENAL FAILURE

A1. (a), (c), but (b) 40% to 75%, (d) prerenal, and (e) has not decreased
A2. (a) Prerenal
  (b) Postrenal
  (c) Intrinsic (intrarenal)
  (d) Intrinsic (intrarenal)
  (e) Prerenal
A3. (a) Decrease; 25:1; not
  (b) 20; tubules; tubules; concentrate
A4. (a) Nephrotoxic
  (b) Nephrotoxic
  (c) Intratubular obstruction
  (d) Ischemia
  (e) Ischemia
A5. (b) (maintenance phase): his urinary output is low, and he has azotemia and hyperkalemia—all signs of low GFR
A6. Uncorrected ARF has a high mortality rate, and reversal of injury requires early intervention. Older people are likely to have reduced renal reserves.
B1. (a) A high level of
  (b) (1), (2), and (3)
  (c) Improved
  (d) Serum creatinine level; creatinine is not reabsorbed into the renal tubule so whatever is filtered in glomeruli will show up (and can be measured) in urine
  (e) 8–25; 800

(f) 0.5–1.0; 10
(g) 125
B2. DRR → RI → RF → ESRD
  (a) Renal insufficiency
  (b) Diminished renal reserve
  (c) Renal failure
B3. Both involve high BUN and high creatinine levels in blood, but uremia involves other multisystem signs or symptoms of renal failure. Uremia occurs when more than two thirds of the nephrons have been destroyed.
B4. GFR falls, leading to fluid retention, edema, and hypertension. However, kidneys may also experience tubulointerstitial damage that causes inability to concentrate urine, polyuria, and dehydration.
B5. (a) $\uparrow$ or $\downarrow$
  (b) $\uparrow$
  (c) $\uparrow, \downarrow, \downarrow$
  (d) $\uparrow$, decreasing
  (e) $\downarrow, \downarrow$
  (f) $\downarrow, \uparrow, \downarrow$
  (g) $\downarrow$
B6. (a) Inversely; PO_4^{-3}; Ca^{2+}
  (b) Hyper (see Question B5[e and f])
  (c) Decreased; over
  (d) Softer; low; decreases; vitamin D; H^+; dialysis; aluminum (Al)
B7. (a) Neurologic
  (b) Neurologic
  (c) Integumentary
  (d) Reproductive
  (e) Immune
  (f) Gastrointestinal
  (g) Cardiovascular (increased heart rate and left ventricular hypertrophy as compensatory mechanisms for hypoxia associated with anemia and decreased oxygen supply to the myocardium)
  (h) Hematologic, cardiovascular
B8. (a) To increase red blood cell count: failing kidneys do not produce adequate erythropoietin and blood is lost through blood testing or dialysis; anorexia may be another factor leading to iron deficiency anemia
  (b) To treat hypertension; also if on hemodialysis. See Question B11(d).
  (c) Kidneys do not eliminate drugs effectively, so blood levels of drugs tend to increase.
  (d) Milk is high in phosphates and CRF patients typically have hyperphosphatemia.
  (e) Aluminum-containing antacids can contribute to osteodystrophy.
B9. Technology and funding for treatments such as dialysis and transplantation have dramatically improved.
B10. (a) H
  (b) P
  (c) H
  (d) H

B11. (a) Low; no, because she needs some sources of protein
 (b) They contain potassium; these patients already have hyperkalemia.
 (c) Yes
 (d) The renin-angiotensin-aldosterone mechanism contributes to thirst, and her daily intake of fluid is probably restricted to 2 to 3 cups a day.
 (e) 6 (13 lb ÷ 2.2 lb/liter)

C1. (a) More; bone growth should be rapid because epiphyses are still open
 (b) Nutrition
 (c) Continuous ambulatory peritoneal (dialysis); does
 (d) He will be receiving immunosuppressants, and these reduce his defenses to infection.

C2. (a) Does; greater
 (b) Is not; because of decreased muscle mass, serum creatinine levels (which derive from creatine in muscle) tend to be lower to start with
 (c) Younger
 (d) Altered immune function (decreased T-cell count) that decreases transplant rejection

Chapter 26

DISORDERS OF URINE ELIMINATION

A1. Micturition
 (a) Trigone; ureters; 12; do not; normally, because of the oblique position of ureters as they enter the trigone, the rise in pressure during micturition prevents backflow (reflux) at the vesicoureteral junction
 (b) Urethra; males
 (c) Has folds known as rugae
 (d) Serous membrane (continuous with peritoneum), muscle, submucosa, mucosa
 (e) Detrusor; great; stimulated; "go"; internal; flow out of
 (f) External; stay within; continence; restrict micturition to appropriate locations (such as a bathroom)

A2. (a) Sympathetic; in; detrusor; is not; adrenergic or anticholinergic (*Hint:* Remember *S* for sympathetic, *S* for stop urination.)
 (b) S2 to S4; pelvic; "go" (*Hint:* Remember *P* for parasympathetic, *P* for "pee."); cholinergic; anticholinergic
 (c) Voluntary; pudendal; decreased
 (d) Motor; all three types; pons; detrusor; external sphincter; cerebral cortex

A3. Sympathetic; trigone and internal sphincter; does not (see Question A2[a])

A4. 150–250; 50

A5. (a) Excretory urography
 (b) Postvoided residual volume (PVR)
 (c) Ultrasound bladder scan
 (d) Cystoscopy

A6. (a) 12 oz = ([5 mL/year × 2] + 2); 336 mL (= 12 oz × 28 mL/oz)
 (b) 90 to 95 (%), 80 to 85 (%)
 (c) See text.

B1. (a) Urinary obstruction with retention or stasis
 (b) Incontinence with involuntary loss of urine. Structural changes in urinary tract or adjacent organs; neurologic disorders

B2. (a) Damage to sacral nerves interferes with normal sphincter function.
 (b) This STD can irritate the lining of the urethra, narrowing the lumen.
 (c) The enlarged rectoanal area presses anteriorly against the urethra.
 (d) Enlarged prostate encroaches on the urethra.

B3. (a) Hyper; fatigue; frequent; stasis and infection; hydroureter and hydronephrosis
 (b) Hyper; bladder spasms and urgency, as well as overflow incontinence

B4. See Chart 26-1.

B5. (a) Stroke, Parkinson disease, or tumors
 (b) Empty; flaccid; at; a
 (c) Higher; T6 to T7; spinal cord (because pathways between brainstem and S2–S4 control levels are cut off); hyper
 (d) Diabetes and multiple sclerosis
 (e) Constricts; increase
 (f) 3
 (g) Catheterization (intermittent or indwelling); adequate fluid intake to reduce risk of UTIs but not overfill the bladder; bladder retraining including manual methods; medications; or surgery such as urinary diversion or implantation of electrodes that stimulate bladder contractions

B6. (a) P; flaccid bladder
 (b) S; inhibits
 (c) S; incontinence

B7. (a) Overflow
 (b) Stress
 (c) Overflow
 (d) Other cause (unfamiliarity with surroundings and confusion)
 (e) Urge (overactive bladder)
 (f) Other cause (medications)

B8. See text.

B9. Elderly. With aging, detrusor function declines, leading to larger postvoided residual (PVR) volumes; elderly women are more likely to have given birth to more children, leading to weakened pelvic support; older men have higher incidence of benign prostatic hyperplasia (BPH); elderly people are more likely to be taking diuretic therapy; may avoid drinking fluids (because of incontinence), which increases risk of constipation and related urinary obstruction; conditions such as failing vision or arthritis interfere with getting to the bathroom fast enough.

C1. (b), (d), (e); but (a) the most common and (c) 94%

C2. (a) Painless hematuria; frequency, urgency, and dysuria (difficult or painful urination)
   (b) Backflow of urine into ureters (hydroureter) and kidneys, leading to renal damage
   (c) Electrocautery; urinary bladder; cystectomy; ileum

Chapter 27

STRUCTURE AND FUNCTION OF THE GASTROINTESTINAL SYSTEM

A1. (a) Intake, digest, and absorb foods; produce enzymes, hormones, and vitamins; eliminate wastes
   (b) Food or wastes pass through the GI tract but not through accessory organs (salivary glands, pancreas, liver, and gallbladder), which contribute secretions.
   (c) The hollow opening in the GI tract through which foods and wastes pass
A2. (a) Mouth, pharynx, esophagus, and stomach; pharynx
   (b) 10; lower; cardiac
   (c) Great; pyloric
   (d) Duodenum → Jejunum → Ileum
   (e) Cecum → Ascending colon → Transverse colon → Descending colon → Sigmoid colon → Rectum → Anus
   (f) Cecum
A3. (a) Mucosa → Submucosa → Muscularis → Peritoneum
   (b1) Peritoneum
   (b2) Mucosa
   (b3) Submucosa
   (b4) Muscularis
A4. (a) Visceral; parietal; ascites
   (b) Mesentery; lesser
B1. (a) Smooth; rhythmic
   (b) Submucosal
   (c) Parasympathetic; vagus; pelvic; overexcite
   (d) Decrease; inhibit; stimulate; decrease
   (e) Are located within; sensory
B2. (a), (b); but (c) brainstem (or pons and medulla) and (d) esophageal
B3. The pressure exerted by the lower esophageal sphincter normally is greater than pressure within the stomach.
B4. (a) 3 to 5; 20
   (b) Pyloric sphincter, sympathetic nerves, and hormones CCK and GIP
   (c) Atony and retention
   (d) Segmentation waves; they mix chyme with digestive enzymes
   (e) Ileocecal
   (f) Auscultation of (listening to) the bowel with a stethoscope pressed against different regions of the abdomen
   (g) Within the (haustra of the) colon
   (h) Large; several times a day

B5. (a) Rectum; sacral; parasympathetic; internal
   (b) External
C1. Seven; local, neural, and hormonal; parasympathetic
C2. (a) Secretin
   (b) Cholecystokinin
   (c) Gastrin
   (d) Cholecystokinin (CCK)
   (e) Glucose-dependent insulinotropic polypeptide (GIP)
   (f) Ghrelin
   (g) Gastrin and ghrelin (both produced by cells in the stomach wall)
C3. (a), (d); but (b) starch, (c) parotid, and (e) intestinal, mucus
C4. (a) Gastrin
   (b) Pepsinogen
   (c) Intrinsic factor
   (d) Mucus
   (e) Hydrochloric acid and intrinsic factor
   (f) Ghrelin
C5. (a) Small intestinal wall
   (b) Salivary glands
   (c) Stomach
   (d) Large intestine
D1. (a) They must be broken down into smaller pieces before they can be absorbed into blood or lymph.
   (b) Small intestine; large (250 m²) surface area provided by circular folds, villi, and brush border
   (c1) Produce mucus
   (c2) Enterocytes secrete brush border enzymes, which have direct access to disaccharides or dipeptides that can be digested and then absorbed "on the spot."
   (d) These lymph capillaries absorb fatty acids resulting from fat digestion.
D2. (a) Mouth; salivary glands and pancreas
   (b) Glucose and galactose; in lactose intolerance (cause by lactase deficiency), lactose cannot be absorbed—it remains within the gut, attracting water and microbes, and contributing to diarrhea and flatulence
   (c) Glucose and fructose; fructose; glucose
   (d) Pancreas; jejunum; bile; A, D, E, K
   (e) Fat; inadequate digestion or absorption of fats (as in cystic fibrosis)
   (f) Inactive; before activation, they are moved away from organs that produce them so that they do not digest the organs themselves
   (g) Pepsinogen and pepsin; trypsinogen and trypsin
   (h) (1), (2)
E1. Loss of appetite; (a) emotional factors, such as fear, depression, frustration, and anxiety; (b) certain drugs or foods; (c) disease states, for example, uremia (the accumulation of nitrogenous wastes in the blood), or distention of the intestinal wall as by backup of blood into abdomen by a failing heart

E2. Anorexia and/or nausea may precede vomiting, they may occur simultaneously, and they have many common triggers.
 (a) Hypothalamus, medulla
 (b) Sympathetic responses: pallor caused by vasoconstriction, sweating, and tachycardia
 (c) Vomiting; both will decrease (vasovagal responses)
 (d) Good news: vomiting serves as a protective signal of disease and helps to eliminate ingested noxious agents; bad news: potentially fatal alterations in fluids and electrolytes and, if chronic, may cause damage to esophagus and teeth by exposure to acidic gastric contents
 (e1) Motion sickness may involve emesis; anticholinergics such as Dramamine, Antivert, and Bonine decrease such nausea.
 (e2) Hypoxia caused by shock, decreased cardiac output, or increased intracranial pressure can trigger vomiting.
 (e3) Visceral afferent neurons transmit such changes in the GI tract.
 (e4) Dopamine stimulates the vomiting center; Compazine (a dopamine antagonist) inhibits vomiting.

Chapter 28

DISORDERS OF GASTROINTESTINAL FUNCTION

A1. (a) Total economic burden
 (b) 60 to 70
A2. (a) Diverticulum
 (b) Achalasia
 (c) Aspiration
 (d) Odynophagia
 (e) Dysphagia
A3. (a), (c), (e); but (b) are not, (d) do, and (f) is not
A4. (a) Narrowing of the esophagus by scar tissue, spasm, and edema
 (b) Metaplastic response to acid irritation in which the superficial squamous epithelium is replaced by more protective columnar epithelium
A5. See text.
A6. Common; an infant has a small esophagus, frequent regurgitation (with burping), and may eat in a reclining position
A7. Esophageal bleeding lowers red blood count; as a result, oxygen and nutrient supply to growing organs will be reduced.
A8. (a), (b), (e)
A9. Dysphagia; late; poor
B1. Tight junctions between mucosal cells and a protective mucus layer with lipid that prevents passage of ionized, water-soluble chemicals
B2. (a) Because aspirin and other NSAIDs are both lipid soluble, they can enter mucosal cells, directly injuring them; they also inhibit synthesis of prostaglandins (PGs), which are needed for normal mucus and bicarbonate production and adequate gastric blood flow.

 (b) Alcohol (lipid soluble) also injures cells; smoking vasoconstricts.
B3. 9 PM; acute
B4. *Helicobacter pylori* is the major microbe involved with chronic gastritis and peptic ulcer and also is linked to stomach cancer.
 (a–b) Both help *H. pylori* move through the mucosa.
 (c) This enzyme helps *H. pylori* survive in the acid gastric environment.
 (d) They recruit and activate neutrophils.
B5. (a) Endoscopy with biopsy test for urease and/or stool specimen test for this bacterium, blood test for antibodies to *H. Pylori*
 (b) A
B6. Parietal cells (text Figure 27-9) normally secrete both intrinsic factor (needed for vitamin B_{12} absorption required for red blood cell production) and HCl. Injury to parietal cells leads to both achlorhydria and pernicious anemia.
B7. (a), (b); but (c) men than in women, (d) has not
B8. (a) *H. pylori* and use of aspirin or other NSAIDs; 70; 10 to 20
 (b) (2), (4) (between meals and during the night); weekly or monthly
 (c) Bleeding with hypovolemic shock
 (d) Signs of peritonitis (see text)
 (e) See text.
B9. (a) Curling ulcer
 (b) Zollinger-Ellison syndrome
 (c) Cushing ulcer
B10. (a) Decreasing; common (the major cause of cancer death)
 (b) Late
 (c) Subtotal gastrectomy
C1. (d), (e), (f); but (a) 1 in 5 to 10 , (b) is not, and (c) is
C2. (a) Both
 (b) Both
 (c) CD
 (d) CD
 (e) UC
 (f) Neither
 (g) CD
 (h) UC
C3. (a), (c); but (b) is and (d) dilation with stasis and absorption of toxic chemicals
C4. Anti-inflammatory drugs, including corticosteroids; also immunosuppressants
C5. (a) *E. coli* O157:H7 infection
 (b) *C. difficile* colitis
 (c) Diverticulosis
 (d) Rotavirus
C6. (a) *C. difficile* is a spore-forming, toxin-producing bacterium that colonizes the colon after antibiotics have eradicated much of the normal flora there.
 (b) More, because smooth muscle tone of the colon may be lost, possibly causing dilation and perforation of the colon.
 (c) Discontinue, and then start other drugs that eliminate *C. difficile*

C7. (a) Nursing homes, day care settings, and hospitals
(b) Hemolytic-uremic syndrome and thrombotic thrombocytopenic purpura; both can lead to renal failure
(c) Treatment is symptomatic because no antibiotics work; prevention by public education is most effective.

C8. (a) More; related to less dietary fiber
(b) Diverticulitis; (1) (lower left quadrant, site of sigmoid colon)
(c) Vesicosigmoid fistula connecting the bowel to the bladder
(d) Increasing; day

C9. (a) Common; young
(b) Colicky; LRQ; increase
(c) Pain that occurs when pressure is applied and then released
(d) Appendectomy (surgical removal)

C10. (a) Wall of the intestine; parasympathetic
(b) 200 to 300; diarrhea; large-volume
(c) Sometimes; acute; acute
(d1) Small volume: infectious
(d2) Small volume: inflammatory
(d3) Large volume
(e) Is not; when prolonged in infants, elderly, or otherwise ill persons, who are especially vulnerable to dehydration and electrolyte imbalances
(f) Should; oral replacement therapy; (1), (2), (3)
(g) They reduce intestinal motility and stimulate water and electrolyte absorption.

C11. (a) Varies for different people (and their views of what should be normal): possibly daily to twice a week
(b1–3) See text.
(c) Response to the urge to defecate, especially after a meal; intake of water and fiber; exercise; avoidance of regular laxatives or enemas

C12. (a) Volvulus
(b) Paralytic ileus
(c) Strangulation
(d) Intussusception
(e) Borborygmus

C13. Anaerobic; mechanical; removal of gas from the bowel (decompression) by nasogastric suction or surgery

C14. This serous membrane lines the entire abdominopelvic cavity and forms the outside layer of the wall of most abdominopelvic organs (such as stomach, intestine, liver, uterus, bladder); normally a membrane free of microorganisms, a small area of infection can "spread like wildfire" over this large membrane.

C15. Any condition that introduces microbes into the normally sterile peritoneal cavity, such as rupture or perforation of the GI wall, pelvic inflammatory disease (PID), abdominal trauma, or surgery. (See text for more.)

C16. (a) (2)
(b) (2)
(c) (1)
(d) (1)

C17. (a) To replace fluids and electrolytes lost by "weeping" from the inflamed peritoneum
(b) To decompress the GI tract and reduce weeping into the peritoneal cavity and related abdominal distention

C18. (a) Lymphatic obstruction
(b) Maldigestion
(c) Transepithelial transport disorder

C19. (a) Barley, rye, wheat
(b1) Because of their high fat content
(b2) He is likely to have less absorption of fat-soluble vitamins, including vitamin K, which is required for clotting.
(b3) Inability to absorb amino acids limits muscle growth and activity.

C20. (a) Common; benign; attached by a stalk
(b) Mucosa; deficient; does

C21. (a) Common (second leading cause of cancer death)
(b) (1), (2), (3), (5), (7). Not risk factors: (4): her husband's cancer is not part of her family history, although it could be relevant if it is related to the environment or diet that Mildred and he share; (6): these medications actually appear to reduce risk of colorectal cancer.
(c) Bleeding from the bowel; change in bowel habits (frequency, urgency, consistency); no pain until later stages
(d) Later

Chapter 29

DISORDERS OF HEPATOBILIARY AND EXOCRINE PANCREAS FUNCTION

A1. (b), (d); but (a) cannot; if it can, may indicate hepatomegaly and (c) hepatic artery and portal vein

A2. Stomach, small intestine, large intestine, pancreas, and spleen; lacks. Blood backlogging from the heart (in heart failure) follows this route: inferior vena cava → valveless hepatic veins → liver. Hepatomegaly, a classic sign of right-sided heart failure, can result.

A3. (a) Kupffer cells
(b) Lobules
(c) Hepatocytes
(d) Sinusoids

A4. Bile canaliculi → Right and left hepatic ducts → Common hepatic duct → Ampulla of Vater → Sphincter of Oddi

A5. (a) Ketone
(b) Amino acid
(c) Urea
(d) Bile
(e) Albumin
(f) Glycogen
(g) Amino acids
(h) Amino acids, lactic acid, and glycerol

A6. (a) Liver cells metabolize ("chew up") virtually all drugs and many of the body's hormones, especially if they are lipid-soluble. The more drugs to which the liver is exposed, the more potential damage to the drug-metabolizing "machinery" of liver cells. A damaged liver can leave high levels of unaltered drugs or their intermediates in blood.

(b) Transformations
   (b1) Inactivated
   (b2) Lipid, water, kidneys

(c) Insulin, thyroid hormones, and steroids such as estrogens, testosterone, cortisone, and aldosterone; increase; refer to Question B11(c) regarding Mr. Nardella's increase in the normally minimal amount of estrogens in the male body.

(d) Intake of numerous drugs can overchallenge the liver and lead to increased levels of these drugs (and their toxic metabolites) in circulating blood; this is especially a problem in elderly patients, who are more likely to have impaired hepatic function and to take a variety of medications.

A7. (a) Passes through the duodenum, jejunum, and ileum, where it is absorbed into blood that passes into the portal vein and then back to the liver to start the cycle again (or is excreted in feces); enterohepatic

(b) Decrease in bile flow; obstruction within the liver (intrahepatic) or by obstruction of bile ducts (extrahepatic, as in last four structures of Question A4)

(c) Pruritus is most common; also, accumulations of cholesterol in skin (xanthomas), high blood levels of lipids including cholesterol, high serum levels of ALP, nutritional deficiencies of fat-soluble vitamins, and possibly signs of liver damage or failure.

A8. Hemoglobin → Biliverdin → Free bilirubin → Conjugated bilirubin* → Urobilinogen**

A9. Bilirubin
(a) (3), (4)
(b) (4)
(c1) Posthepatic
(c2) Intrahepatic
(c3) Prehepatic
(c4) Prehepatic
(c5) Intrahepatic or posthepatic

A10. Damaged cells release their normal contents, including enzymes such as ALT or AST; ALT (alanine aminotransferase)

B1. Drugs including alcohol, toxins, infection or inflammation, immune responses, metabolic disorders, and tumors

B2. Inflammation
(a) All
(b) They are all caused by different viruses, such as hepatitis A virus (HAV).

B3. (a) B
(b) E
(c) D, B
(d) C
(e) A, E
(f) B, C, D
(g) 90%; 25%; HBV DNA.
(h) Is; all children younger than 18 years and anyone else in a high risk category (see Study Guide Table 29-1).

B4. (a) Induction of immune responses against viral antigens
   (a1) Does; does
   (a2) Fewer; leads to a chronic or carrier state; sometimes; B, C, and possibly D

(b) Jaundice
   (b1) Preicterus; malaise; myalgia; severe anorexia; nausea, vomiting, diarrhea; high serum levels of liver enzymes (AST and ALT)
   (b2) Jaundice, high blood bilirubin, severe pruritus
   (b3) Sense of well-being, hearty appetite

(c) 2; 4

B5. (a) 6
(b) B, C, D; D
(c) Are, can; B, C, D (the same types that can be chronic)
(d) Are not
   (d1) Interferon, such as alfa-2b or an antiviral nucleoside analogue (lamivudine)
   (d2) Liver transplantation

B6. Rapidly; HBV

B7. Genetic predisposition and an environmental agent that triggers an immune response against liver cells

B8. (a) PSC
(b) PBC
(c) SSC
(d) Both PBC and PSC

B9. Ten million; 10 to 15

B10. Fatty liver disease → Alcoholic hepatitis → Cirrhosis
(a) Yellow; steatosis; are
(b) Obesity, type 2 diabetes, the metabolic syndrome, hyperlipidemia, rapid weight loss, parenteral nutrition
(c) Binge drinking or an increase in alcohol intake; (1), (2), (4), (5); but (3) compression of hepatic veins by nodules occurs with alcoholic cirrhosis; 10 to 30
(d) Small; as they enlarge (combined with fibrous bands), they block portal blood flow (leading to portal hypertension) and bile flow (cholestasis); yes, it signals end-stage liver disease

B11. 80% to 90%
(a) Viral hepatitis, toxic reactions to drugs, biliary obstruction (including tumors), and iron or copper deposits within liver
(b) Hepatomegaly indicates interference with blood flow through the fibrotic liver, backing up blood into the portal vein (portal hypertension);

ascites occurs when portal vein blood backs up into veins of the abdomen, seeping fluid into the peritoneal cavity; the extra fluid leads to anorexia and also masks weight loss; ankle edema is associated with decreased plasma protein (albumin) synthesis by the failing liver and decreased liver metabolism of the hormone aldosterone, which causes water retention.

(c) Gynecomastia results from an increase in female hormones that are normally present in small amounts in males, but the unhealthy liver does not destroy these.

B12. (a) Portal hypertension backlogs blood into esophageal veins, dilating them and increasing risk for rupture into the stomach (see Question B15[e]); a tendency to bleed exacerbates the condition.

(b) Like Mr. Nardella, he has ascites, but to such a degree that fluid presses on his diaphragm, causing dyspnea; diuretics reduce his fluid retention, and repeated paracentesis draws off abdominal fluid.

(c) The failing liver is not producing adequate clotting factors; splenomegaly (from backup of blood caused by portal hypertension) removes excessive numbers of platelets and red blood cells from blood; folic acid deficiency (from poor diet) may lead to megaloblastic anemia.

(d) Jaundice is a late manifestation of liver failure; clubbing results from chronic hypoxia associated with anemia and possible heart failure related to effects of toxic chemicals on myocardium.

(e) Caused by backup of portal vein into rectal veins (anorectal varices)

B13. See text.

B14. (a) Posthepatic
(b) Intrahepatic

B15. (a) Caput medusae
(b) Fetor hepaticus
(c) Asterixis
(d) Azotemia
(e) Esophageal varices (see Question B12[a])

B16. (a) 0.5 to 2; developing countries
(b) Hepatocytes; cirrhosis (and alcohol); HBV, HDV, and especially HCV (see Question B3[d])
(c) Cancer of the bile ducts; is not
(d) Late; 1
(e) Metastatic; colorectal, breast, lung, or urogenital

C1. (a) Concentrate
(b) Cholecystokinin (CCK)
(c) Cystic
(d) Small (duodenum)

C2. (a) Cholesterol; bilirubin
(b) Abnormalities in composition of bile, cholestasis, and inflammation of the gallbladder
(c) (3), (4), (5), (6), (8), (9)
(d) When bile flow is obstructed; right shoulder and back (via right phrenic nerve)
(e) Large

C3. (a) Cholelithiasis
(b) Choledocholithiasis
(c) Cholangitis
(d) Cholecystitis

C4. (a) Is
(b) Fatty meals
(c) Colicky
(d) (3)
(e) Cholangitis; if the duct ruptures, acute pancreatitis and possibly peritonitis (which may be fatal) may result (see Question C8 also).

C5. (b)

C6. Rare; insidious

C7. (a) Duodenum; spleen; only when changes are great because the pancreas has functional reserve and can expand greatly without exerting undue pressure on other organs.
(b) The main pancreatic duct, which unites with the common bile duct to form the hepatopancreatic ampulla, which empties into the duodenum
(c) Many; starch; fats
(d) Pancreatic enzymes are secreted in an inactive form and activated once they are in the duodenum; in addition, the pancreas produces a trypsin inhibitor.
(e) Alkaline; acid

C8. (a) Gallstones in the common bile duct or an alcoholic binge
(b) Alcohol stimulates pancreatic secretions that can block the passageway into the duodenum (sphincter of the bile duct), and it also is known to cause constriction of the sphincter of the pancreatic duct.
(c) The pain associated with this condition is aggravated when the person is lying supine; it is less severe when the person is sitting and leaning forward.
(d) Life-threatening; pancreatic enzymes can digest and necrose the pancreas and other abdominal tissues; this is acute necrotizing pancreatitis.
(e) These are compensatory mechanisms that accompany hypovolemia related to shift of fluid through inflamed abdominal tissues with pooling in the abdominal cavity or retroperitoneally.
(f) Amylase and lipase (because most of these are produced by pancreas cells); damage to pancreatic cells will release the normal contents of these cells into blood where the enzymes are then detected.
(g1) To replace those he is "third-spacing"
(g2) To decompress the distended bowel and inhibit secretion of pancreatic enzymes
(g3) To prevent infection of necrotic tissue resulting from inflammation

C9. (a) Thick mucus combined with protein plugs can block the passageway into the duodenum. Enzymes pass retrograde from duodenum into pancreas, digesting part or all of it.
(b) See Chapter 22, Question B18.

(c) The pancreas makes more than 80% of the body's lipases, especially in response to fatty foods. Lowering fat intake lowers lipase levels, which will help prevent digestion of fat in/on any abdominal organs and also reduce fat in the stool (steatorrhea).

(d) These enzymes help replace pancreatic enzymes that are "stuck" in the pancreas because of mucoprotein plugs.

C10. (a) 1%; elderly; after

(b) Diet high in calories, fat, meat, salt, dried foods, refined sugar, and soybeans

(c) Smoking and family history of some other cancers, such as melanoma and breast or colon cancers

(d) Insidious; pain, jaundice (if cancer of the head of the pancreas—which blocks bile ducts), weight loss, dull epigastric pain or back pain which are worse in the supine position

(e) Protective factors include a diet rich in vitamin C, fresh fruits and vegetables and other sources of dietary fiber; also avoidance of smoking, and other factors listed in C10(b).

Chapter 30

ORGANIZATION AND CONTROL OF THE ENDOCRINE SYSTEM

A1. See text.

A2. (a) Estrogen exerts effects on the uterus, breasts, ovaries, hypothalamus, pituitary, and bones.

(b) Increase of blood glucose is regulated by epinephrine, glucagon, cortisone, and growth hormone.

A3. Auto; juxta; blood plasma

A4. (a) Fatty acid derivatives

(b) Amines or amino acids

(c) Steroids

(d) Peptides, polypeptides, glycoproteins, and proteins

(e) Amines or amino acids

A5. (a) Smooth; peptide, polypeptide, or protein; rough

(b) Protein; Golgi

(c) Inactive; aldosterone, cortisone, estrogen, thyroid hormone (thyroxine)

(d) 99; aspirin competes for thyroxine's carrier and will lead to release of thyroxine into the unbound (active) state; this can exacerbate an already elevated thyroid hormone level (as in thyrotoxicosis)

(e) Days

A6. (a) Either degrades the hormone into an inactive form or activates some hormones

(b) In the liver or at the site of the hormone's receptor

(c) MAO (monoamine oxidase) or COMT (catechol O-methyltransferase)

(d) They are conjugated in the liver, which inactivates them, and are then eliminated in bile.

A7. Hormones bind to cells that have specific receptors for the hormone (much like locks into which only one type of key fits).

(a) As many as 100,000

(b) Increase; induction; up-regulation

(c) Water; cannot; surface; first; cAMP; second; second

(d) Can (because they are lipid); intracellular

A8. (a) Hypothalamus

(b) Anterior pituitary

(c) Anterior pituitary

(d) Adrenal cortex

(e) Posterior pituitary (note that these are synthesized in hypothalamus)

(f) Kidney

(g) Testes and adrenal cortex

A9. (a) Calcitonin

(b) Insulin

(c) Releasing hormones such as CRH, GnRH, and TRH

(d) Catecholamines including epinephrine (adrenalin) and norepinephrine

(e) GH

(f) Gastrin

B1. (a) Blood vessels; hypothalamus; anterior pituitary; releasing

(b) Anterior; thyroid; thyroid hormone (T_3T_4); negative or opposite; decrease

(c) Cortex; cortisol; glucose; exo; decrease; suppression

(d) Anterior pituitary

(e) Insulin and glucagon (by glucose), calcitonin and PTH (by Ca^{2+}), and aldosterone (by blood levels of Na^+ and K^+)

B2. (a) IRMA and RIA

(b) See text.

(c) They provide information about the size of endocrine glands for diagnosis of tumors or follow-up monitoring.

Chapter 31

DISORDERS OF ENDOCRINE FUNCTION

A1. Hypo; see text

A2. (a) 3° if hypothalamus is destroyed or 2° if the pituitary is destroyed by radiation

(b) 1°

(c) 2°

B1. (a) ACTH: adrenocorticotropic hormone

(b) FSH: follicle-stimulating hormone

(c) LH: luteinizing hormone

(d) TSH: thyroid-stimulating hormone

(e) GH: growth hormone

(f) PRL: prolactin

(a), (b), (c), and (d)

B2. (a), (e), (f); but (b) hypothalamus, (c) 70% to 90% and (d) sometimes

B3. GH → LH → FSH → TSH → ACTH (*Hint:* remember the mnemonic "Go Look For The Adenoma.")

B4. (a) GH, insulin, T_3T_4, androgens
  (b) (1), (2); but (3) indirectly by stimulation of the liver to produce IGFs and (4) increases use of fats and decreases use of carbohydrates

B5. (b), (c), (e); but (a) throughout life, (d) inhibited, and (f) increase

B6. (a) Actual height, velocity of growth, and parental height
  (b) Is
  (c) These techniques can assess the size and shape of the pituitary gland within the sella turcica of the sphenoid bone.
  (d) Short; normal; recombinant DNA
  (e) Male children: 6'1"; female children: 5'8"

B7. (a) Laron-type dwarfism
  (b) Psychosocial dwarfism
  (c) Genetically short stature
  (d) Panhypopituitarism
  (e) Constitutional short stature
  (f) Congenital GH deficiency

B8. (a) Somatopause
  (b) Acromegaly
  (c) Gigantism

B9. (a) Is not; growth plates in his long bones closed decades ago
  (b) Rare; insidious; benign
  (c) Organs (including the heart) grow abnormally large; cardiomegaly is likely to lead to cardiac ischemia. Excessive GH also causes release of free fatty acids from adipose tissue; possible acromegaly-related diabetes also would increase cardiac risk.
  (d) His enlarged pituitary increases pressure on his optic nerves, blood vessels, and meninges.
  (e) A transsphenoidal approach accesses the pituitary through the nose.

B10. (a) Thelarche
  (b) Menarche
  (c) Isosexual precocious puberty

C1. (a) Larynx; follicles; thyroglobulin
  (b) Tyrosine; iodide; triiodothyronine (T_3); three
  (c) Protein; TBG; free
  (d) De; in (see Chapter 30, Question A5[d])

C2. See Chapter 30. Inhibit; triggers; hypothalamus

C3. All major; increases
  (a) De
  (b) In
  (c) De; in
  (d) In; in
  (e) De; in; de
  (f) In
  (g) In; de

C4. (a–e) All hypo

C5. (a) Goiter
  (b) Cretinism
  (c) Myxedema
  (d) Myxedema
  (e) Hashimoto disease
  (f) Thyroid storm
  (g) Graves disease

C6. (a), (d); but (b) the most common and (c) an acute

D1. (a) On top of the kidneys
  (b1) M
  (b2) C
  (b3) C
  (b4) C

D2. (a) Aldosterone
  (b) Aldosterone
  (c) Dehydroepiandrosterone (DHEA)
  (d) Cortisol

D3. Varies with time of day; ACTH (and consequently, cortisol) are higher in the morning and lower at night. This pattern is reversed for night workers and is altered with Cushing syndrome.

D4. (a) Increases
  (b) Breakdown
  (c) Gluconeogenesis
  (d) Decreases
  (e) Decreases
  (f) Decreases
  (g) Anti-inflammatory

D5. (a) Glucocorticoids affect parts of the brain that alter mood and behavior.
  (b) Exogenous cortisone inhibits her production of CRH and ACTH, causing atrophy of her adrenal gland.
  (c) This is dangerous because her atrophied adrenals cannot suddenly begin making cortisol; gradual weaning from steroids can prevent this problem; recovery may take a year or more.

D6. (a) 24-hour urinary free cortisol test
  (b) Administration of a high level of (exogenous) dexamethasone (synthetic glucocorticoid) normally exerts a negative feedback effect to suppress ACTH production.

D7. (a) Is; cortisol
  (b) Increases; increases; increases; virilizing effects of her external genitalia

D8. (a) Secondary adrenal cortical insufficiency
  (b) Secondary adrenal cortical insufficiency (she may have developed iatrogenic Cushing syndrome)
  (c) Adrenogenital syndrome
  (d) Addison disease
  (e) Cushing disease (a form of Cushing syndrome)
  (f) Cushing syndrome (ectopic)

D9. (a) Primary (because the problem lies in the thyroid gland itself); 10%
  (b) (1) and (3) (due to deficiency of aldosterone); but (2) a sign of Cushing syndrome, (4) hypoglycemia and lethargy, and (5) bronzed skin because his high ACTH levels mimic high melanocyte-stimulating hormone (MSH)
  (c) Will; should

D10. Excessive; (b) (moon face and buffalo hump), (c) (purple striae); but (a) opposite, (d) osteoporosis, and (e) hypertension related to the effects of steroids on fluid retention

Chapter 32

DIABETES MELLITUS AND THE METABOLIC SYNDROME

A1. Its high incidence (more than 18 million persons) and effects on so many systems (cardiovascular, renal, and special senses, especially eyes); its prevalence is greater among minority populations such as Hispanics and African Americans.

A2. (a) Carbohydrates
(b) Fats
(c) Fats
(d) Fats
(e) Proteins
(f) Carbohydrates and fats

A3. Islets of Langerhans
(a) Glucagon, increases
(b) Insulin, decreases; amylin
(c) Somatostatin; insulin, glucagon; decreases

A4. Effects of hormones that trigger release of insulin after a high-carbohydrate meal; glucagon-like peptide-1 (GLP-1) and glucose-dependent insulinotropic polypeptide (GIP); small intestine; mimics

A5. (a) 76; 36
(b) (1), (3)
(c) (3); liver
(d) (1)
(e) Cortisol, epinephrine, glucagon
(f) (2)
(g) Lacks. This enzyme is required for catabolism of stored glycogen sufficient to allow products to pass through the cell membrane and enter the circulation; therefore, glycogen stored in muscles cannot be directly used as an energy source for the body. However, use of stored glycogen by muscle cells does permit other glucose sources to be available to tissues such as the brain.
(h) Increases; insulin; blood into cells, stimulates, glycogen (glycogenesis); lowers
(i) All except insulin; insulin; increases

A6. (a) Protein; C
(b) Glucose; GLUT-2; preformed (followed by release of newly synthesized insulin)
(c) Portal vein; 15
(d) Adipose and skeletal muscle; insulin; 1; does not
(e) Amino acids; protein; fatty acids; lysis
(f) Inhibit, antagonizes; increase
(g) Excessive GH (in acromegaly) and cortisol (in chronic stress or in Cushing syndrome) both lead to chronic increase in blood glucose (Figure 32-1, *A* and *B*) and overstimulation of beta cells, which can lead to diabetes.

B1. (a), (c); but (b) sweet, related to sugar in urine and
(d) Fewer

B2. (a1) C
(a2) A
(a3) D
(b) 1A; immune-mediated; insulin; do; juvenile
(c) Inhibits; 1; ketones or ketoacids (diabetic ketoacidosis or DKA)

(d) Is; 95
(e) Beta cells are destroyed; 85%
(f) Honeymoon period
(g) Few; idiopathic (no known cause)

B3. (a1) Resistance
(a2) Abnormal (increased and then decreased as beta cell exhaustion occurs)
(a3) Increased
(b) Obese, high; diabesity, metabolic syndrome; can

B4. See text.

B5. (a) Obesity
(b) High, low
(c) Increased, increased
(d) Hypertension, increased

B6. Cause
(a) Gestational diabetes mellitus
(b) Endocrine disorder
(c) Drug disorders

B7. (a), (b), (d), (f), (i) ; but (c) older women, (e) more than five pregnancies, (g) obese, and (h) glucosuria

B8. Even mild maternal hyperglycemia can be injurious to the developing fetus; are

B9. (a) 2
(b) Increased; high blood glucose (hyperglycemia) "spills over" into urine and "pulls" water (osmotically) into urine; decreased circulating blood can lead to hypotension, hypoxia, and fatigue
(c) Polydipsia (clients "dip into water" as cells are dehydrated by polyuria)
(d) 1; cells cannot access glucose, fats, or proteins
(e) 1; fluid loss (polyuria), depletion of cellular fat and protein as these are "burned" for fuel, and possibly vomiting with episodes of ketoacidosis
(f) More; glucose in skin and mucus "invites" microbes, including *Candida;* loss of sensation reduces awareness and early treatment of infection
(g) High blood glucose can pull fluid from the lens

B10. (a) Oral glucose tolerance test
(b) Fasting blood glucose test
(c) Casual blood glucose test
(d) Glycated hemoglobin (A1C) test
(e) Self-monitoring test

B11. (a) Blood; checks for ketones that can detect ketoacidosis for type 1 or pregnant diabetics
(b) Nutrition, exercise, and antidiabetic agents (oral hypoglycemic medications), along with education for self-management and problem solving
(c) Does not; consistent
(d) See text.

B12. 2
(a) ISC, IHC
(b) IHC, ISC (so may be toxic to liver)
(c) SBC, ISC

B13. (a) Insulin (required for individuals with type 1 diabetes); insulin is a protein and would be destroyed by gastric acid and enzymes
(b1) Short-acting

    (b2) Long-acting

    (b3) Intermediate-acting

    (c) Is

C1. (a) Hypoglycemia

    (b) Diabetic ketoacidosis (DKA) (See Study Guide Figure 32-1, C.)

    (c) Hyperglycemic hyperosmolar state (HHS) and diabetic ketoacidosis

    (d) Hypoglycemia

    (e) Diabetic ketoacidosis and hypoglycemia

    (f) HHS

    (g) HHS

    (h) HHS

C2. 260

    (a) (1), (2), (3), (4)

    (b) Ketones; acids; decrease; decrease

    (c) Fruity smell of her breath as blood with ketones passes through her lungs; ketones can be detected in her urine by a "dip stick" method; she may exhibit signs of DKA.

    (d) Decrease; tachy; hyperglycemic blood leads to polyuria with low circulating blood volume; heart rate increases (tachycardia) as a compensatory mechanism for low blood pressure.

    (e) Rapid and deep (Kussmaul respirations); acidosis (and related hypercarbia) will stimulate respiratory centers.

    (f) Lower blood glucose and increase fluids (IV) gradually to prevent cerebral edema; raise blood pH; correct Na^+ and K^+ imbalances

C3. (a) (2), (3), (4)

    (b) (1), (2), (5); but (3) may occur as a parasympathetic response and (4) may occur if sympathetic responses dominate causing vasoconstriction and sweating

    (c) (2); but (3) or (4) once he is conscious

C4. (a) Increase

    (b) Hypo

    (c) Increase; epinephrine, glucagon, cortisol, and growth hormone

    (d) Somogyi; hypo, hyper

    (e) Morning; exacerbate

C5 (a), (e); but (b) kidneys, (c) common, and (d) glomeruli

C6. (a) Feet and hands; proximally; "stocking-glove"; bilateral

    (b) Loss of sensation can lead to burns and exacerbations related to lack of awareness of infection; weakness can result in falls that injure joints.

    (c) (3), (4), (5), (6); but (1) and (2) signs of peripheral neuropathies

    (d) (1), (2), (3), (4), (6)

    (e) Heart (heart attack), brain (stroke), feet and legs (peripheral vascular disease with ulcerations)

    (f) His inability to sense on the plantar surface of his foot; loss of sensation of pain and muscle sense (proprioception) that can lead to foot injuries and increased risk of infection related to hyperglycemia

    (g) Retinopathy; (1) (because onset of type 1 DM is likely to be early in life) and (2); (3) and (4) somewhat because they contribute to stress and related hyperglycemia

C7. Tight control of blood glucose levels, maintenance of normal lipid levels, and control of hypertension

Chapter 33

ORGANIZATION AND CONTROL OF NEURAL FUNCTION

A1. See Chapter 1, answers to Questions D10–D11.

A2. Peripheral

    (a) Myelin; white

    (b) Insulator; increases; lacking; saltatory

    (c) Is; neurons lacking myelin will die, possibly because the myelin sheath secretes neurotrophic compounds

    (d) Regeneration; central; may account for the fact that CNS neurons do not regenerate well

A3. (a) Astroglia

    (b) Astroglia

    (c) Ependymal cells

    (d) Microglia

    (e) Oligodendroglia

    (f) Satellite cells

    (g) Satellite cells, Schwann cells

A4. (a) 2; 20; hyper

    (b) Cannot; glial cells do store glycogen, and ketones can provide small amounts of energy

    (c) No; death is likely to begin after 4 to 6 minutes of anoxia

    (d) Hypoglycemia deprives the brain of a constant supply of glucose.

B1. Action potential

    (a) Negative

    (b) Sodium; negative; is; depolarization

    (c) Potassium; negative; hyper

B2. (a) Electrical

    (b) Chemical

B3. (b) → (c) → (a) → (e) → (d)

D4. (a) Each neuron may be involved in thousands of synapses between different parts of neurons; the excitatory and inhibitory effects are additive.

    (b) Transmission at chemical synapses requires only 0.3 msec (thousandths of a second).

    (c) These include a myriad of neurotransmitters, hormones, neuromodulators, and growth factors.

B5. (a) Dopamine, norepinephrine, serotonin

    (b) Endorphins and enkephalins, substance P

    (c) Acetylcholine

B6. (a) ADH (vasopressin)

    (b) Neuromodulator

    (c) Neurotropic

C1. (a) Cognition; regulation of breathing

    (b) Central; skeletal; vertebral column

    (c) Meninges, vertebrae, muscles, and skin; spina bifida with meningomyelocele

(d) Forebrain

(e2) Ectoderm

(e3) Mesoderm

(e4) Mesoderm

(e5) Mesoderm

(e6) Mesoderm

(e7) Endoderm

(e8) Endoderm

(f) 33; 10

(g) 2; dorsal; sensory; IA; dorsal

(h) Output; motor; lower; output association; ventral

(i) Internuncial

C2. (a) SSA

(b) GSE; GSA

(c) SVA; PE; GVE; GVA

C3. White; outer

(a) Archi; shortest

(b) Paleo; middle

(c) Neo; brainstem and cerebrum; approximately 6 years of age; adequate myelination is required before a child can achieve bladder control or fine, coordinated movements.

D1. (a) Shorter; L1 or L2; cauda equina (horse's tail)

(b) At L3 or L4; this site is inferior to the lower end of the spinal cord, so the cord is not injured during the procedure

(c) Gray; ventral; motor; lower; skeletal

(d) C5 and lumbar to upper sacral, which are origins of nerves that supply arms and legs

(e) Denticulate ligaments and filum terminale (both pia mater) and spinal nerve roots

D2. (a) 32; Cervical: 8; Thoracic: 12; Lumbar: 5; Sacral: 5; Coccygeal: 2+

(b) Sensory; motor; mixed

(c) Branches of spinal nerves, and all are mixed; ventral because they form plexuses that supply all except small regions posterior to the vertebrae

(d) Axons of sympathetic nerves en route to sympathetic ganglia

(e) Both sensory and motor; (2), (1), (3), (4)

D3. (a) L2–S1 (and portions of S2–S4)

(b) C5–C8 (and T1)

(c) C1–C4

D4. (a) Cerebrum, hypothalamus, thalamus

(b) Midbrain

(c) Cerebellum, medulla, pons

D5. Fore(brain); recent; more

D6. (a) Pons

(b) Medulla

(c) Midbrain

(d) Cerebellum, medulla, and pons

(e) Midbrain

(f) Thalamus and hypothalamus

D7. (a) IX–XII (9–12)

(b) V–VIII (5–8)

(c) III–IV (3–4)

(d) XI (11)

D8. (a) Oculomotor, III, L

(b) Spinal accessory, XI, R

(c) Facial, VII, L

(d) Hypoglossal, XII

(e) Facial, VII; note that glossopharyngeal (IX) would affect saliva (but not tear) production

(f) Trigeminal (mandibular branch), V

D9. (a) H

(b) T

(c) T

(d) H

D10. (a1) Corpus callosum, W

(a2) Basal ganglia, G

(a3) Internal capsule, W

(b1) Temporal

(b2) Occipital

(b3) Parietal

(b4) Frontal

D11. (a) Limbic system

(b) Premotor area (6)

(c) Primary auditory cortex (area 41)

(d) Auditory association area (22)

(e) Somatosensory association cortex (5 and 7)

D12. (a) Dura mater, arachnoid, pia mater

(b) Pia mater

(c) Dura mater

D13. Cranial bones; meninges (including the falx cerebri and tentorium cerebelli that limit shifting of cerebral hemispheres) and CSF

D14. (a) Capillaries of the choroid plexuses located in the four ventricles

(b) 0.5 to 0.75 (Note: 1 cup = 237 mL)

(c) Lateral ventricles → (Interventricular foramina of Monro) third ventricle → cerebral aqueduct → fourth ventricle → (Foramina of Luschka and Magendie) subarachnoid space → arachnoid villi → superior sagittal sinus

D15. (a) Tight junctions of endothelial cells, basement membrane, and astrocytes

(b) All except epinephrine (a catecholamine)

(c) Ependymal

(d) CO_2, H_2O, O_2

E1. Subconscious regulation of viscera

E2. (a) S (Memory aid: S for Stress)

(b) P (Memory aid: P for Peace)

(c) S

(d) P

(e) P

(f) P

(g) S

(h) P

(i) S

E3. (a), (d); but (b) opposing and (c) parasympathetic

E4. (a) III, VII, IX, and X

(b) Solid; P

(c) S

(d) S; many

(e) S; S

(f) S

(g) P

(h) Adrenal medulla, blood vessels of skin, hair muscles of skin, sweat glands

E5. (a) See text.

(b) See text.

E6. (a) Acetylcholine

(b) Acetylcholine

(c) Norepinephrine (or other catecholamines)

(d) Acetylcholine

(e) Norepinephrine (or other catecholamines)

E7. (a) Acetyl CoA + choline; nicotinic and muscarinic; muscarinic

(b) AChE

(c) Tyrosine (an amino acid) $\rightarrow$ DOPA $\rightarrow$ Dopamine

(d) Norepinephrine; epinephrine

(e) Active reuptake (recycling) by the presynaptic neuron, enzymatic destruction by the enzymes MAO or COMT, or diffusion of the neurotransmitter into tissues surrounding the synapse

(f) Adrenergic

(f1) (3)

(f2) Increases; decrease

(f3) Relax; dilate

(f4) Contract; constriction; increase

Chapter 34

DISORDERS OF SOMATOSENSORY FUNCTION AND PAIN

A1. (a) Three; peripheral; dorsal root; C6–C8

(b) Do; anterolateral; left

(c) Cerebral cortex; left; parietal; homunculus; (3)

(d) (1)

A2. (a) Anterolateral pathway

(b) Dorsal column-medial lemniscal pathway

(c) Dorsal column-medial lemniscal pathway

(d) Anterolateral pathway

(e) Dorsal column-medial lemniscal pathway

(f) Dorsal column-medial lemniscal pathway

(g) Anterolateral pathway

A3. (a) Thoracic

(b) C5 to C7

(c) L2 and L3

A4. (a) Touch, heat, pain, pressure, tickle, itch, muscle or joint awareness (proprioception), vision, hearing, taste, smell

(b) Selective sensitivity of receptors to specific forms of physical or chemical energy

A5. (a) Meissner corpuscles

(b) Pacinian corpuscles

(c) Free nerve endings

(d) Hair follicle end-organs

(e) Ruffini end organs

A6. (a) Lips; fingers

(b) Do not; sensation of temperature change is protective

(c) Awareness of body position and movement

(d) Dynamic

B1. It is a warning signal of tissue injury but is also "a pain."

B2. (a) Common

(b) Virtually all; pattern

B3. (a) Fast; slow; Melzack, Wall

(b) Multiple factors, many including the brain, genetics, and culture, influence perception of pain. See text.

B4. Pain

(a) Skin, teeth, periosteum, meninges, and internal organs

(b1) Mechanical: intense pressure, muscle contraction, or stretching of tissues

(b2) Heat or cold

(b3) Chemical: release of chemicals (such as prostaglandins, leukotrienes, histamine, or bradykinin) is associated with trauma, inflammation, or ischemia

(c) Aδ

(d) Aδ; vasodilation; chronic

(e) Neo; fast; paleo

(f) Such stimulation affects Aδ sensory fibers, depressing pain signals from the same area.

B5. (a) Thalamus

(b) Somatosensory area of parietal cortex

(c) Association areas of parietal cortex

(d) Limbic cortex

B6. (a), (d), (e); but (b) initiate and prolong and (c) midbrain and leads to analgesia (pain relief)

B7. They are the body's own (endogenous) pain-killing chemicals; enkephalins, endorphins, and dynorphins

B8. Tolerance; threshold

B9. (a) Deep somatic; sharp, bright

(b) Visceral; splanchnic; autonomic nervous system (ANS) nerves are activated

(c) (1)

(d) Is not; see text

(e) Referred; pain from visceral receptors (in ischemic heart) enters dorsal roots at the same level as somatic afferents (from skin in left arm and chest)

(f) Right; neck; these organs lie just inferior to the diaphragm, which developed embryologically in the neck with its nerve supply at C3 to C5

(g) Acute; 6; anxiety, muscle spasms, and sympathetic responses

(h) Acute; it serves as a warning signal and points to possible diagnoses, whereas chronic pain extends beyond a period of usefulness and can deplete resources.

(i) Chronic

B10. (a) (1)

(b) Questions or scales that describe quality, severity, duration, location, pattern, radiation of pain; questions about factors that trigger or relieve pain; Ms. Templeton's reaction to pain

B11. (a), (d); but (b) less, (c) less, and (e) not all

B12. (b), (c)

B13. (a), (d); but (b) sensitize and (c) reverse

B14. Without

(a) Codeine, morphine

(b) Aspirin, nonsteroidal anti-inflammatory drugs (NSAIDs)

(c) Acetaminophen

(d) Serotonin reuptake inhibitors

B15. (c), (d); but (a) euphoria, a decrease and (b) and for

C1. (a) Paresthesia

(b) Hyperalgesia

(c) Hyperpathia

(d) Allodynia

(e) Athermia

C2. (a) Nerve compression or entrapment or specific neuralgias (trigeminal or postherpetic)

(b) Diabetes mellitus, chronic alcoholism, hypothyroidism, renal alterations, and neurotoxic drugs

C3. (a) Treat the underlying cause, such as diabetes or hypothyroidism.

(b) Palliative pain medications ease pain without curing the underlying cause (such as cancer).

C4. Severe, often repetitive pain along cranial or spinal nerves

(a) Trigeminal; cranial nerve V; unilateral; severe, lightning-like; light touch along the face; see text

(b) Zoster; shingles; chickenpox; more because of decrease in numbers of large nerve fibers and decreased immunity

(c) Sympathetic nerves are involved, and these affect blood vessel diameter and sweat glands.

C5. 70%. See text.

D1. (a), (b); but (c) some but not most and (d) without

D2. Sudden onset of severe, intractable (not responsive to treatment) pain; also those that disturb sleep, occur with exertion, or are accompanied by drowsiness, changes in vision or mental status; or a new headache in children under 5 years or adults over 50 years

D3. Factors that trigger, exacerbate, or relieve the headache, including meals, alcohol, stress, exercise, menstrual cycle, and medications

D4. (a) Tension-type

(b) Tension-type

(c) Migraine

(d) Migraine

(e) Cluster

(f) Tension-type

(g) Temporomandibular joint (TMJ) syndrome

(h) Cluster

D5. (a) 5 to 20 minutes

(b1) Double vision related to paralysis of eye muscles

(b2) Mixed type of migraine that is combined with tension-type or chronic daily headache

(c) Can; (3), (4), (5)

(d) Are not; trigeminal; does; dilate

(e) Nonpharmacologic; avoidance of triggers (including certain foods, possibly chocolate and aged cheese), regular patterns of eating and sleeping; stress

E1. Research indicates that neonates respond to painful heel sticks, children as young as 3 years accurately report and remember pain, and the prevalence of pain increases among elderly.

E2. (a) Show pictures of faces with smiley or hurting expressions or show outlines of bodies on which Jewel can indicate location of pain

(b) Numeric or word graphic codes, and the child's self-report of pain

E3. Before; positive self-talk, imagery, modeling, and rehearsal

E4. To maintain a steady blood level of the medication in an attempt to prevent pain

E5. They may not want to be a burden or to experience testing or treatment or related costs.

E6. (a) Decreased absorption of drugs from stomach or intestine, related to decreased perfusion and motility of these organs, may lead to inadequate blood levels of the drugs

(b) Decreased metabolism and elimination of medications by decreased liver or kidney function may increase blood levels of drugs

E7. (a) Elderly persons may already be taking a number of medications (polypharmacy) for other health conditions.

(b) Some elderly persons may not take proper dosages of drugs related to confusion, forgetfulness, impaired mobility, or cost of the drugs.

Chapter 35

DISORDERS OF NEUROMUSCULAR FUNCTION

A1. C → B → A

A2. A lower motoneuron (LMN) and the muscle fibers it innervates; thousands; small

A3. (a) Supplementary motor cortex

(b) Primary motor cortex

(c) Premotor cortex

(d) Primary motor cortex

A4. (b) → (a) → (d) → (c) → (f) → (e)

A5. (d), (e); but (a) hands and face, (b) face, and (c) left

A6. (a) Pyramidal

(b) Extrapyramidal

(c) Extrapyramidal

A7. (a) Afferent (sensory) neuron → synapse → efferent (motor) neuron

(b) By stretching of the tendon of a muscle; knee-jerk reflex

(c1) Belly; intrafusal; 1a, rapidly

(c2) Dorsal

(c3) Alpha, extrafusal; flexion

(c4) Hamstrings; known as reciprocal innervation, relaxation of opposing (antagonistic) muscles enhances speed and efficiency of movements by prime movers (in this case, the quadriceps).

(c5) They monitor the functional status of muscle fibers from moment-to-moment as muscles shorten or lengthen.

(d) Proprioception

(e) Inhibited; crossed-extensor

A8. (a) Less than normal
(b) Increased; inhibit
(c) Paresis; para; hemi
(d) LMNs; hypertonia or spasticity

A9. (a) (1)
(b) UMNs, below
(c) Complete use; spasticity (because regions below T6 still have spinal cord reflexes because LMNs are intact there)
(d) Is; may (by first level reflexes involving tactile stimulation but not by psychic or visual stimuli because spinal pathways are severed)

A10. (a) LMNs; hyper; tetany
(b) LMNs; flaccid; atrophy

A11. L4; right

B1. (a) Duchenne muscular dystrophy
(b) Denervation atrophy and disuse atrophy
(c) Myasthenia gravis
(d) Disuse atrophy
(e) Polyneuropathy
(f) Mononeuropathy

B2. (a) Males, because DMD is an X-linked disorder. (DMD occurs rarely in females by spontaneous mutation.)
(b) Muscular; dystrophin
(c) (1), (4)
(d) High; shows muscle cell destruction with leakage of contents into blood
(e) Chorionic villi sampling
(f) Is not; cardiovascular (heart), respiratory (diaphragm)

B3. (a) Acetylcholinesterase
(b) Physostigmine and neostigmine
(c) Curare
(d) *Clostridium botulinum* toxin
(e) Malathion

B4. (a) Women
(b) (1), (2), (3); but (4) more distal movements are less affected and (5) myasthenia gravis is a neuromuscular junction disorder, not a sensory disorder
(c) Physostigmine and neostigmine
(d) Antibodies that may be attacking her neuromuscular junctions (NMJs)
(e) Respiratory failure

B5. (a) (3), (4)
(b1) Segmental demyelination
(b2) Axonal degeneration
(c) Far away from
(d) Endoneurial tube; Schwann cells
(e) Less; axons

B6. (a) (1), (2); but (3) hyperthyroidism
(b) (2), (3); but (1) numbness in thumb, index finger, and middle finger
(c) Can be

B7. Poly

B8. Common; 90%; (a), (c), and (d)

B9. (a) Herniated; (soft inner) nucleus pulposus; posteriorly, because ligamentous support is weakest there

(b) L4–L5 (the greatest weight-bearing region); common
(c) Pain; rare

C1. (a) Cerebrum
(b) Putamen; caudate nucleus
(c) Nigra; dopamine
(d) Do; these connections modulate voluntary movements, posture, and muscle tone, leading to efficient, balanced, graceful movements.

C2. (a) Chorea
(b) Athetosis
(c) Ballismus
(d) Tardive dyskinesia
(e) Tic
(f) Dystonia

C3. (a) After; before
(b) Idiopathic; after long-term use of antipsychotic drugs or severe carbon monoxide poisoning, after stroke, head trauma, or encephalitis
(c) Is; 80%; tremor, rigidity, and bradykinesia; unilateral
(d1) Bradykinesia
(d2) Cog-wheel movements
(d3) Tremor
(d4) Masklike face
(d5) Dysphagia
(d6) Autonomic manifestations
(e) Five
(f1) Drug that increases dopamine levels
(f2) Decrease levels of (excitatory) ACh to balance low levels of (inhibitory) dopamine

C4. Inferior; tentorium cerebelli
(a) Helps to produce smooth movements, especially in skilled movements that require repeated practice
(b) Compares and evaluates the actual movement with the intended movement

C5. Stroke or trauma that leads to ischemia; tumor; chronic alcoholism

C6. (a) Truncal ataxia
(b) Intention tremor
(c) Dysdiadochokinesia
(d) Over- and under-reaching
(e) Dysarthria
(f) Nystagmus

D1. (a) Lou Gehrig; few; older; 2 to 5
(b1) Shrinkage of muscles related to destruction of
(b2) Lateral corticospinal tracts (axons of UMNs) in the spinal cord
(b3) Hardening caused by scar tissue (gliosis) in lateral corticospinal tracts
(c) (2), (4), (6), (7)
(d) An antiglutamate drug (riluzole)
(e) By blinking eyelids or moving eyes

D2. (a) Before; women; is
(b) CNS; plaques; decreases; oligodendrocyte; both
(c) Multiple demyelinated areas of axons become hardened plaques with scar formation (gliosis) composed of proteins, enzymes, and various cells that indicate inflammation.

(d) Is; T cells and antibodies may induce oligodendrocyte damage.

(e) (3), (4)

(f) See text.

(g) (1), (3)

(h) See text.

D3. (d)

D4. (a) Flexion: the head is struck from behind or the person falls backward on the back of the head; extension: the neck is hyperextended, for example, by a fall on the chin or face

(b) Compression: by a severe blow to the top of the head or a forceful landing on the feet; axial rotation: tearing of vertebral ligaments by a twisting fall

(c) Primary: irreversible injury (compression, shearing, fracture, dislocation, or penetration) that occurs at the time of the trauma; secondary: tissue necrosis that follows the initial injury, for example, by severing of blood vessels, vasospasm, inflammation and edema, or spinal shock

D5. Tetraplegia (or quadriplegia) refers to loss of function in all four extremities, trunk, and pelvic organs; in paraplegia, use of the arms and upper trunk is retained.

D6. (a) I

(b) C

(c) I

(d) I

D7. (a) B

(b) Left; contralateral; ipsilateral

(c) Arms; the elderly

(d) Arms; cauda equina; is

(e) Primary; is not; secondary (see Question D4[c])

D8. (a) To preserve residual neurologic function and prevent additional neurologic damage

(b) To maintain circulation to the injured cord (and to the rest of the body)

(c) To reduce inflammation and edema that could impede blood flow and exert pressure on injured tissues

D9. (b), (c), (e); but (a) more; and (d) is not because tenodesis (natural finger flexion when wrists are hyperextended) requires use of arms and wrists as with C6 or lower SCIs

D10. (a) Is; spastic

(b) A; absent; positive

D11. C3 to C5; intercostal muscles receive innervation from T1 to T7, and abdominal muscles from T7 to T12; both of these sets of muscles are required for coughing and deep breathing needed to clear mucus from lungs.

D12. Low

(a) Persist (because it arises from the medulla, which is not injured in the SCI); its slowing effect on the heart is not counterbalanced by sympathetic impulses.

(b) Ann; because her injury is so high (C3) that more of her sympathetic nerves (all those originating below her injury) are deprived of their regulation from the brainstem. Sympathetic nerves (from about levels T1–T5) to the heart do not stimulate the heart (which also receives less venous return from paralyzed lower extremities); nerves from T1–L2 do not vasoconstrict blood vessels to maintain blood pressure; excessive blood in dilated skin vessels gives up heat, which lowers the body temperature.

(c) Suctioning stimulates afferents of vagus nerves and leads to bradycardia (vagovagal response).

(d) Postural (orthostatic) hypotension; gradual elevation to the sitting upright position and wearing of compression hose

D13. (a) Ann and Mr. Tenley; their injuries are high (T6 or above) with large areas (below injury) of unregulated sympathetic nerves

(b) Full bladder or rectum or painful episodes (see others in text)

(c) Exaggerated; pallor; high

(d) Flushing; dilation; brady

(e) Lower; upper; is

D14. (a) Immobility leads to edema, stasis of blood, and increased risk of clot formation.

(b) See text.

(c) Once the period of spinal shock (areflexia) is over, persons with UMN disorders experience lack of awareness of bladder filling and have spastic bladder (micturition when bladder is full); persons with LMN lesions cannot void voluntarily or involuntarily because of the flaccid bladder.

(d) Spastic bowel if the lesion is above S2 to S4 of the cord, and flaccid bowel if below S2 to S4 of the cord

(e) See text.

(f) See text.

Chapter 36

DISORDERS OF BRAIN FUNCTION

A1. (a) 2; 20

(b) Ischemia; hypoxia

(c) They depend on anaerobic metabolism.

(d) Focal; cardiac arrest, circulatory shock

(e) 2 to 4; formation of blood clots and blood sludging with high blood viscosity and increased resistance to flow; possibly vasoconstriction following acidosis

(f) Ionic gradients; Na^+ and water enter brain cells, causing them to swell (cerebral edema); prolonged ischemia can lead to cell death (cerebral infarction).

(g) (3), (4) and (5).

(h) Distal; see text.

A2. (a) Glutamate

(b) Memory, cognition, movement, and sensation

(c) Stroke, severe hypoglycemia, and neurodegenerative disorders such as Huntington disease, amyotrophic lateral sclerosis (ALS), and Alzheimer dementia.

(d) NMDA receptors for the neurotransmitter glutamate allow excessive calcium to enter cells; the resulting calcium cascade leads to release of intracellular enzymes that can injure and kill brain cells.

(e) They interfere with glutamate-NMDA pathways.

A3. (a) Vasogenic

(b) Cytotoxic

A4. (a1) Brain; brain tumor or cerebral edema resulting from trauma or surgery

(a2) Cerebrospinal fluid (CSF); excessive CSF production or obstructed outflow

(a3) Cerebral blood; hemorrhage or obstructed venous outflow

(b) Brain (edema); blood (hemorrhage and possible obstruction to outflow by clot formation); and possibly CSF (by obstruction of outflow caused by brain edema, bleeding, and clots)

(c) Dramatically

(d) Decreased level of consciousness (LOC), evidenced by lethargy and confusion

(e) Her MABP is 110 + 30 = 140 mm Hg. Her CPP is MABP − ICP = 140 − 55 = 85; normal although both MABP and ICP are high.

(f) Increased; systolic; constriction; widened

(g) Brady; ischemic (triad); late

A5. (a) Dura; vertically; the two cerebral hemispheres; cingulate, anterior; medial; leg

(b1) A horizontal section of dura mater, it separates cerebral hemispheres from cerebellum; transtentorial or central

(b2) Opening or "notch" in the tentorium through which the midbrain passes; uncal

(c) Blindness, respiratory arrest, dilated pupil; posturing (decorticate or decerebrate); possibly death by compression of vital structures in the medulla

(d) Decorticate

(e1) Infratentorial

(e2) Brainstem

A6. (a) CSF

(b1) NC

(b2) C

(c) Infants; because sutures are still open

(d) (2), (3), (4)

(e) Ophthalmoscopic observation of the optic nerve

A7. The skull and CSF normally do offer protection, but the skull cannot expand to accommodate swelling or bleeding of the brain; fractured skull bones can inflict injury on the brain; excess CSF can exert pressure on the brain.

A8. (a) Accidents involving vehicles and pedestrians; comminuted

(b) Concussion, contusion, and diffuse axonal injury

(c) Concussion, contusion; do

(d) Diffuse axonal injury

(e) Posterior

(f) Ischemia

A9. (a1) Epidural; rapid

(a2) Right; left

(a3) Is

(b1) Subacute

(b2) Arachnoid membrane; veins; slowly

A10. (a) Medulla, midbrain, hypothalamus, pons, thalamus

(b) Ascending reticular activating system (ARAS); cerebral cortex

(c) Hypothalamus; limbic system

A11. (b), (d), (f), (g); but (a) focal, (c) is not, (e) delirium, and (h) move and rotate

A12. High; eye opening (E), motor response (M), verbal response (V)

A13. Rostral; caudal

(a) Midbrain

(b) Medulla

(c) Diencephalon

A14. Related to advances in scientific knowledge and technology; see text.

A15. See text.

B1. (a) Vertebral arteries; basilar artery

(b) Internal carotid arteries; middle cerebral arteries; language difficulties (aphasia) and loss of fine motor skills

(c) Anterior cerebral arteries

(d) Posterior communicating arteries; posterior cerebral arteries

B2. (a) Superficial; because of their location on the surface of the cerebral cortex

(b) Dura; internal jugular

B3. (a) 15; deep; local; auto; 60 to 140

(b) (1), (3), (5)

(c) Depresses; increased perfusion "flushes out" excessive H^+

B4. (a) Vascular disorders that injure and destroy myocardial and brain tissue, respectively; in both cases impairment may be limited by rapid emergency treatment.

(b) Both are warning signs of decreased perfusion; treatments of angina and TIA may reduce the risk of infarctions in these organs. TIAs are of shorter duration (maximum of 1 hour) than strokes and do not involve infarction of tissue.

(c) Ischemic strokes are due to thrombi or emboli and account for 88% of all strokes; hemorrhagic strokes, due to bleeding into brain tissue, are less common but more fatal.

B5. (a) African American

(b) 75

(c) Hypertension

(d) History

B6. (a) Blood sludging during a crisis increases risk of clot formation.

(b) Stasis of blood in the left atrium increases the risk of cardiogenic emboli to the middle cerebral arteries.

(c) Polycythemia leads to sluggish flow (with possible clot formation) and hypertension.

B7. Smoking cessation, avoidance of alcohol and cocaine, lowering blood cholesterol levels and weight (if obese), increasing exercise (if sedentary), control of hypertension and diabetes

B8. (a) The "halo" of brain tissue surrounding the core of the dead or dying cells resulting from a stroke

(b) Rapid emergency treatment can increase perfusion to penumbral cells and allow them to survive unimpaired.

B9. (a), (c); but (b) usually are not and (d) focal (less widespread) effects, such as clumsy hand syndrome

B10. (b); active; older age, hypertension, aneurysm, trauma, or drugs

B11. (a) L; middle cerebral artery

(b) R; anterior cerebral artery

(c) Posterior cerebral artery

B12. (a) Is not; because symptoms have lasted more than 1 hour and her manifestations are global rather than focal.

(b) Is; slurred speech; she cannot maintain her balance, posture, and muscle tone.

(c) Because ischemic (thrombotic) and hemorrhagic strokes require very different treatments, and early treatment may salvage penumbral areas.

(d) Magnetic resonance imaging

(e) Ischemic

(f) See text.

B13. (a) Dysarthria

(b) Nonfluent aphasia

(c) Wernicke aphasia

(d) Anomic aphasia

(e) Babinski sign

(f) Apraxia

(g) Hemineglect

(h) Agnosia

B14. (a), (b); but (c) more and (d) is

B15. (a), (c), (d), (e); but (b) severe headache

B16. (a) Involves narrowing of the cerebral artery; leads to gradual brain deterioration

(b) Occurs especially within the first 24 hours after rupture; rapidly deprives the brain of blood flow

(c) Related to blockage of reabsorption of CSF into arachnoid villi

B17. (a) Capillary beds are lacking, so veins are subjected to higher pressure blood from arteries (rather than lower pressure from capillaries); therefore they are at higher risk for rupture.

(b) Are; do

C1. (a) Encephalitis; myelitis

(b) (2), (3)

(c) Rapidly, through CSF around brain and cord

(d1) B

(d2) V

(d3) B

(d4) B

(e1) Nuchal rigidity

(e2) Petechiae

(f) Glucocorticoids (steroids); see text

(g) Viral; do

C2. (a) Neuroglia: astrocytes, neuroglia: oligodendroglia; neurons (in infants and children)

(b) Meningeal cells, pineal cells, pituitary cells

(c) Breast cancer cells, prostate cancer cells

C3. (b), (c); (f); but (a) can, based on location and size, (d) benign, slow, and (e) less

C4. The brain does lack pain receptors, but headache associated with brain tumors is related to stretching of dura mater or blood vessels.

C5. (a), (c); (e); but (b) less and (d) almost always

D1. Abnormal electrical discharges from cerebral cortex neurons, causing signs and symptoms; a type of motor seizure involving the whole body; common; before; vary according to the location of cells affected and degree of spread to other parts of the brain; sensory, motor, and autonomic changes; confusion, hallucinations, and loss of consciousness

D2. (b), (c), (e); but (a) common and (d) secondary

D3. (a) Is

(b) See text.

(c) Does not; one

(d) Do; both; common

(e1) A

(e2) S

(e3) M

(e4) M

(f) An aura is considered to be a simple partial seizure involving a small part of the brain; it can serve as a warning sign of more complex partial seizures; is

(g) Clonic

D4. (a) Tonic-clonic

(b) Atonic

(c) Absence

D5. (a) Are

(b) Protect the patient from injury, try to abort or prevent seizure activity, and treat the underlying disease.

(c) Avoids drug interactions and additive side effects

D6. Seizures that do not stop spontaneously and, if not treated, may be fatal

E1. Depression is one sign of dementia; antidepressants may be introduced for a differential diagnosis: they relieve depression but not the cognitive changes associated with dementia.

E2. (a) Cortical atrophy

(b) Sundown syndrome

(c) Neurofibrillary tangles

(d) Senile plaques

(e) Acetylcholine

(f) Amyloid precursor protein

E3. High; the APP gene is located on chromosome 21, and almost all persons with Down syndrome have three (trisomy) of chromosome 21 (and thus more APP gene)

E4. (a) Second

(b) First

(c) Third

E5. A matter of ruling out other diseases; see text

E6. (a) Pick disease
    (b) Wernicke-Korsakoff syndrome
    (c) Huntington disease
    (d) Creutzfeldt-Jakob disease
    (e) Vascular dementia

Chapter 37

DISORDERS OF SPECIAL SENSORY FUNCTION: VISION, HEARING, AND VESTIBULAR FUNCTION

A1. (a) Sclera → Uveal tract (or vascular layer) → Retina
    (b) Cornea → Anterior cavity → Lens → Posterior cavity
    (c) Bony orbit, eyelids and eyelashes, tears, conjunctiva, and extraocular muscles

A2. (a) Bacterial (because of the mucopurulent discharge) because bilateral
    (b) Pinkeye; hyperacute; is; is
    (c) Antibiotics specific to the causative microbe and good eyelid hygiene to prevent further infections

A3. (a) Minimal; watery
    (b) Exposure to adenoviruses by respiratory infections accompanied by sore throat and fever, inadequately chlorinated swimming pools, and crowded military or school sites
    (c) Unilateral; antivirals (Antibiotics are not effective and corticosteroids are not recommended because they can activate the virus.)
    (d) *C. trachomatis* A to C; vaginal delivery; 12
    (e) (3)

A4. Cause: hay fever (rhinoconjunctivitis) is an IgE-mediated hypersensitivity reaction; symptoms: bilateral tearing, itchy, red eyes; treatments: avoidance of allergens, use of cold compresses, oral antihistamines

A5. (a) Is not; blood vessels do not block light rays from passing through the cornea, but the cornea must depend on adjacent tissues and fluids (such as sclera, aqueous humor, and tears) for oxygen and nutrients; because of its avascularity, the cornea can be transplanted with minimal risk of rejection.
    (b) Highly; prolonged wearing of hard contact lenses, acute glaucoma, or blunt trauma
    (c) In addition to causing severe pain, a traumatized or inflamed cornea can lead to altered light transmission, visual impairment, and possible blindness.
    (d) Keratitis
      (d1) Infections such as syphilis or tuberculosis or a viral infection; lupus
      (d2) Conjunctivitis that moves into the cornea, exposure to trauma, and extended-wear contact lenses
    (e) Common (the most common form in the United States); 1; 2
    (f) Irritation, burning, and photophobia

    (g) Shingles or chickenpox
    (h) Does not

A6. Ciliary processes → Posterior chamber (of anterior cavity) (then around iris) → Anterior chamber (of anterior cavity) → Trabeculae and canal of Schlemm

A7. (a) Aqueous humor; obstructed outflow
    (b) On an eye screening provided at his work site; this condition typically is asymptomatic
    (c) 10 or 17; increase
    (d) Wide; (2) (3) (4) (5)
    (e) Alteration in the trabecular meshwork that should empty aqueous humor into the canal of Schlemm
    (f) A leading cause of blindness; the increased intraocular pressure leads to degeneration of the optic nerve
    (g) Pharmacologic; outflow, production

A8. (a) Small
    (b) Narrow; dilation; any condition that dilates the pupil: sympathetic responses, night vision, or dilator (mydriatic) drugs used to better visualize the retina
    (c) All (1–5)
    (d) Removal of part of the iris (iridectomy) to enhance flow of aqueous fluid

A9. (a) Refraction; they pass from air (low density) into the conjunctiva and cornea (higher density), then through varying densities in aqueous humor, lens, and vitreous humor. As a result, the image of something much larger than your eye (bird or bird feeder) can be focused on a tiny spot (fovea) on your retina.
    (b) Rounded or convex; ciliary; accommodation
    (c) Anterior; myopia; near; biconcave
    (d) Constriction or miosis; iris (constrictor); narrowing
    (e) Thicker; presby

A10. (a) Lens; older; common
    (b) Aging, genetics, diabetes, long-term exposure to UVB radiation (sunlight), trauma, and use of corticosteroids

A11. Slowly; the lens enlarges as new fibers form and old ones are altered and fill with vacuoles; concentrations of several electrolytes increase; proteins become less soluble, unfold, and cross-link; the lens yellows and has decreased transparency

A12. Blurred vision with glare and loss of visual acuity for both near and far vision

A13. (a) Strong bifocals, good lighting, visual aids such as magnifying lenses
    (b) Fragmentation and extraction of the lens followed by a lens implant

A14. (a) C
    (b) R
    (c) R (because needed for formation of rhodopsin)
    (d) R

A15. Posterior; macula lutea; does not; cones; point of sharpest vision

A16. (a) Choriocapillaris of the choroid
    (b) Central retinal artery branches

A17. (a) Retinal blood vessels are the only vessels in the body that can be observed directly, and they reflect health of brain vessels because the retina is an embryonic outgrowth of the brain.
(b) Anterior protrusion of the optic cup (of optic nerve) when high intracranial pressure collapses retinal veins and backs up fluid into the optic papilla (papilledema)

A18. (a) (2)
(b) Is
(c) Photocoagulation using argon laser

A19. Proliferative; new vessels grow and leak blood into the vitreous anterior to the retina; they also tightly connect the vitreous to the retina and may pull on the retina and detach it.

A20. (a) Hypertensive retinopathy
(b) Cotton-wool spots or exudates on the fundus
(c) Papilledema
(d) Detached retina
(e) Macular degeneration

A21. Area 17 is the end point of visual pathways for visual reception; association areas ascribe meaning to what has been seen.

A22. (a) One; both
(b) Do not (*Note:* axons do not terminate until they reach the thalamus); nasal
(c) Right; both

A23. (a) Homonymous
(b) Heteronymous
(c) Anopia
(d) Quadrantanopia
(e) Hemianopia

A24. By focusing images from the same spot on this page onto corresponding points of the two retinas, you can read with clear, binocular (not double) vision.

A25. (a) Superior rectus (inferior oblique is somewhat synergistic)
(b) Medial rectus (reciprocal contraction)
(c) Lateral rectus with some help from superior oblique and inferior oblique
(d) Levator palpebrae superioris
(e) All except lateral rectus (cranial nerve VI) and superior oblique (cranial nerve IV)

A26. (a) Diplopia
(b) Strabismus
(c) Amblyopia
(d) Hypertropia
(e) Cyclotropia
(f) Esotropia

A27. (a) Concomitant (nonparalytic)
(b) Concomitant (nonparalytic)
(c) Nonparalytic; childhood; months
(d) Paralytic; strokes, inflammation or tumor of the central nervous system

A28. Lazy eye; before age 6 years

B1. (a) External ear, middle ear
(b) External ear
(c) Middle ear
(d) Middle ear
(e) Inner ear
(f) Inner ear
(g) Middle ear

B2. Moist ears (swimming, bathing), allergies (hay fever), irritation (wearing earphones), and scratching itchy ears

B3. (b), (d), (e); but (a) negative and (c) warm

B4. (a) Equalize pressure on the two sides of the eardrum, drain middle ear secretions into the throat, and protect the middle ear
(b) Air at higher altitudes (such as in an airplane) exerts less pressure on the outside of the eardrum, so the eardrum gets "stuck" in the outward position. Relief is provided as you yawn or swallow and low-pressure (high-altitude) air enters the eustachian tube and middle ear, equalizing the pressure on the two sides of the eardrum.
(c) Closed; contraction of the tensor veli palatini (TVP) muscles, such as occurs during swallowing or yawning
(d) Lack of tube stiffness (related to limited cartilage development) or weakness of TVP muscles; also inflammation within the tube or external compression (caused by, for example, enlarged adenoids)
(e) Functional
(f) The eustachian tubes of infants are shorter, wider, and more horizontal; infants spend more of their day lying supine.

B5. His age, gender, being bottle fed, attending a large day-care center, having a sibling with a history of OM, and Evan's own recent history of AOM with antibiotic therapy

B6. (a) (4)
(b) Do; from nasopharynx through eustachian tube to the middle ear
(c) (2), (3), (5)

B7. (a) Because of dramatic increase in drug-resistant *S. pneumoniae* in persons who take antibiotics frequently
(b) A prophylactic approach that is an alternative to antibiotics
(c) To relieve pressure and prevent ragged scarring that would accompany a spontaneously perforated eardrum
(d) Placement of "tubes in the ears" to relieve pressure resulting from recurrent OM infections; keeping head out of water to prevent entrance of microbes or fluid into tubes

B8. (c), (d); but (a) 6 months or 4 episodes in 1 year and (b) absent

B9. (a) To develop well linguistically, children need to hear sounds as they watch lips or read words.
(b) Repeated episodes of reduced hearing by the presence of fluid in the middle ears; damage to the eardrum by pressure or perforation; adhesions of ossicles that cause conductive hearing loss
(c) Cholesteatoma formed from debris from the injured eardrum, and mastoiditis or infection of other cranial bones by spread of OM microbes

B10. (a) Autosomal dominant
 (b) Resorption of bone → Bone becomes spongy and soft → Overgrowth of hard bone develops
 (c) Stapes; stapedectomy with reconstruction of a stapes
 (d) Is; is (because otosclerosis typically is at least partly a conductive deafness)
B11. (a) Temporal
 (b) Oval
 (c) Cochlea
B12. (a) External ear canal → Tympanic membrane → Malleus → Incus → Stapes → Oval window → Perilymph of the scala vestibuli
 (b) Scala vestibuli containing perilymph → Vestibular membrane → Cochlear duct containing the organ of Corti and endolymph → Basilar membrane → Scala tympani containing perilymph
 (c) Tectorial membrane → Hair cells → Cochlear nerve fibers
B13. (a), (c), (d) but (b) VIII and (e) temporal
B14. (b), (c) but (a) common (objective tinnitus is rare) and (d) "hard of hearing"
B15. (a) Left; auditory association
 (b) (3)
 (c) Receptive
B16. (a) Sensineural deafness
 (b) Conduction deafness
 (c) Sensineural deafness
 (d) Sensineural deafness
 (e) Sensineural deafness
 (f) Presbycusis (a form of conduction deafness)
 (g) Sensineural deafness
B17. All answers
B18. (a) Common; denial related to social embarrassment about hearing aids
 (b) (2)
 (c) Family or friends who are aware of his hearing losses; history of ear trauma and infections, environmental noise exposure, use of toxic drugs, and past use of hearing aids
 (d) Tuning forks
B19. Position yourself so your face is in the light; directly face the person as you speak, and articulate clearly in a setting with low background noise; keep your voice tones low (not a high-pitched yell).
B20. (a) Hearing influences language development
 (b) Safety issues, avoiding social isolation and depression
C1. (a) Recover and maintain a stable body and head position (equilibrium) and maintain a stable visual field when the head moves
 (b1) Facilitate smooth, coordinated movements needed for posture
 (b2) Control eye movements as the head is moved
 (b3) Lead to nausea and vomiting with excessive vestibular stimulation
C2. (a) Semicircular canals
 (b) Saccule, utricle
 (c) Saccule, utricle
 (d) Saccule, utricle
 (e) Semicircular canals

C3. (a) Nystagmus
 (b) Motion sickness
 (c) Ménière disease
 (d) Benign paroxysmal positional vertigo (BPPV)
C4. (a), (b), (d), (e); but (c) peripheral, such as inner ear
C5. (a) Reduce the volume of the endolymphatic space.
 (b) Head positioning maneuvers can relocate debris in semicircular canals.
 (c) Alcohol may trigger episodes of vertigo.
C6. Brainstem ischemia, cerebellar tumor, or multiple sclerosis
C7. (a) Romberg test
 (b) Electronystagmography
 (c) Caloric stimulation
 (d) Rotational tests
C8. (a) Antidopaminergics
 (b) Anticholinergics
 (c) Antidopaminergics
C9. See text.

Chapter 38

DISORDERS OF THE MALE GENITOURINARY SYSTEM

A1. Produce androgens such as testosterone; produce, transport, and ejaculate sperm (Urine is also eliminated through the urethra.)
A2. (a) Generation of spermatozoa (or sperm)
 (b) Conversion of spermatocytes to sperm
A3. All answers (a–d)
A4. (c) → (b) → (e) → (a) → (d); (b)
A5. (a) Two; posterior; fructose; prostaglandins
 (b) Seminal vesicles
A6. (a) Gonadotropin-releasing hormone (GnRH)
 (b) Follicle-stimulating hormone (FSH), luteinizing hormone
 (c) Follicle-stimulating hormone
 (d) Inhibin
 (e) Luteinizing hormone (LH)
 (f) Testosterone
 (g) Estradiol
 (h) Testosterone
A7. (a) Differentiates male genitalia and regulates descent of testes
 (b) Develops secondary sex characteristics such as changes in hair, skin, and voice; facilitates full maturation of sperm
 (c) Maintains secondary sex characteristics and promotes and maintains musculoskeletal growth
A8. (a) Glans; prepuce; circumcision
 (b) Corpora (or corpus, singular); spongiosum
A9. (a) Parasympathetic; sacral; pelvic
 (b) (1); corpus cavernosa and corpus spongiosum
 (c) Sympathetic; detumescence
 (d) cGMP; relaxation; erect
 (e) At the base; squeezing of the penis during ejaculation
A10. (a) Mixed; organic
 (b) Diabetes mellitus, which diminishes neuronal function

(c) Cigarette smoking and hypertension cause vasoconstriction; hypercholesterolemia is related to arteriosclerosis.

(d) Aging, use of antidepressants, depression regarding psychosocial issues such as divorce, and history of alcohol abuse

(e) Does

(f) Testosterone and prolactin

(g) Increases cGMP that leads to vasodilation in the penis (see Question A9[d]); also increases blood flow into the cavernous regions of the penis

B1. (a) Be retracted over

(b) Balanoposthitis

B2. (a) Peyronie disease

(b) Smegma

(c) Balanitis xerotica obliterans

(d) Priapism

B3. (a) True urologic emergency; fibrosis of penile tissue leading to erectile dysfunction, possibly as soon as a day or two after onset; low-flow (stasis)

(b1) Trauma, infection, or neoplasms

(b2) Sickle cell disease, stroke, spinal cord injury, and medications (including injection therapy for erectile dysfunction)

(c) Stasis of blood in cavernous sinuses during erection leads to deoxygenation, sickling, and additional stasis of blood there.

B4. (a) Middle-aged; highly; embarrassment

(b) Poor hygiene, HPV infection, UV radiation (including tanning salons), HIV (especially with Kaposi sarcoma) or other causes of immunosuppression

(c) Carcinomas; erythroplasia of Queyrat; Bowen disease

B5. (a) Dennis may have "undescended testes" (cryptorchidism). Testes develop in the abdominal cavity (near kidneys) and normally descend into the scrotum during the last 2 months of fetal life. Cryptorchidism increases risk for testicular cancer and can lead to infertility because sperm require the cooler temperature of the scrotum for normal development.

(b) As testes descend, their blood and lymphatic vessels are pulled down with them. So testicular cancer cells enter lymphatic pathways that accompany testicular veins and ascend to nodes parallel to the aorta at about the level of the kidneys (where testes originally developed).

(c) When testes descend into the scrotum, they exert pressure on the inguinal canal, which may not close completely; females have no such descent so are much less likely to develop inguinal hernias.

B6. (a) Vaginalis; albuginea; vaginalis

(b) Dartos; cremaster

(c) Veins; do

B7. (a) Hematocele

(b) Hydrocele

(c) Varicocele

(d) Spermatocele

B8. (a), (b), (f); but (c) do not, (d) from 15 to 35, and (e) left, right

B9. Injury, inflammation, lymph obstruction, germ cell tumor, or side effect of irradiation

B10. (a) Scrotal palpation of a varicocele is compared to the feel of a "bag of worms."

(b) The varicocele disappears in the recumbent position as blood moves from testes into spermatic and renal veins and on into the inferior vena cava.

B11. (a) Spermatic artery, veins, lymphatics, nerves, and vas deferens

(b) Neonates

(c) More; can

B12. (a) Within the scrotum, posterior to testes; serve as sites for storage, maturation, and transport of sperm

(b) *Neisseria gonorrhoeae;* young men

(c) Pressure from the infected site causes backflow of infection into the ejaculatory duct and the vas.

(d) Infection carried by lymphatics or blood vessels (septicemia)

(e) Days; common; yes, because the causative microbe is *Chlamydia*

(f) Bed rest; to encourage lymphatic drainage out of the epididymis by gravity; antibiotics, antipyretics, and analgesics; discouraged

(g) One or both testes

B13. Mumps (infection of parotid gland[s])

(a) Both involve pain and swelling in the scrotal area and commonly include fever; orchitis does not involve dysuria or urethral discharge.

(b) About 20% to 35%

B14. (a) Testicular

(b) It was the first type of cancer linked to a specific occupation (chimney sweeps); poor hygiene, HPV infection, or exposure to UV light

(c) 15 to 35; is

(d) Cryptorchidism (see Question B5[a]); seminiferous; men in their 30s; highly

(e) (1); but (2) and (3) both signs of metastasis

(f) Alpha-fetoprotein, human chorionic gonadotropin, lactic dehydrogenase

(g) All; orchiectomy

B15. (a) Mucosal; main; alkaline; 6.0 to 6.5

(b) Muscle; ejaculation; serves as a sphincter preventing urine from passing from bladder into urethra (or semen from urethra to bladder) during ejaculation

B16. (a) Chronic prostatitis/chronic pelvic pain syndrome (the inflammatory type)

(b) Acute bacterial prostatitis

(c) Chronic bacterial prostatitis

B17. (c), (d); but (a) inferior, (b) inner periurethral, and (e) make it worse; 5α-reductase inhibitors are likely to improve BPH

B18. All except Japanese descent

B19. (a) Obstruction of urine outflow with retention of urine in the bladder

(b) Infection of urine retained in the bladder leading to UTIs; overflow incontinence with related urgency; development of bladder hypertrophy with ischemia and infected

diverticula; back pressure into ureters with possible hydronephrosis and renal failure
- (c1) Surrounding
- (c2) Greater
- (c3) Decreased
- (d1) Indicate UTI probably related to urinary stasis
- (d2) Negative screening for prostate cancer
- (d3) Higher than normal volume indicates urinary stasis in bladder (see Chapter 26, Question A5)
- (d4) Compromised renal function because creatinine level is twice normal

B20. Moderate, because score falls in the range of 8 to 20.

B21. (a) Is not; transurethral resection (of the) prostate
- (b) Nonsurgical procedure to temporarily widen the urethra to allow urinary flow

B22. (b), (c); but (a) common—the leading male cancer and second leading cause of cancer deaths and (d) late—is often asymptomatic until after metastasis

B23. (a) Pressure of the prostatic tumor that impedes urinary outflow
- (b) Metastases to lungs
- (c) Metastases to vertebrae and pelvis

B24. Digital rectal palpation of a hard mass; PSA (positive in 30% of prostate cancers but also in some cases of BPH); transrectal ultrasonography for identifying small masses

B25. Poorly; prostatectomy or radiation

C1. (a) Hypo; 300; cryptorchidism; ambiguous genitalia may occur as chromosomal aberrations; 9 months
- (b) Less; location of the urinary bladder outside of the abdominopelvic cavity (exstrophy)

C2. (b), (d); but (a) is not so the foreskin can be used for surgical repair and (c) should not to avoid infection, scarring, or paraphimosis

C3. (a) Failure of one or more testes to descend into the scrotal sac
- (b) Common (one third of premature boys); rare (3% to 5%); unilateral; 7th to 9th
- (c) Birth to 3
- (d) A retractable testis is palpable at birth but retracts into the inguinal canal because of the exaggerated cremaster muscle action.
- (e) To enhance potential for fertility, reduce risk for testicular cancer, and for cosmetic appearance
- (f) Years; is; orchiopexy; 95

C4. (b), (c), (f); but (a) less, (d) smaller, and (e) typically do not change in size

C5. (a) Symptoms in aging men related to decreased androgen levels
- (b) Increases lean mass and decreases bone loss, but may have side effects such as acne, enlargement of breast tissue, exacerbation of sleep apnea (if present), decrease in HDLs

Chapter 39

DISORDERS OF THE FEMALE GENITOURINARY SYSTEM

A1. Clitoris, urinary opening, vaginal orifice, anus

A2. (a) Introitus
- (b) Clitoris
- (c) Urinary meatus
- (d) Vestibule
- (e) Labia majora

A3. (c), (e); but (a) external genitalia (but not the vagina), (b) recesses surrounding the cervix, and (d) cervix

A4. (a) Fundus, body, cervix
- (b) Rectum, uterus, bladder
- (c) (2)
- (d) Endometrium, myometrium, perimetrium
- (e) Myo

A5. (a) Proliferative
- (b) Secretory
- (c) Menstrual

A6. (a) Fallopian (uterine) tubes
- (b) Uterus
- (c) Fallopian (uterine) tubes
- (d) Ovaries

A7. (a) GnRH
- (b) FSH, LH, prolactin
- (c) Estrogen, progesterone

A8. FSH, LH

A9. (a), (b); but (c) just before ovulation and during the postovulatory (luteal) phase and (d) estradiol

A10. (a), (b), (d), (e), (f); but (c) decrease and (g) ductile growth and development

A11. This hormone decreases myometrial contractions.

A12. Do; ovaries and adrenal cortex

A13. PF → SF → ODF → IF → LH → CL → CA

A14. (a), (d); but (b) theca interna and (c) pain accompanying ovulation

B1. External
- (a) Essential vulvodynia
- (b) Cyclic vulvovaginitis
- (c) Leukoplakia
- (d) Bartholin gland cyst

B2. (c), (d); but (a) less and (b) is a precursor to

B3. (a) Normal flora; glycogen; 4.5
- (b) Decreased; alkaline; increases. Estrogen replacement helps regenerate the vaginal lining and increase the population of Döderlein bacteria; after using the toilet, it is advisable that a woman wipe from front to back to avoid fecal contamination of vagina or urethra.

B4. (a) No, they indicate infection.
- (b) Antibiotics can destroy the normal flora, allowing yeast to proliferate; stress can lower Sally's resistance to infection.

B5. (a) Rare; 60; daughters of women who took DES, and young women exposed to human papillomavirus (HPV)
- (b) To prevent miscarriage; 1940–1971; benign
- (c) Abnormal vaginal bleeding
- (d) Local excision, laser, loop electrode excision procedure (LEEP), radical surgery, and/or radiation

B6. (a) (1); (2)
- (b) 1 becomes 2; transformation

(c) Metaplasia; normal for the body but not for this region; can

(d) Trauma and infections (such as HPV)

(e) Nabothian; no, but they may have to be removed if they excessively enlarge the cervix

(f) Polyps; benign

B7. (a) C

(b) A

B8. (a) Years; cervical cells become increasingly abnormal (dysplastic) over an extended period

(b) Better

(c) There is a strong link between HPV and cervical cancer, especially if women have multiple sexual partners.

(d) Smoking, HPV, and multiple sex partners

(e) Common (the number one); is; decreased; gynecologic examinations with Pap smears can identify early stages of dysplasia

(f) Screening; colposcopy

B9. (a) Uterus (endometritis); Fallopian tubes (salpingitis); ovaries (oophoritis)

(b) *Neisseria gonorrhoeae, Chlamydia trachomatis*; they ascend from the vagina, are harbored in the sloughing endometrium in the uterus, and may then ascend to tubes and ovaries

(c) (3), (4); but (1) 16–24 years and (2) single, nulliparous women

(d) Extremely painful cervix, lower abdominal pain that may start after a menstrual period, pelvic tenderness, C-reactive protein in the blood; increase; is

(e) Antibiotics

B10. (a) (2), (3), (4)

(b) Endometrial tissue in her ovaries; old blood that resembles chocolate syrup; rupture may lead to peritonitis and adhesions

(c) Retrograde movement of endometrium through fallopian tubes, spread of immature cells during embryonic life; passage of cells via blood or lymph, or genetic or immune factors

(d) Cyclic rise in estrogen stimulates endometrial tissue to grow wherever it is located.

(e) Pain during sexual activity (dyspareunia) and infertility

(f) Observation by laparoscopy; surgery; high

B11. (a) Leiomyoma

(b) Adenomyosis

(c) Endometritis

(d) Endometriosis

B12. (a) More; older than

(b) (1), (3), (4), (5); but (2) unopposed estrogen

(c) (1), (2); but (3) painless and (4) not in early stages

(d) (4)

(e) 90%

B13. (a) (3)

(b) (1)

(c) Gravity, pregnancy, childbirth, aging, coughing, lifting, or straining with defecation

(d) (3) (*cyst* prefix means bladder)

(e) (2)

(f) (3)

B14. Do; Kegel exercises or use of pessary in the vagina to support the uterus

B15. (b), (d), (f); but (a) the most common form, (c) high (LH) and normal (FSH), and (e) benign (well-differentiated)

B16. (a) (2), (3)

(b) Frequently; after; vague; gastrointestinal

(c) Are no; CA-125; is

C1. (a), (b); but (c) is not and (d) 28 days

C2. Is; fat is a source of estrogens; all

C3. (a) Metrorrhagia

(b) Menorrhagia

(c) Amenorrhea

(d) Oligomenorrhea

C4. (a) Thinner

(b) Thicker; fails to

(c) Low; heavy; is not; teenagers and perimenopausal women

(d) History (including bleeding pattern) and physical examination

(e1) S

(e2) P

C5. Dys; secondary

C6. (d), (e), (f); but (a) is not, (b) late 20s and early 30s and (c) probably multifactorial

C7. See text.

C8. (a) Peri

(b) Diminished; even if her ovaries have stopped producing estrogen, the adrenal cortex and fat tissues continue to produce some of the hormone

(c) Hot flashes

(d) Hot flashes, night sweats, and insomnia directly related to hormonal changes

(e) Increased; bone resorption occurs at a rate faster than bone formation

(f) Can

D1. (a) Alveoli

(b) Cooper ligaments

(c) Areolar tissue

D2. (a) Mastitis

(b) Ductal ectasia

(c) Papilloma

(d) Fibrocystic disease

D3. (a) 30 to 50; are

(b) Ultrasound

(c) Avoided; these foods contain xanthines, which are linked to fibrocystic disease.

D4. (a) Common (second leading cause of cancer deaths among women); 8; increased; more women take part in screening

(b) (2), (4), (5); but (1) older women and (3) women who have been nulliparous until at least age 30

(c) (2)

D5. Monthly breast self-examination (BSE), annual mammogram, physical examination by physician

(a) 1 mm; 1 cm; painless

(b) Fine needle aspiration biopsy, excisional biopsy, ultrasound, estrogen and progesterone receptor analysis

D6. (a), (d), (e); but (b) less and (c) first

Chapter 40

SEXUALLY TRANSMITTED DISEASES

A1. (a) More
(b) Is
(c) Increasing

A2. Mouth, vagina and surrounding tissue of the vulva, urinary meatus (urethral opening), rectoanal area, and skin

A3. (a) (4)
(b) 100; is
(c) Cervical; smoking, immunosuppression such as by HIV, and hormonal changes as with oral contraceptives or pregnancy
(d) August 31 (6 weeks to 8 months); itching of the vulva, results of Pap smear, colposcopy, or biopsy
(e) There are no treatments that eradicate HPV once the infection occurs, although some medications and surgeries can provide symptomatic relief (see text).
(f) Type 16; helps reduce the risk of cervical cancer

A4. Nine; chickenpox; shingles; simplex
(a) 2; fever blisters; also can
(b) 50 million; women; women have a larger surface area of genital mucosa
(c) Dorsal root (sensory) ganglia; sacral; neurotropic; are not
(d) Do not; do not; epidemic proportions
(e) Women: vulva, vagina, cervix; men: penis, scrotum; either gender: urethra or anus
(f) All answers
(g) Malaise, myalgia, headache, fever, swollen lymph nodes
(h) Vesicles or pustules

A5. (a1) A
(a2) Primary; some immunity is built up after the initial infection
(a3) 7 to 10
(a4) Is no known; they can reduce the incidence and severity of recurrent infections and decrease viral shedding and contagion during sexual activity.
(a5) HSV can infect the corneas and lead to blindness.
(b1) A
(b2) Cesarean

A6. (a) Virus
(b) Bacteria
(c) Bacteria
(d) Virus

A7. Genital warts (condyloma acuminata) and herpes simplex; all answers (a–d)

B1. Moniliasis, thrush, yeast infection

B2. (c), (e), (f); but (a) three of four, (b) usually not, and (d) commonly

B3. In warm, moist folds of skin under breasts, under abdominal flap, or in inguinal folds; also in organs such as esophagus in immunosuppressed persons

B4. (a) Has an; over 6.0
(b) Metallic; contraindicated; gastrointestinal; cardiovascular

(c) Is; is

B5. (a), (c); but (b) minimally (d) are not because it is not highly inflammatory, and (e) is not

B6. (a) and (c)

C1. *Chlamydia;* these three STDs are likely to exert widespread systemic effects.

C2. (a) Primarily
(b) Are many types; elementary; reticulate
(c) Quite similar; *Chlamydia;* 50%; cases go undiagnosed and untreated and may lead to more serious conditions such as pelvic inflammatory disease (PID), infertility, or cervical cancer.
(d) Conjunctiva, joints, and mucosa
(e) Eye

C3. (a) 600,000; days; oropharynx (throat), eyes of neonates
(b1) Pain or burning upon urination
(b2) Pain upon intercourse or other sexual activity involving the vulva
(b3) Inflammation has spread to her fallopian tubes
(c) Orogenital sexual abuse

C4. Syphilis; treponemal; gummas; cardiovascular and nervous; penicillin

C5. See completed Table 40-1 on page 356.

Chapter 41

STRUCTURE AND FUNCTION OF THE SKELETAL SYSTEM

A1. (a) Provides protection, support, stability, shape, mineral storage, and blood-forming tissue
(b) Axial: skull, hyoid, thorax, and vertebrae; appendicular: bones of shoulders, hips, and extremities
(c) Bone, cartilage, tendons, and ligaments

A2. (a) E
(b) C

A3. (a) Hyaline
(b) Hyaline
(c) Elastic
(d) Fibrous

A4. (a) Chondro; perichondrium
(b) Do not; by diffusion from vessels in the perichondrium

A5. (a) Two; calcium; collagen
(b) Cancellous; compact
(c) Osteogenic cells → Osteoblasts → Osteocytes
(d) Osteoblasts; alkaline phosphatase
(e) Osteocytes; lacunae; lamellae
(f) Osteon or haversian system; blood vessels; canaliculi permit communication between lacunae and blood vessels
(g) Vessels in periosteum travel across bone via Volkmann canals to reach haversian systems.
(h) Clasts; monocytes; PTH

A6. It is bound to calcium and can cause discoloration and deformity in the teeth of the developing child.

A7. (a) Contains blood vessels and serves as the point for anchoring tendons and ligaments

Table 40-1   Comparison of Sexually Transmitted Diseases

Name of STD	Causative Microbe	Description
(a) **Condyloma acuminata**	**HPV virus**	Genital warts, pruritis; increased risk of cervical cancer; rapidly growing STD in the U.S.; treatments cannot cure but reduce symptoms
(b) **Trichomoniasis**	Protozoan: pear-shaped with flagellae	**Copious green or yellow discharge with odor; can be cured; usual medication (metronidazole) leaves metallic state; 5 million cases annually in the U.S.**
(c) **Chlamydia**	**Intracellular parasite smaller than most bacteria**	The most prevalent reportable STD in the U.S.; no symptoms in 90% of cases; women may have mucopurulent discharge; spread to fallopian tubes can cause infertility; can cause blindness in infected neonates and Reiter syndrome (of eyes) in adults
(d) Chancroid	**Gram-negative bacteria: *Haemophilus***	**Highly infectious; painful ulcers and buboes (lymphadenopathy); rare in U.S. but common in Africa and parts of Asia**
(e) **Gonorrhea**	*Neisseria* bacteria (gram-negative diplococci)	**Creamy yellow discharge with urethral pain in men; can spread to other genitalia or systemically; can cause blindness in infected neonates**
(f) **Bacterial vaginosis**	**Possibly *Gardnerella vaginalis* and other anaerobic bacteria**	Thin gray-white discharge with foul, fishy odor; "clue-cells" seen on slides; very common; **minimally inflammatory**
(g) **Syphilis**	Spirochete bacteria *Treponema pallidum*	**Painless chancres in primary stage; rash and flu-like symptoms may occur in secondary stage; multisystem tertiary stage may occur 20 years later**
(h) Genital herpes	**HSV-2 (or HSV-1):** neurotropic virus	**Prodromal paresthesia; painful vesicles in acute stage, especially in primary infections; no cure but antivirals can reduce duration and frequency of recurrences**
(i) **Candidiasis**	***Candida (Monilia)***	Most women have this infection at least once; thick, cheesy, odorless discharge; antifungals can cure

(b) Site of osteogenic cells for new bone growth and remodeling

(c) Lines the inside of haversian canals, the marrow cavity, and spaces in spongy bone; formed of osteogenic cells that remodel and repair bone

A8. (a) Mesoderm
    (b) (3) → (1) → (2)
    (c) Third
    (d) Epiphesial; cartilage; C; D
    (e) Periosteum; endosteum
A9. (a) Parathyroid hormone; vitamin D; calcitonin
    (b) Parathyroid hormone; calcitonin
    (c) All three do

(d) Calcitonin
(e) Parathyroid hormone; calcitonin
A10. Bones, intestine (especially the jejunum via stimulating kidney activation of vitamin D), and kidneys (by reabsorption)
A11. (a) Steroid; fish, liver, irradiated milk
    (b) Skin; liver, kidneys
    (c) May have reduced kidney and liver function; if immobile or institutionalized, they may not have skin exposed to sunlight; and may not ingest dairy products containing the vitamin
    (d) (3)
    (e) Stimulate; inhibits
    (f) Decreased

A12. (a) Are no

(b) Paget disease because it involves overactive osteoclasts

B1. (a) Irregular

(b) Short

(c) Long

B2. (a) Epiphysis

(b) Diaphysis

(c) Metaphysis

B3. (a) Children

(b) Ligaments; tendons; tendons; limited

(c) Synarthroses; synchondrosis

(d) Diarthroses; synovial; freely movable

B4. See Figure 41-6 in *Essentials of Pathophysiology.*

B5. (b), (c); but (a) is not and (d) poorly

B6. A case of referred pain because the hip receives some branches of nerves that cross the hip en route to supply the knee joint.

B7. A bunion is a bursa over the metatarsophalangeal joint of the great toe (MTP-1).

Chapter 42

DISORDERS OF THE SKELETAL SYSTEM: TRAUMA, INFECTION, AND CHILDHOOD DISORDERS

A1. 70; bones, joints (including capsule, cartilage, tendons, and ligaments), and muscles

A2. (a) Common; high-speed motor accidents

(b) Falls; more; vertebrae, humerus, and proximal femur (hip joint)

(c) Contusions; strains, and sprains; stress fractures

A3. (a) Laceration

(b) Contusion

(c) Puncture wounds

(d) Hematoma

A4. (a) Bones; muscles

(b) Muscles or muscle–tendon units; strains; all answers

(c) Cold

(d) Ankle; in; 3 and 4 (See Figure 42-1 in *Essentials of Pathophysiology.*)

(e) To reduce pain, swelling, and the risk of muscle contractions pulling injured ends apart

(f) Partial; more; hip and knee

(g) Pieces of cartilage and bones

A5. (a) Shoulder; baseball; tennis; supraspinatus, infraspinatus, teres minor, and subscapularis; supraspinatus

(b) Knee; cartilage; deepen the tibial socket that receives femoral condyles, lubricate and nourish the joint

(c) Cartilage is avascular; to avoid total joint replacement

(d) Skiing and tennis; immobilization or bracing, muscle-strengthening exercises, and antiinflammatory drugs

(e) Softening

(f) Is; is

(g) Proximal femur; all answers except Male

A6. (a) Pathologic fracture

(b) Fatigue (stress fracture)

(c) Sudden injury fracture

A7. (b), (c), (e); but (a) sudden injury, (d) proximal, and (f) children and partial break

A8. (a) Decrease (reduction) of space between broken bone ends so that the bony pieces are returned to their original locations; transverse

(b) Swelling, bleeding (with open fractures), loss of function, deformity, abnormal mobility involving the fractured bone

(c) Angulation, shortening, and rotation; muscle pull on bone fragments

(d) A grating sound as bone fragments rub against each other

(e) Nerve function often is lost temporarily (local shock).

A9. Reduction, immobilization, and preservation or restoration of function; immobilization

(a) Open

(b) Should

(c) (1) and (2) with medical guidance

A10. Hematoma → fibrocartilaginous callus → ossification → remodeling

(a) Hematoma

(b) Fibrocartilaginous callus

(c) Ossification

(d) Remodeling

A11. (a) (1)

(b) (2)

(c) (2)

(d) (1)

(e) (2)

A12. (a) Delayed union

(b) Nonunion

(c) Malunion

A13. (a) Fat embolism syndrome

(b) Fracture blisters

(c) Reflex sympathetic dystrophy

(d) Compartment syndrome

(e) Fat embolism syndrome (possibly leading to PE)

A14. (a) Scar tissue from burns; tight dressing; limb compression in accident or unconscious state

(b) Trauma to extremity, including fractures and bone surgeries; postischemic swelling; excessive IV fluids

A15. (a), (c) because major arteries are located outside of compartments, (e); but (b) is and (d) is not, because BP in that extremity would fall owing to gravity

A16. (a) Subtle changes in behavior, disorientation

(b) Rapid pulse, sweating, and pallor

(c) That does not blanch upon application of pressure possibly because of the presence of emboli in skin capillaries and thrombocytopenia as platelets stick to fatty globules

A17. (a)

B1. (a) Marrow; difficult to cure

(b) By extension of an open fracture or wound; by spread via the bloodstream; from skin infections in persons with poor circulation

(c) Bone contamination from an open wound

(d) *Staphylococcus aureus;* these microbes can bind to bone and they can enter osteoblasts where the microbes are sheltered from antibiotic effects

(e) Children; at growing points (metaphyses) of long bones; vertebrae, wrists or ankles

B2. (a) Chronic; osteomyelitis is considered chronic at 1.5 to 2 months after the initial infection.

(b) Sequestrum; involcrum; are

(c) To remove drainage or release pressure and possibly replace a prosthetic device involved with the infection

B3. Poor circulation to his lower extremity, which leads to the skin infection and ulcer and then to spread of infection to his bone

B4. *Mycobacterium;* vertebrae (by direct spread from lungs)

B5. (a) Death; blood

(b) Subchondral regions of epiphysis and medullary (marrow) cavity of metaphysis, which have a limited blood supply; cortical bone is likely to have collateral circulation.

(c) Yes: the femoral head is composed mostly of spongy bone, and it has poor collateral circulation.

(d) Often; no known cause; fracture or hip surgery, steroid therapy, injury to vessels as by radiation; also sickle cell, Legg-Calvé-Perthes disease, lupus, or rheumatoid arthritis

(e) Rheumatoid arthritis and corticosteroid usage

(f) Pain at the site

(g) Joint (hip) replacement; 10

B6. Medullary necrosis releases both fat and calcium, which form the "soap"; bone lacks the ability to "clean up" the soapy material.

C1. (a) Metastatic

(b) Benign

(c) Benign; common

(d) Benign, do

(e) Poorly

C2. Is not; presence of a mass that can interfere with normal movement.

C3. (a) Adolescents, elderly, 35 year olds

(b) The most common; is

(c) Sudden

(d1) Warm, shiny, and stretched over the tumor

(d2) Restricted range of motion

(e) Lungs

(f) A surgery in which malignant bone and surrounding tissue is excised; the bone is replaced with a combination of donor (cadaver) bone, the client's own bone, and metal plates or rods.

C4. (a1) (3)

(a2) (1), (4)

(a3) Because fever and weight loss may accompany Ewing sarcoma and may suggest other diagnoses.

(b1) (2)

(b2) (2)

(b3) (1), (2)

(b4) (1)

C5. (a) 50%

(b) (2)

(c) Breast, lung, prostate

(d) Stretching of the periosteum or pressure of the tumor on nerves

(e1) This enzyme and this electrolyte are both likely to increase.

(e2) Palliative therapy (to reduce pain and try to prevent fractures)

(e3) Stabilize bones that are weakened by cancer

D1. (a) Flexion; flexion; months

(b) Ligaments typically are lax in the newborn and are affected by intrauterine position as well as by sleeping or sitting positions of infants. Also, familial tendencies.

(c) Common; often

(d) Intoeing; outtoeing; is

(e) Internal; anteversion; *W*; exacerbates

D2. (a) Bowlegs; varum (*Hint:* Draw a large capital *R* for vaRum in the wide space between the child's bowlegs in Figure 42-16 in *Essentials of Pathophysiology.*); very common; sometimes

(b) Knock-knees; valgum (*Hint:* A capital *R* is too large, but a lower case *l* as in valgum, would just about fit into this narrow space between the knees of the child on the right side of Figure 42-16 in *Essentials of Pathophysiology.*); medial; rarely

(c) These may lead to osteoarthritis or other disorders; early treatment reduces risk of such sequelae.

(d) Proximal epiphysis; bowlegs; large; early; uni (see Figure 42-17 in *Essentials of Pathophysiology*)

D3. (a), (c); but (b) presence of an extra finger or toe

D4. (a) Fragile; dominant; recessive, II; is no

(b) Inward; varus; not smoking

D5. (a) She is a first-born white female; was born breech; joint laxity

(b) Quite common (1 in 100); more

(c) Dislocated; dislocatable

(d) Waddling (gait)

(e) Abducted

D6. (a) Osteogenesis imperfecta, developmental dysplasia of the hip, and congenital clubfoot

(b) Developmental dysplasia of the hip

(c) Congenital clubfoot

(d) Osteogenesis imperfecta

(e) Developmental dysplasia of the hip, Legg-Calvé-Perthes disease, and slipped capital femoral epiphysis

(f) Legg-Calvé-Perthes disease

(g) Osgood-Schlatter disease

(h) Slipped capital femoral epiphysis

(i) Blount disease; Osgood-Schlatter disease

D7. (a) (1), (2), (3)

(b) Uni; yes, in 85% of cases

(c) To reduce deformity of the femoral head; abduction

(d) Greater because he has more time for remodeling of the femoral head

D8. Lateral; convexity

(a) Girls; 1,000

(b) Postural; structural

(c) Not known (idiopathic); laxity; (1)

(d) High shoulder or scapula on the right side (see Figure 42-22 in *Essentials of Pathophysiology*) with uneven sleeves and hemline, or right shoulder hump when Suzannah bends forward

(e) Bracing; surgery

Chapter 43

DISORDERS OF THE SKELETAL SYSTEM: METABOLIC AND RHEUMATIC DISORDERS

A1. (a) Clasts; blasts (*Hint:* Remember *C* for *C*hew up bone, and *B* for *B*uild up bone); progenitor

(b) Months; resorption

(c) Blasts; immobilization

(d) C; D

(e) PTH; 6; Paget

(f) Calcitonin (also estrogens)

(g) The RANK ligand on osteoblasts binds to the RANK receptor on osteoclast precursors, leading to production of osteoclasts that resorb bone.

(h) OPG prevents this binding, therefore inhibiting formation of osteoclasts required for excessive bone resorption occurring in osteoporosis.

(i) Penia; osteoporosis, osteomalacia, certain malignancies, or thyroid disorders

A2. Porous; fine porcelain vase; increases

(a) Common; 44 million

(b) Primary; 14 (0.7% per year × 20 years since peak at age 30 years); 34 (1% per year × 20 years since age 50)

(c) (2), (4), (5), (7); but (1), (3), and (6) are factors that lower risk

(d) Early; increased; trabecular; vertebrae, and the head of femur ("broken hip")

(e) (1), (2), (3)

(f) Secondary

(f1) Gina is well on her way to the "female athlete triad" of disordered eating (including low intake of calcium and vitamin D), leading to amenorrhea (with decreased estrogen) and OP; phosphates in diet soda deplete calcium.

(f2) These antacids and steroids increase calcium excretion. Her HRT will offset effects of her oophorectomy.

(f3) High protein (steak and cheese), high alcohol and lack of exercise are risk factors, and cigarette smoke constricts vessels into bone.

(g) No, not unless fractured; pain resulting from fractures, including vertebral compression fractures

(h) This increased concavity of the thoracic spine is related to osteoporotic wedging of thoracic vertebrae.

(i) Decreases; (2)

(j) A = age, B = bulk, and ONE = never on estrogen

(k) Bone mineral density (BMD) via DXA; measurement of serial heights; refinement of risk factors

(l) Weight-bearing exercise, dietary calcium (1000–1,500 mg/d) and vitamin D (400–800 IU/d); also decrease of other modifiable risk factors

(m1) Calcitonin

(m2) Bisphosphonates

(m3) Estrogen

A3. (a) Minerals; calcium; phosphate; softer; rickets

(b) Anticonvulsants, diuretics, sedatives, muscle relaxants, tranquilizers

(c) Bowlegs, muscle weakness, pain; severe hypocalcemia (leading to secondary) hyperparathyroidism

(d) Vitamin D- and calcium-rich diet; exposure to sun

A4. (a) Fat; skin; calcium

(b) Impaired absorption; northern China, Japan, northern India

A5. (a) Activation

(b) Less; more; hypo; increased; resorption; renal

(c) Phosphate; long-term use of antacids that bind phosphates within the GI tract and thus prevent their absorption from foods

A6. (a) Softened; de; 6 months to 3 years

(b) Lack of vitamin D, calcium or phosphate, or inability to absorb these chemicals

(c1) Short body with protruding abdomen

(c2) Prominent rib cartilages in abnormally shaped thorax

(c3) Enlarged with delayed closure of fontanels

(c4) Causes tetany or convulsions and eventual weakness and lethargy

(d) Same as for osteoporosis: vitamin D-rich diet, exposure to sun

A7. A progressive disease involving excessive bone breakdown (by osteoclasts) and abnormal formation of bone (by osteoblasts)

(a) Adults

(b) Thickened skull bone that may compress vessels or nerves. (*Note:* It is thought that Beethoven's deafness, significant by age 28, may have been related to Paget disease.)

(c) Softening of the femoral neck as well as sacrum and iliac bones

(d) Fractures that occur in diseased bones that can break with even minimal stress

(e) Heart failure related to vasodilation of vessels in bone and the overlying skin; this increased circulating blood volume forces the heart into overload. Also, she is at increased risk for development of sarcoma.

(f) Yes, if multiple bones are involved in this breakdown-growth process.

B1. (a), (c); but (b) the leading and (d) many

B2. (a) Women; middle age

(b) Is not; most

(c) Reacts with; complex; the answer is not known, but possibly a microbe alters the IgG so it is regarded as foreign as occurs in autoimmune disorders, or there may be a genetic predisposition for this alteration

B3. (a) Immune complex (formation)

(b) Phagocytosis

(c) Pannus formation

(d) Ankylosis

(e) Extra-articular changes

B4. (a) RA only; destructive to

(b) Pain in

(c) Small, such as in hands and feet; bilateral

(d) Distal interphalangeal

(e) Thumbs (see Figure 43-7 in *Essentials of Pathophysiology*); dislocation; knee

(f) Cervical; neck; knee; quadriceps

(g) Nodules, swelling of at least three joints for at least 6 weeks, x-ray changes of hand joints (note that other common signs of RA include anemia, cloudy synovial fluid, and elevated ESR, but these are not included in the ARA criteria)

B5. Reduce pain and inflammation, maintain or restore joint function, and prevent bone and cartilage destruction

B6. (a) Infliximab

(b) NSAIDs

(c) Corticosteroids

(d) Methotrexate

B7. (a) Arthroplasty

(b) Synovectomy

B8. (a) Higher; androgens; African Americans and Asians; family history, immune and environmental factors such as drugs and exposure to UV light, and viruses

(b) Excessive; autoantibodies; nuclear components; autoimmune

(c) Antigens; immune complexes lead to inflammatory responses and tissue injury

(d) Injury within so many different systems mimics the effects of other diseases that affect these systems; joints, skin, kidneys, lungs, heart, and brain

(e) Both have symmetric effects on joints and affect small joints of the hands.

(f1–f2) Destruction of red blood cells and platelets by autoantibodies that attack surfaces of these components of blood; fatigue can also result from cardiopulmonary complications of SLE.

(f3) Renal involvement such as nephrotic syndrome occurs in 50% of persons with SLE.

(f4) Vasculitis or hypertension affecting cerebral vessels

(g) Face (cheeks and nose), areas that are especially photosensitive

(h) Many; antinuclear antibodies (ANA)

B9. All answers

B10. (a) Scleroderma

(b) SLE

(c) DSLE

C1. Vertebrae; stiffness of joint

(a) Axial (including the spine); ligaments that insert into bone; are (indicated by "–itis")

(b) Is not; negative; B27

C2. (a–b) The sites where ligaments insert into bone are eroded by inflammation, followed by ossification. As ligaments convert to bony "belts" connecting vertebrae, the spine takes on the bamboo-like appearance; see Figure 43-9 in *Essentials of Pathophysiology*.

(c1) His posture, possible osteoporosis, and diminished vision related to posture (head down) and AS-linked uveitis

(c2) Crowding of his heart and lungs (a reason to get a flu shot to prevent infections) by thoracic joints and posture

(c3) Involvement of his sacroiliac joint and lumbar vertebrae; maintenance of his abnormal posture and gait may have led to injury of his hip joints.

(c4) Caused by pain (which is worse when resting or immediately after he arises), stiffness, and muscle spasms

(d) (1), (2) (4), (6); but (3) warm bath or heat applications and (5) he is already underweight

C3. (a) Reiter syndrome; also in 25% to 30% of persons with ankylosing spondylitis

(b) Ankylosing spondylitis

(c) Psoriatic arthritis

(d) Ankylosing spondylitis

(e) Enteropathic arthritis

(f) Psoriatic arthritis, Reiter syndrome

C4. (a) Bacterial infection; negative

(b1) *Salmonella* or *Shigella*

(b2) *Chlamydia*

(c) Eyes (uvea = iris and ciliary body), intestine, skin, or heart

D1. (a) Metabolic

(b) Idiopathic

(c) Anatomic

(d) Neuropathic

(e) Post-traumatic

D2. (a) RA

(b) OA

(c) OA

(d) RA

(e) RA

(f) RA

(g) OA

D3. (a) Articular cartilage

(b) Provides a smooth weight-bearing surface that decreases friction; as cartilage deforms (Figure 43-11), it transmits the load to bone.

(c) Chondrocytes; water, ground substance (a hydrated, semisolid gel), proteoglycans that provide elasticity and some stiffness, and collagen that provides tensile strength and support

    (d) Increases, decreases; decreased; weaker

    (e) IL-1 (and) TNF, protein; proteoglycans

    (f) Sclerosis, eburnation; osteophytes, crepitus

    (g1) Activity overload decreases deformation and damages cartilage.

    (g2) Lack of mechanical loading deprives the avascular cartilage of motion required to squeeze fluids between synovial fluid and chondrocytes, a mechanism that provides nutrients and removes wastes.

D4. Both large and small

    (a) Hip joint, knee joint

    (b) Cervical vertebrae, lumbar vertebrae

    (c) First carpometacarpal joint, first metatarsophalangeal joint

D5. Is not; weight loss (if obese), strengthening exercises alternated with rest, and modification of activities and tasks by supporting joints with splints and possibly using a cane or walker

E1. (a), (c); but (b) middle-aged to older men, (d) monosodium urate or uric acid, and (e) not all

E2. (a) Has no; is; primary; (2), (3), (4)

    (b) Monosodium urate crystals cause an inflammatory response as the crystals attract white blood cells; the joint becomes swollen, red, and painful; chemicals released in the inflammation attack cartilage and subchondral bone; repeated gout attacks lead to chronic arthritis and formation of tophi.

    (c) Monosodium urate; about 10 years

    (d) One; may not occur for years; toes and other parts of feet and hands; crystals deposit in synovial fluid where these crystals are less soluble than they are in plasma and most often in regions of the body with cooler temperatures.

E3. (a) Joint inflammation (which can lead to rapid joint destruction); NSAIDs

    (b) They increase renal elimination of uric acid.

    (c) This treatment of gout decreases production of uric acid.

    (d) Purines; organ meats such as liver, kidney, and sweetbreads (thymus and pancreas) as well as certain fish (sardines and anchovies)

F1. To address developmental needs of the child and family issues

F2. (a) Pauciarticular arthritis

    (b) Polyarticular arthritis

    (c) Systemic JRA

    (d) Pauciarticular arthritis

F3. (a) First-line

    (b) Good

    (c) Sometimes

    (d) Sometimes

    (e) Joints of extremities

    (f) Renal

    (g) Muscles and skin; calcifications

F4. Common; osteoarthritis; see text.

F5. Increase; pseudogout

F6. (a) Month; higher

    (b) Days

    (c) Will

F7. They are both forms of the same disease; blood vessels (arteries); blindness

Chapter 44

STRUCTURE AND FUNCTION OF THE SKIN

A1. See text.

A2. (a), (d); but (b) epidermis and (c) epidermis

A3. (a) Merkel cell

    (b) Langerhans cell

    (c) Melanocyte

    (d) Keratinocyte

A4. Germinativum, spinosum, granulosum, lucidum, corneum

    (a) Corneum

    (b) Lucidum

    (c) Germinativum

A5. (a) Tyrosinase

    (b) Sebum

A6. (a), (d); but (b) do not migrate but instead send out extensions between keratinocytes and deposit melanin in that way and (c) faster

A7. (a) Thicker; connective; vascular

    (b) Present antigens to immune cells

    (c) Dermis

    (d) Does

    (e) Arrector pili muscles

    (f) Sympathetic

    (g) Eccrine; apocrine

    (h) Sebaceous; sebum

    (i) Bulb; melanosomes

    (j) Stratum corneum; continuously

B1. (a) Elevated and fluid-filled

    (b) Elevated and fluid-filled

    (c) Elevated and solid

    (d) Flat with color change

B2. (a) Petechiae

    (b) Hyper

    (c) Erythematous

    (d) Excoriation

    (e) Dilated blood vessels

B3. (a), (b); but (c) induce and (d) does not heal although may give temporary relief

B4. Lower; melanin; dry; acne, sunburn, or other injuries to skin; less

Chapter 45

DISORDERS OF THE SKIN

A1. In

A2. (a) Superficial; other humans, animals, or soil

    (b) Keratin

    (c1) Less

    (c2) More, because of systemic effects

    (d) More, because feet have less exposure to air

A3. Ringworm or superficial mycoses or dermatophytoses; fungal
    (a) Nails
    (b) Scalp or head
    (c) Body (trunk, back, or buttocks)
    (d) Foot
    (e) Hand

A4. (a) Griseofulvin
    (b) Potassium hydroxide
    (c) Corticosteroids
    (d) Acyclovir
    (e) Isotretinoin or tretinoin

A5. (a) The antibiotic "wipes out" not only the agent (*Streptococcus*) that is causing the respiratory problem but also much of the "normal flora" on any mucous membrane, so *Candida* can then proliferate.
    (b) Frank lacks the CD4$^+$ cells that would normally target *Candida*.

A6. (a) Children; superficial; beta-hemolytic
    (b) Oil; bacteria *(Propionibacterium acnes)*; blackheads; common; androgens; keratolytic agents and antibacterial agents
    (c) Benign; thicker; papilloma; can
    (d) Sensory; burning or tingling (paresthesia); fluid-filled vesicles; do
    (e) (1); (2)
    (f) Is not; acyclovir (or similar antiviral drugs); can

A7. (a) Zoster (or varicella); chickenpox; elderly; immunosuppressed
    (b) Uni; weeks
    (c) Can be; blindness; months
    (d) Use of an antiviral agent, particularly within three days of rash development; also analgesics and antidepressants

A8. (a) Plantar warts
    (b) Acne conglobata
    (c) Rosacea
    (d) Atopic eczema
    (e) Nummular eczema

A9. (a) Urticaria
    (b) Toxic epidermal necrolysis
    (c) Psoriasis
    (d) Pityriasis rosea
    (e) Lichen planus

A10. (a) Plaque-type
    (b) Guttate

A11. Is not; (a), (b), (c), (d), (e); see text.

A12. (a) Bacteria
    (b) Fungi
    (c) Virus
    (d) Virus (warts)
    (e) Virus

B1. Increased
    (a) (2)
    (b) (1)
    (c) Dilate, erythema; increase (this is the basis of tanning)
    (d) DNA; immune
    (e) (1)

B2. (a) (2)
    (b) (1)
    (c) (2)
    (d) (1)

B3. Flame and smoke inhalation; scalding fluids; chemical, electrical, or radiation burns

B4. (a) (4), (2), (3), (1)
    (b) (1)
    (c) (3)
    (d) (2)
    (e) (4)

B5 (a) Yes, because some areas will have second-degree burns that are painful.
    (b) About 42% (18% of each lower extremity plus 6% for about one third of his posterior trunk); major.
    (c1) 3, because much of plasma seeps out of burned blood vessels into interstitial spaces, so less circulating blood, a condition known as *burn shock*.
    (c2) Increased. The stress of burn injury triggers release of epinephrine and cortisol.
    (c3) Increased. Blood is thicker (polycythemia) related to fluid loss; compensatory vasoconstriction occurs in response to burn shock.
    (c4) Increased, because reflex vasoconstriction of vessel into gastrointestinal organs causes gastric mucosa to be ischemic and vulnerable to Curling ulcer
    (c5) Decreased, because reflex vasoconstriction of vessels into kidneys reduces urine formation
    (c6) Interstitial (between cells) areas. Low urinary outputs contributes to edema, but most of the edema comes from seeping of fluid (and proteins) from burned vessels into spaces between cells.
    (c7) Decreased. Injured and possibly infected airways and lungs cannot function adequately to oxygenate blood, and his hypermetabolic rate increases his need for oxygen.
    (c8) Increased. The body's first line of defense has broken down.
    (d) Enormous amounts of replacement fluids because he is "third-spacing," and nutrients are needed for healing his injured body

B6. See the text.

B7. (a) Decubitus ulcers, decubiti, or bedsores; ischemia of skin and underlying tissues by forces that impair blood or lymph flow
    (b) Over bony prominences in the lower part of the body, such as sacrum and coccyx, ischial tuberosities, and greater trochanters
    (c) Immobilizing conditions such as spinal cord injury or stroke; diminished mental capacity such as Alzheimer disease or coma; malnourishment, dehydration, edema, compromised circulation, and incontinence of bowel or bladder
    (d) Sliding of one tissue over another with stretching and damage of skin, underlying tissues, and blood vessels

B8. (a) Reposition in bed every 2 hours; avoid applying shearing forces; assist with fluid and nutritional intake; observe skin while cleansing it and applying moisture barriers, keep bed linens and pads clean, dry, and wrinkle free.

(b) Reposition in the wheelchair or move to bed every hour with padding that cushions bony prominences; especially observe skin over ischial tuberosities. Other interventions as in B5(a).

B9. (a) Stage III

(b) Stage I

C1. (a), (b); but (c) melanocytes, (d) well, and (e) dysplastic

C2. Increased; fair, red or blonde; increased sun exposure, especially intense, intermittent exposure on weekends and vacations, and thinning of the ozone layer so that UV rays reach the earth more readily

C3. Malignant melanoma → Squamous cell carcinoma → Basal cell carcinoma

(a) Basal cell carcinoma

(b) Squamous cell carcinoma

(c) Malignant melanoma

C4. (a) Red hair, freckles on upper back, working outdoors for three or more adolescent years,

family history; having a nevus that has changed and visiting tanning salons also increase her risk; 20

(b) A (asymmetry), B (borders uneven), and D (diameter more than 6 mm), and E (evolved, or changed, recently)

(c) Common; are; is

(d) 60; is

C5. Protect against exposure to sun; detect early by regular, thorough self-examination

D1. (b), (d); but (a) potentially malignant melanomas and (c) strawberry hemangiomas

D2. (a) Widely distributed macules to beefy, red, excoriated skin surfaces

(b) Moist

(c) Infrequently

D3. (a), (c)

D4. See text.

D5. Macules on trunk, spreading to extremities and head → Vesicle formation → Scab formation

D6. (a) Roseola based on his age, fever, and lack of lymph node involvement

(b) Hard measles (rubeola) based on nature of rash, slight elevation in temperature, and probable myalgia

D7. See text.